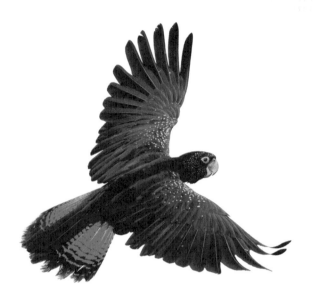

AUSTRALIA'S
RURAL, REMOTE
and
INDIGENOUS HEALTH 3e

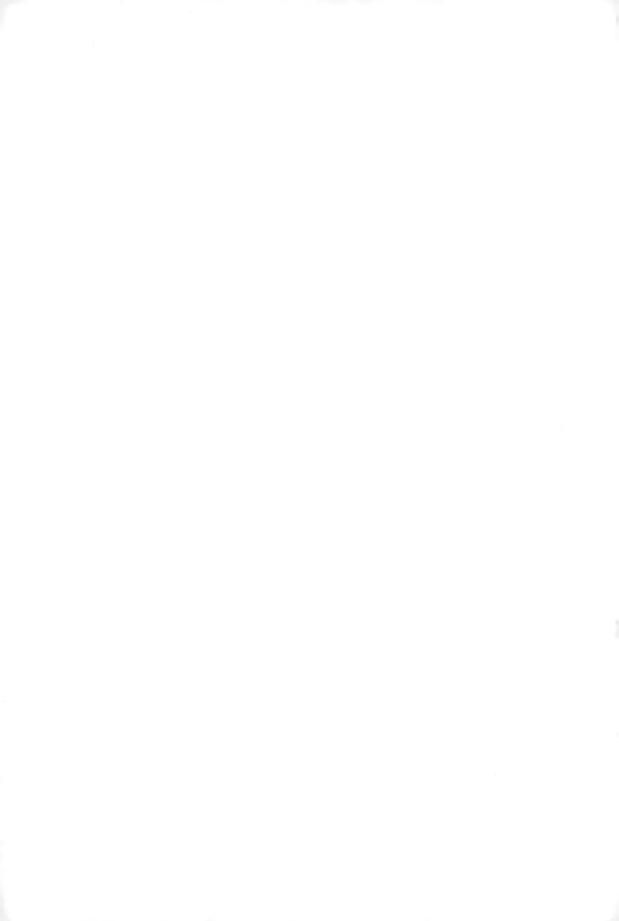

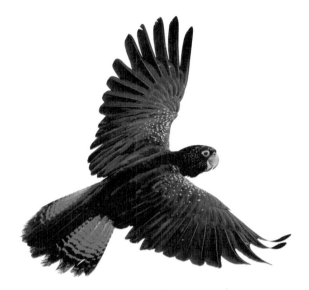

AUSTRALIA'S
RURAL, REMOTE
and
INDIGENOUS HEALTH 3e

Janie Dade Smith

Professor of Innovations in Medical Education
Faculty of Health Sciences and Medicine
Bond University
Gold Coast, Queensland, Australia

President, CRANA*plus*

ELSEVIER

ELSEVIER

Elsevier Australia. ACN 001 002 357
(a division of Reed International Books Australia Pty Ltd)
Tower 1, 475 Victoria Avenue, Chatswood, NSW 2067

Notice

This publication has been carefully reviewed and checked to ensure that the content is as accurate and current as possible at time of publication. We would recommend, however, that the reader verify any procedures, treatments, drug dosages or legal content described in this book. Neither the author, the contributors, nor the publisher assume any liability for injury and/or damage to persons or property arising from any error in or omission from this publication.

National Library of Australia Cataloguing-in-Publication Data

Smith, Janie Dade, author.

Australia's rural, remote and Indigenous health / Janie Dade Smith.
3rd edition.

9780729542418 (paperback)

Includes index.

Rural health services–Australia.
Aboriginal Australians–Medical care.
Aboriginal Australians–Health and hygiene.

362.1042570994

Content Strategist: Larissa Norrie
Content Development Specialist: Lauren Santos
Senior Project Manager: Karthikeyan Murthy
Edited by Linda Littlemore
Proofread by Antonietta Scaffidi
Index by Robert Swanson
Cover and internal design by Natalie Bowra
Typeset by Toppan Best-set Premedia Limited
Printed and bound in Australia by the SOS Print + Media Group.

TABLE OF CONTENTS

VIDEO CONTENTS

PREFACE

It has been nine years since the second edition of this book was published, and many things have changed and improved in rural and remote Australia during that time, which is very pleasing. This edition is therefore a considerable rewrite, with several new chapters written collaboratively with five other authors from whom I have learnt so much.

During these nine years rural turned into regional, the profile of rural health increased, the government invested more and the landmass experienced more drought and flooding rains. The First World got fatter, the Third World got thinner and diabetes and chronic disease increased. National organisations such as Health Workforce Australia and the Australian National Preventive Health Agency were birthed and then closed down along with many other health organisations as a result of the controversial 2014 budget. During this time the Australian Government intervened into Aboriginal communities in the Northern Territory, the then Prime Minister the Hon Kevin Rudd made the historic Apology to Indigenous Australians and the Close the Gap Campaign commenced to measure the impact of these initiatives. Some things, however, did stay the same: Australia's focus on terror, fear and international events, which left floods of refugees fleeing for their lives.

Writing this third edition was a reflective and liberating process. I found myself in a privileged position that gave me time to reflect and find a louder voice about remote, Indigenous and rural health education. Many universities prescribe this book as a core text for undergraduate and postgraduate medical, nursing, pharmacy, occupational therapy, allied health and Indigenous health subjects, and I thank them for their encouragement to get on and write the third edition.

This third edition is restructured into four sections for easier accessibility and is also available as an eBook for the first time, which has been quite an educational process for me. It has two new chapters on clinical practice coauthored by an Aboriginal GP and a remote area nurse that, I am sure, will become student favourites. In addition, the eBook includes a variety of electronic links, videos, audio files, photos and colour that make it come to life. I also changed the title so that it better reflects the strong Indigenous content.

Life for me has always been a series of everyday events punctuated by moments of absolute bliss and those few critical moments that remove us from the ordinary life path that our mothers always thought we might follow. For me, undertaking a one-week student placement on Bathurst Island in the Northern Territory became one of those critical moments in my career, as it took me down a different life path – a rural, remote and Indigenous health path. For many years this path took me over completely. It challenged my values and priorities in life and my worldview. At times it made me think I was between worlds, and that I never really fitted into either. I loved it, I hated it and, 30 years later, I remain absolutely fascinated by it. This book brings together some of those critical moments and combines those experiences with the current literature available in the field. Once I found my voice, which was amazingly rural, the pages seemed to take on a life of their own. Rural, remote and Indigenous health work can be enormously rewarding. To make it such, the rural and remote health workforce need to be adequately prepared for the adventures and the realities that they face. This book aims to meet that need.

Enjoy and have no fear!

Professor Janie Dade Smith

FOREWORD

Before we learnt to recite the words of Judith Wright's *A Sunburnt Country*, and before Albert Namatjira painted his ghostly gums at the outskirts of Alice Springs, remote Australia had been a permanent part of our national identity. Regrettably, this has not always flowed through to our social policies.

It must strike an outsider as strange that this part of the nation, which is so central to our national psyche, has not been central to the way health care is planned or delivered.

This can be measured with precision. The inequality of health outcomes is well known and documented. The further you live from a capital city, the more likely you are to die younger, suffer a chronic disease or suffer a serious and avoidable illness without access to medical care. It is precisely these parts of our country where health professionals are most needed and where we have struggled to attract and retain staff.

This is changing. New models of practice, a greater focus on prevention, and new schemes to train, attract and retain workers in rural and remote Australia are making a difference. We know that, to succeed in retaining staff and improving health, our health professionals need to understand and be part of the communities they serve.

In 2008, Prime Minister Rudd brought the nation together and delivered the National Apology to the Stolen Generations. It will be properly remembered as one of the great and unifying moments in Australian history and a key point on our journey to reconciling black and white Australia. Since that moment, each parliament has committed to reporting on Closing the Gap in a handful of social and health indicators – from life expectancy to employment. This Closing the Gap project serves as a reminder to the Australian Parliament and peoples about what works and what is still to be done, and is the score card of the litany of invariably failed and sometimes well-intentioned policies before it. An important factor will be Aboriginal control over Aboriginal health care to achieve a reconciled future.

This book makes an important contribution to closing this gap. It is as much a practical guide to remote and rural health practice as it is a collation of stories that bring life to the key themes. It harnesses the power of storytelling and ties together the key economic, social and political forces that have, and will continue, to shape health care in rural and remote Australia.

Hon Stephen Jones MP
Federal Member for Throsby
Shadow Assistant Minister for Health

ACKNOWLEDGEMENTS

Developing the third edition of this book has been an enjoyable, collaborative, though largely solitary task that provided me with opportunities for reflection and learning…my two favourite things. This edition has provided me with the pleasure of working with five other writers in four of the chapters – Jacinta Elston from Townsville, Sue Lenthall from Alice Springs, Robyn Williams from Darwin and Shannon Springer and Regan Jane Sharp from the Gold Coast. It has been a great privilege to work closely with these like-minded and highly skilled thinkers. They have added a great depth and richness to this third edition, with their four chapters being pretty much a rewrite to reflect their innovative thinking and ways of seeing the world.

I would also like to thank those at my workplace in the Faculty of Health Sciences and Medicine at Bond University who greatly assisted in kind by listening to me ramble on and provide ideas, time and support; as well as my research assistant Thanya Pathirana who very competently dealt with the detail. I also thank the CEO of CRANA*plus*, Christopher Cliffe, and Professor Sabina Knight who kindly read some of the chapters and provided constructive feedback, and Anne-Marie Bouchers from CRANA*plus* who greatly assisted with photographs. A special thank you to the Hon Stephen Jones MP, Assistant Shadow Minister for Health, who very generously wrote the Foreword to this book. And to my friend and mentor, Professor Richard Hays.

I would like to thank the students and academic reviewers who provided timely and constructive feedback on the various chapters. This feedback is essential for all authors and the great majority of your suggestions and insights have been used to improve the book to make it more accessible for students as they learn about rural, remote and Indigenous health. Thank you.

I want to acknowledge and thank the wonderful staff at Elsevier who made this book and the eBook so accessible and beautiful. I particularly want to thank the publisher, Larissa Norrie, and the Content Development Specialists, Neli Bryant and Lauren Santos, from the Sydney office for their exemplary guidance, ideas, support and for keeping me on track. Thanks to Karthikeyan Murthy, the Senior Project manager in Chennai, India, for his enduring patience and eye for detail; I will miss our email exchanges. Sarah Thomas, the permissions editor, who dealt so well with my many odd requests and always came up with something better, and Linda Littlemore for her great copyediting. I must say I have dealt with a few publishers over the years and this experience has been a continuously wonderful, respectful and collaborative experience. My sincerest thanks to you all.

Janie Dade Smith

LIST OF
REVIEWERS

Terrance Cox *PhD*
Lecturer, Centre for Rural Health, School of Health Sciences, University of Tasmania, Tasmania

Jonathan Newbury *MBBS, MD, FACRRM*
Professor of Rural Health, School of Population Health, University of Adelaide, South Australia

Margaret Lesjak *BSc(Hons), MSc(Community health), PhD, Grad Dip Appl Epi, Grad Cert*
Senior Epidemiologist, Public Sector Management, Far West and Western New South Wales Local Health Districts

Michael Douglas *MBBS, FAFPHM, FACRRM, MPH, IDHA, DipRACOG, MA*
Deputy Director, University Centre for Rural Health, NSW

Margaret Stebbing *PhD, MPH, Dip App Sci Nursing*
Adjunct Senior Lecturer, Monash University School of Rural Health, Victoria

Carolyn Lloyd *MPH, PG Cert Child Youth & Family Health, BN, B App Sci (Health Promotion), RN*
Lecturer, College of Public Health, Medical and Veterinary Sciences, James Cook University, Queensland

Judith Nicky Hudson *BMBS, MSc, PhD*
Director, Department of Rural Health, University of Newcastle, New South Wales

Sabina Knight *RN, MTH, FACN, F CRANAplus, ARLF, GAICD*
Professor and Director, Mt Isa Centre for Rural and Remote Health, James Cook University, Queensland

Christopher Cliffe *RN, Dip Nursing Science, MPH, Grad Cert Rural Leadership*
CEO, CRANAplus, Queensland

Raymond Blackman *MBBS, FRACGP*
General Practitioner, The Palm Island Children and Family Centre, Queensland

Somer Wrigley *RN, M Nursing*
Lecturer, First Peoples Health Unit, Griffith University, Queensland

DEDICATION

This book is dedicated to the love of my life, my late husband Philip Charles Witts. Philip was a professional writer, playwright and screenwriter. He edited every word I wrote in the previous two editions, which always made me look a better writer than what I actually was. I have greatly missed his advice in this edition, though I keep hearing him say as I write…'less is more darling, less is more'.

This book is for you my darling man. You made me laugh out loud every day and I feel so privileged to have been your wife. Philip died suddenly in July 2011; he was 63 years young.

ABOUT THE AUTHOR
JANIE DADE SMITH

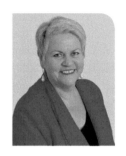

Janie Dade Smith was born in rural Queensland in the year television came to Australia and has lived rurally for most of her life. Being a middle child in a large family, she developed a strong sense of 'a fair go' early on. This formed the foundation for a life driven by humanist values, a social justice agenda and an ability to think outside the square.

Janie is a highly experienced health educationalist and project manager who has worked extensively in national curriculum develop-ment, program accreditation, educational resource development, policy development, organisa-tional review, Indigenous health, as a clinician and in research. She has worked across all health disciplines – medicine, nursing, pharmacy, allied health, and with Aboriginal and Torres Strait Islander health practitioners.

Janie's passion for justice, remote and Indigenous health and plain English writing meant that she has often found herself sitting on an island by herself, struggling to fit into impractical and bureaucratic systems. Therefore, in 2004 she established her own rural health consulting company, RhED Consulting Pty Ltd, and undertook consultancies, developed curricula, and pro-vided program evaluations and reviews for health departments, universities, professional colleges and government and not-for-profit organisations.

Since 2012 Janie has worked for the Faculty of Health Sciences and Medicine at Bond Uni-versity and is the Professor of Innovations in Medical Education. Janie coordinates the Master of Clinical Education Program, leads the development of the Doctor of Medicine program and works on the Indigenous and rural and remote curriculum. She is well published and has won many awards for her work, the most recent being the prestigious *2015 Australian Office of Learning and Teaching Award for University Teaching Excellence* with the Indigenous health team for their work on the Indigenous medical curriculum. Janie is the President of CRANA*plus*, the peak body for all remote health in Australia, and previously sat on the Council of the National Rural Health Alliance.

ABOUT THE
CONTRIBUTING
AUTHORS

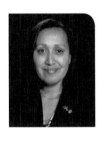

JACINTA ELSTON

Jacinta Elston is an Aboriginal woman from Townsville in North Queensland. She is Professor and Associate Dean, Indigenous Education and Strategy, in the Division of Tropical Health and Medicine, and Co-Director of the Anton Breinl Centre for Health Systems Strengthening at James Cook University. In this role she provides Indigenous leadership and strategic advice in health. For over two decades she has worked in higher education on Aboriginal and Torres Strait Islander health, facilitating Aboriginal and Torres Strait Islander health workforce development.

Jacinta is currently on the Board of the Breast Cancer Network of Australia and the Aboriginal and Torres Strait Islander Women's Legal Service North Queensland. She has previously served on the Advisory Council of Cancer Australia and the NHMRC Research Committee. Jacinta holds a Master of Public Health and Tropical Medicine and is currently completing her PhD.

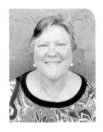

SUE LENTHALL

Sue Lenthall has worked extensively in remote communities in Queensland and central Australia in the Northern Territory as a remote area nurse prior to educating health professionals – Indigenous Health Practitioners, nurses and medical practitioners. Sue holds a Bachelor of Education, a Master of Public Health and Tropical Medicine and a PhD, which aimed to reduce occupational stress among remote area nurses in the Northern Territory. Sue is Associate Professor and the Academic Leader, Central Australian Remote Health Education, at the Flinders University Centre for Remote Health in Alice Springs. She coordinates the Remote Health Practice program and the Masters of Remote and Indigenous Health. Sue is particularly interested in interprofessional education, best practice in remote areas, occupational stress, client consultation skills, cultural safety and primary health care.

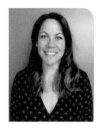

REGAN JANE SHARP

Regan Jane Sharp is a Community Psychologist working in the field of youth mental health. With over 15 years of experience working in community and mental health services, Regan has an eclectic professional background and has previously worked in the alcohol and other drug sector with substance using parents, Indigenous health, prisons, youth work, training and education in Queensland and Western Australia. Regan's specialty areas of practice are LGBTIQ mental health and regional community development.

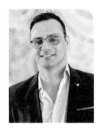

SHANNON SPRINGER

Shannon Springer is an Aboriginal and Australian South Sea Islander from Mackay in North Queensland. After accepting a scholarship to train with the Broncos he completed a Bachelor of Indigenous Primary Health Care to become an Aboriginal Health Worker. However, in 2004 he became one of the first Indigenous doctors to graduate from James Cook University in Townsville, and is now a Fellow of the Royal Australian College of General Practitioners. Shannon has held various positions in Indigenous organisations both at local community level and nationally. Shannon is Associate Professor of Aboriginal and Torres Strait Islander Health and Discipline Lead at Bond University's School of Medicine. He works part-time as a GP for the Aboriginal Medical Services on the Gold Coast and in Charleville.

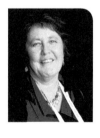

ROBYN WILLIAMS

Robyn Williams has over 35 years' experience working with Indigenous peoples, primarily in the Northern Territory. Robyn coordinates the Bachelor of Health Science at Charles Darwin University. She holds both nursing and education qualifications. Her fields of expertise include cross-cultural curriculum development and program implementation; evaluation of community-based programs; and qualitative research in Indigenous and rural and remote health issues.

In the past Robyn has worked with colleagues at Charles Darwin University to develop a cultural competency framework and a remote health pathway in the Bachelor of Nursing program, as well as intercultural communication workshops for government and Aboriginal Community Controlled Health Organisation staff. Robyn is undertaking PhD studies on exploring preparation for health professionals to be culturally safe and effective practitioners in Indigenous primary health care settings.

INTRODUCTION

Australia's Rural, Remote and Indigenous Health continues to be one of the few books that discusses and applies Indigenous history, health and policy to rural and remote health in Australia, a subject that has now become compulsory in most undergraduate health programs. This text aims to fill this gap by providing the basic information required by any health professional to work in rural, remote and Indigenous Australia.

Australia's Rural, Remote and Indigenous Health is intentionally different from other rural health books, as it is based on a social justice and social determinants framework. Social justice essentially means giving people a 'fair go', a share or a choice. It is the foundation upon which the primary health care approach to health is based. This perspective questions the important issues of human rights, equity, access to services and the appropriateness and affordability of what is provided. The very tenets of primary health care are founded in social and economic justice.

The material is also presented differently, using a variety of plain English forms of writing. These include storytelling, historical accounts, video and audio links and real-life experience, supported by the literature. These approaches apply the realities of everyday human life in rural and remote Australia to professional practice, and provide some useful teaching and learning resources. This makes it easy for the learner and the teacher.

Opposed to a medical evidence-based perspective, this book uses the evidence to support social justice and social determinants arguments. It also questions the very foundation of how we address health in Australia, and why we do not approach it from a more inclusive social justice framework.

Geographically, rural and remote Australia has many more playing fields compared to urban Australia, yet rural people have less access, fewer appropriate fields and fewer affordable ones compared with their city cousins. This affects one of their basic human rights as citizens of this great country: their right to an equal level of health, although theirs is lower on most health indicators. This is particularly so for Indigenous Australians.

This book is aimed particularly at those who are undertaking studies in rural, remote and Indigenous health – in nursing, medicine, pharmacy and allied health, as well as Aboriginal and Torres Strait Islander health professionals; those in sociology, anthropology, cultural studies and education; and at undergraduate as well as postgraduate levels. It will also be of use to those working in policy, social justice and law, and to those with an interest in the area.

COMMONLY USED
TERMS

Aboriginal where 'Aboriginal' is used separately it refers only to Aborigines.

Indigenous refers to Aboriginal and Torres Strait Islander Australians.

indigenous refers to indigenous peoples from countries other than Australia.

primary health care refers to a social approach to health. The World Health Organization, in the declaration of Alma Ata in 1978 (p. 1), defines primary health care as:

> an essential health care based on practical, scientifically sound and socially acceptable methods and technology, made universally accessible to individuals and families in the community through their full participation, and at a cost that the community and country can afford to maintain, at every stage of their development in the spirit of self-reliance and self-determination. It forms an integral part both of the country's health system, of which it is the central function and main focus, and of the overall social and economic development of the community. It is the first level of contact of individuals, the family and community with the national health system, bringing health care as close as possible to where people live and work, and constitutes the first element of a continuing health care process.

regional refers to those areas defined in the ARIA classification scheme. 'Inner regional' refers to large regional cities and centres and 'outer regional' refers to those areas that would have previously been called rural described in Chapter 2.

remote when 'remote' is used alone, it refers only to remote locations as in the classification systems described in Chapter 2.

rural when 'rural' is used alone, it refers only to rurally defined locations as in the classification systems described in Chapter 2.

rural and remote refers to those towns and populations that exist outside major metropolitan and urban areas. Much of the literature does not separate these two factors; in such cases the terms were used together.

rural and remote people the 31 per cent of Australians living outside cities – outer regional, remote and very remote communities.

social justice 'social' refers to society, 'justice' refers to fairness. Therefore, social justice refers to a 'fair society', based on the values and priorities that we, as a society, see as fair and important. It is about giving people a fair share or a choice based on their human rights as determined by the United Nations Universal Declaration of Human Rights (1948).

Torres Strait Islanders where 'Torres Strait Islanders' is used separately it refers only to Torres Strait Islanders.

urban refers to metropolitan areas and cities.

CHAPTER 1

ADVANCE RURAL AUSTRALIA

Janie Dade Smith

I love a sunburnt country,
A land of sweeping plains,
Of rugged mountain ranges,
Of droughts and flooding rains.
I love her far horizons,
I love her jewel-sea,
Her beauty and her terror –
The wide brown land for me!

(DOROTHEA MACKELLAR, 1908)

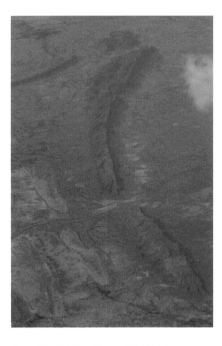

Reproduced with permission from: CRANAplus. Cairns: CRANAplus. <www.crana.org.au>.

In her poem 'My Country', Dorothea Mackellar described the extremes of rural Australia: its moods through drought and flood, its vast distances and the love–hate relationship Australians have with their country.

This first chapter aims to set the rural Australian scene. It explores the rugged history of how rural Australia 'grew up' and the two key ideologies that arose – mateship and country-mindedness. Rural people developed their unique rural culture from these beginnings, which provide a platform for understanding why they love the 'sunburnt country', the place where they belong (Dempsey, 1990). This background is important for health professionals to understand as it underpins the health beliefs and values that many rural and remote Australians hold today.

WHO LIVES IN RURAL AUSTRALIA?

If asked to describe the typical rural Australian, one could be excused for immediately conjuring up a white male image of a suntanned fifth-generation wealthy grazier, dressed in cream moleskins, RM Williams boots and an Akubra, standing in the 45-degree heat with his leg resting on his dusty Toyota four-wheel drive, patiently rolling his 'rollie'* as he squints into the sky looking for any sign of a cloud. He would, of course, be quietly confident, slow to respond, independent, self-reliant, a bit of a larrikin, a real gentleman when ladies were around and a true-blue conservative voter.

*A rollie is a hand-rolled cigarette.

He would enjoy a cold beer on a hot day and would definitely have a loyal dog: his best mate, Bluey.

Nothing, however, could be further from the truth. The populations living in rural and remote Australia are diverse. This diversity is a result of government policy, immigration, post-war trends and geographic isolation. Although the stereotypical wealthy rural farmer still exists, he is becoming an endangered species.

When we read the history of rural Australia it is important to note that most of the written history is by, and about, the white men who explored and discovered this country. Most children educated in Australia will have learnt the stories about Burke and Wills, Captain Cook and John Flynn during their school years. Everywhere they go there are places and roads named after these men; their legends live on, as they should.

This 'his-story',* however, generally excludes the realities and hardships experienced by the many women who contributed enormously to rural Australia. It excludes also the thousands of Aboriginal stockmen and workers who did much of the work to establish and maintain the stations. It also excludes the Aboriginal women who cared for the property owners' houses, wives and children, and who bore a whole generation of 'half-caste' children who were later stolen from them under the government policy of the day. It excludes the soldier settlers – the 'battlers', as they were known – who were granted land after the First World War and the hundreds of thousands of immigrants who brought with them their rich cultures and diverse lifestyles. It also generally excludes the ordinary Australians who live in rural towns: the shopkeepers, farm workers, school teachers, doctors and nurses who provide the country services and make up the strong fabric of rural Australia as we know it today.

The following historical overview aims to give some insight into how rural and remote Australia was put together over the past two centuries. It will link the richness that the various groups brought to this continent with the political forces of the day and explain how two key ideologies arose – mateship and country-mindedness – and how these are now reflected in today's rural culture. Only those historical factors that address these issues will be included, as they contribute to the way in which rural people view their health.

THE FIRST INHABITANTS

There is a perception that Australia is a new country, just over 200 years old, yet it has been the home of one of the most ancient populations in the world. Aboriginal peoples have lived on this continent for over 50 000 years (Australian Bureau of Statistics, 2012b). While there are no accurate records of the size of the Australian population prior to European settlement, in 1930 the anthropologist Radcliffe-Brown estimated a minimum Indigenous population of 300 000 (Australian Bureau of

---

*'His-story' is a feminist term used to refer to recorded history, which was usually written by men and excludes the contributions of women.

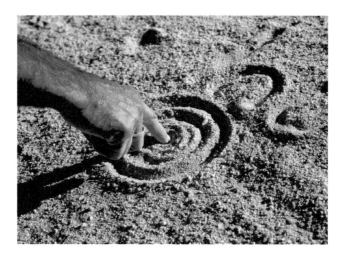

Reproduced with permission from: iStockphoto/Kerrie Kerr.

Statistics, 2012b). Other estimates, based on archaeological findings, have put the figure several times higher (Australian Bureau of Statistics, 2012b). Despite the size of the Aboriginal population before European settlement, it declined dramatically afterwards, due to the impact of new diseases, massacres, repressive and often brutal treatment, dispossession and social and cultural disruption and disintegration. The decline of the Indigenous population continued well into the twentieth century. In 2013 there were an estimated 698 583 Aboriginal and Torres Strait Islander people representing approximately 3 per cent of the population (Australian Bureau of Statistics, 2014c). This is projected to increase by over one-third by 2026 and may exceed 900 000. In outer regional, remote and very remote communities Indigenous Australians make up 43.2 per cent of the population (Australian Bureau of Statistics, 2013b). Due to the importance of Indigenous history and the resulting health status, these are dealt with in separate chapters.

'SETTLING' THE COUNTRY: 1788–1900

The settlement of Australia differed in the various colonies (now states), which contributed towards their diverse multicultural rural development.

When the first thousand convicts arrived in Australia in 1788, 75 per cent were male. Although 24 000 female convicts arrived between 1788 and 1852, they represented only one-seventh of the total number of convicts transported (Moore, 1998). The proportion of men in rural Australia was overwhelmingly higher, as it was usually the men who did the initial exploring, leaving the women to undertake domestic chores in the urban settlements (Moore, 1998).

There was also cultural and religious maldistribution of the various groups of convicts between the colonies. A much smaller percentage of Irish than English convicts went to Van Diemen's Land (now Tasmania) than went to New South Wales, as far fewer ships travelled to Tasmania from Ireland. This resulted in a much higher percentage of Irish Catholics in New South Wales (Hughes, 1988). As a result, mainland Australia was founded on a very strong Irish Catholic male base, while Tasmania was founded on a more Anglo–English Protestant male base. This factor made a considerable difference to the cultural and rural development of the various colonies. The English and Scottish were also largely from urban areas, whereas the Irish were mainly from rural stock (Jupp, 1990).

In 1792 the first land grants were made; 80 per cent went to time-expired convicts (or emancipists) and the remainder went to free settlers. By 1828 one man in three owned land, and a consistent pattern of family ties arose whereby parents applied for land for their sons, and the sons petitioned for land close to their fathers' farms (Hughes, 1988). This pattern continues today, with over 99 per cent of farms being family owned (National Farmers Federation, 2012).

In 1849 the Family Colonisation Loan Society was set up. This organisation lent money to migrants for their passage and found them work in Australia (Hughes, 1988). There was a strong push for yeomen* (who would later dominate) to take up farming. The farms were small landholdings and a push began to 'open up the land' into larger areas to enable a more sustainable living.

The gold rush era, first in Victoria, then in New South Wales and Queensland during the 1850s and 1860s, disturbed the order of Anglo-Australian society and helped create an 'Australian bourgeoisie' or middle class (Hughes, 1988). The gold rush brought with it mass immigration of 'new chums'† and a huge intercolony migration where more farmland was opened and mining men were encouraged to take up farming. In a way it created an 'equality' in that those who never thought they would be wealthy found their place in the 'lucky country'. If they did not drink it all away, many became wealthy men. This factor helped change the traditional English class structures. Here it was possible to become wealthy through hard work; you did not need to be born into money.

The end of the Crimean War in 1855 saw a further influx of immigrants, which resulted from political and economic turmoil in Europe at the time (Jones, 1973). The proportion of unassisted immigrants compounded the huge gender discrepancy: 208 males arrived for every 100 females. Males predominated in pastoralism, agriculture and mining and there was little employment for women apart from domestic work and prostitution. The preferred immigrants were English, German and Scottish – not Irish, as there was a great deal of religious and racial prejudice against them at the time (Jupp, 1990).

---

*A yeoman was the freeholder of a small amount of land, who was in a class below the gentry (*Australian Pocket Oxford English Dictionary*, 1982).
†New chums were newly arrived immigrants or convicts from Britain (*Australian Concise Oxford Dictionary*, 2000).

The shearing circuit in Australia was mostly seasonal. Men and youths started the circuit in Queensland in mid-winter, moved south to Victoria by Melbourne Cup time in November and then to New Zealand by February, returning again to Queensland (Moore, 1998). In the 1850s the trade unions began their battle with rural and urban capital interests and the outback shearers were among the earliest unionised and most militant workers in Australia (Moore, 1998). Unionism flourished, aided by many ex-convicts who had been transported for their union activities. A climax came in 1854 with the Eureka Stockade, in which 30 men were killed and a new Australian identity was born. Attempted shearers' strikes often ended in failure due to the 1890s depression and widespread unemployment, but in Queensland the shearers refused to give up. These activities stimulated the formation of the Australian Labor Party in 1891 and the Australian Workers' Union in 1894.

Growing the state differences

During the 1850s gold rush the population of Victoria increased by 600 per cent. Among the newcomers were thousands of Californians, Chinese, Europeans, ex-convicts from all colonies and an estimated 2660 Italian-speaking Swiss immigrants (Martinuzzi-O'Brien, 1988). Victoria, however, had never been a convict state and took considerable pride in having a free population. It did not take kindly to the 'convict taint' that resulted from the mass migration of ex-convicts, especially the Tasmanians who were seen as the worst of all convicts. To combat this, the *Convicts Prevention Act* was introduced in 1852, whereby people moving to Victoria had to prove that they were unconditionally free. Failure to do so would result in three years' hard labour in irons (Hughes, 1988). This helped to foster the anti-authoritarian, 'sticking-to-your-mate' ethos that is still found among many rural people today.

Queensland differed from the other colonies in that the majority of their immigrants – some 82 per cent – came directly from Europe. Queensland received 261 709 immigrants between 1860 and 1899, more than all of the other colonies combined (Moore, 1998). The predominantly male Queensland rural communities were seen as a haven for adventurous young men, particularly those in their twenties (Moore, 1998). It was also the one-way destination of some 50 000 Melanesian men. They were called 'kanakas', which is a Hawaiian word meaning human being, although their numbers also included South Sea Islanders, Polynesians and Micronesians (*Webster's Dictionary*, 2010). Sugar plantations employed 62 000 young Pacific Islander males and some females between 1863 and 1904 (Jupp, 1990). They were 'recruited' by blackbirders* on labour vessels, were often poorly treated and provided much of the hard labour in the north (Jupp, 1990). There was clear delineation between what was kanaka work and what was not (Jones, 1973), supported by the widely-held belief that Asians and kanakas were more suited than white-skinned people to working in

*Blackbirding was the act or practice of kidnapping Pacific Islanders and selling them for slave labour, mainly for Queensland cotton and sugar plantations (*Australian Concise Oxford Dictionary*, 2000).

the tropics. The White Australia Policy* of the time, based on similar theories, also promoted this attitude (Jupp, 1990).

There were large numbers of Chinese in the mining, shearing and agricultural industries, Japanese on the pearling luggers and Aboriginal workers on properties. Discoveries of coal, copper, silver and tin widened the mining base and young men overwhelmingly populated these industries. The most dramatic example was the Palmer River goldfield in 1877, which attracted 18 000 single Chinese males and a few thousand males of European origin (Moore, 1998). There was a strong anti-Chinese feeling during the gold rush era, which helped bring about the end of free Asian migration and the development of the White Australia Policy (Jupp, 1990). By 1888, Chinese were excluded from all Australian colonies, although those who were already in Australia were not deported. In Western Australia the Chinese were prohibited from working in gold and many became station cooks and hotel workers instead (Jupp, 1990). Racism and class structures were unyielding, and alcohol was freely available to all men except Melanesians and Indigenous Australians (Moore, 1998).

Again, Queensland was unique in that it was the only Australian state populated by both Aboriginal and Torres Strait Islander peoples; ironically, it was also the centre of the White Australia movement (Jupp, 1990). In 1859 Queensland's population consisted of 23 520 mainly British settlers and possibly 100 000 Aboriginal and Torres Strait Islander people. By the turn of the century there were half a million settlers of European, Asian and Melanesian origin and, of concern, around 27 000 Aboriginal and Torres Strait Islander people (Moore, 1998). This different social structure, consisting of large, rurally based European, Asian and Islander male populations and directed by government policies such as the White Australia Policy, had implications for the different ways in which Queensland developed, compared to the other Australian states – and for the different effects on health that resulted.

The White Australia Policy can be traced back to the 1850s. It had a lasting impact on the national and social development of rural Australia. The policy particularly targeted immigration, which is why, for example, many of the darker-skinned Italians were sent to the northern tropics – northern Europeans at the time considered themselves 'genetically unfit to labour in tropical climates' (Kidd, 1997). The way in which the policy was constructed contributed towards the set of cultural values and beliefs that formed the national self-identity of Australians; that is, what they perceived as truly 'Australian' characteristics (Human Rights and Equal Opportunity Commission, 2001b). 'True blue' Australians were, of course, white; and the policy excluded and marginalised groups based on their ethnicity and race. While the final vestiges of the

---

*The White Australia Policy, introduced in the 1890s, was a system of both official and unofficial discrimination whereby immigration policy and citizenship requirements were heavily biased to favour white European migrants, and more specifically Anglo-Saxon migrants, over other races. It was not officially abandoned in Australia until 1973 (Jupp, 1990).

White Australia Policy were removed in 1973 by the incoming Labor Government (Department of Immigration and Border Protection, 2012), it provided a platform upon which to build and perpetuate the stereotypes of other cultural groups that still exist in Australia today.

PAUSE AND THINK

List three stereotypes about rural people that exist in Australia today.

What impact did the White Australia Policy have on the social structure of rural populations in Australia?

What impact has this rural history had on the values and health beliefs of rural Australians today?

The Northern Territory, as the frontier land of Australia, offered its new inhabitants special challenges and had a significant males-to-females discrepancy that existed well into the 1970s. With a landmass that covers one-sixth of the Australian continent, it holds only one per cent of the total Australian population (Australian Bureau of Statistics, 2012c). James (1989) tells us that the Northern Territory was seen as the toughest environment for women. She found that, when the Overland Telegraph was finished in 1872, there were only 172 white males and 12 white adult females, plus large populations of Chinese and Indigenous Australians. The Northern Territory provides some of the greatest documented stories of the women who pioneered it. While they were less visible and greatly outnumbered by the men, they were often the real managers of the Territory, the stabilising influence and the builders of the social structure, and they maintained an almost naïve faith in the Territory when the catastrophes they endured seemed to scream: 'Give up' (James, 1989).

Prostitution

As rural Australia grew organised prostitution became based around Asian and European women. Exploitation of Aboriginal women was colony wide; rape, concubinage and prostitution of Aboriginal women were endemic in rural areas (Moore, 1998). Moore (1998) quotes a report of a station hand at one station in 1898 where 30 to 40 Aboriginal women were at work in the wool sheds as roustabouts or water carriers. These women were divided into three groups for sexual services: the bosses' women, the jackeroos' women and those for the larger group of general hands. At the end of the shearing season these women were often released without payment.

Mateship

In this first century the 'settling' of rural Australia developed from a strong male, convict and immigrant base. It was a rugged history of exploration, hardship, settlement, development and discovery and its systems and infrastructure were built from male ways of thinking. In this environment, if you did not rely on yourself or your mate, you would probably not survive. From the convict era of state-controlled flog-gings, the men learned patterns of physical violence that they commonly adminis-tered to others through rough bush justice (Moore, 1998). These convict floggings confirmed the state's authority and imposed a sense of submission, or a feminisation of the male convicts' masculinity (Moore, 1998). A similar punishment, enforcing submission and masculinisation, was also imposed on female convicts, who had their heads shaved.

As a result, colonial manhood was violent, racist and sexist (Moore, 1998, p. 10). These traits would later influence how masculinity would be viewed in Australia. From this experience, a uniquely Australian social behaviour arose that would remain in the very ethos of being an Australian male, and particularly a rural male: the idea of 'mateship'.

Robert Hughes (1988), in his epic book about the convict era, *The Fatal Shore*, argues that those features that best describe most Australian male bush virtues – intransigence, strong anti-authoritarianism, sticking to your mate, distrust of the judge and unpolished self-reliance – were due to the Irish influence in New South Wales and not the convict system per se. He claims Tasmanian convicts 'had little sense of the frontier and hence no context in which the "bush ethos" could flourish' (Hughes, 1988, p. 594).

In 1966 Russell Ward described the 'typical Australian' as:

A practical man, rough and ready in his manners and quick to decry any appearance of affection in others. He is a great improviser, ever willing 'to have a go' at anything, but willing too, to be content with a task done in a way that is 'near enough'.... He swears hard and consistently, gambles heavily and often, and drinks deeply on occasion. Though he is 'the world's best confidence man', he is usually taciturn rather than talkative, one who endures stoically rather than one who acts busily. He is a 'hard case', scepti-cal about the value of religion, and of intellectual and cultural pursuits generally. He believes that Jack is as good as his master but, at least in principle, probably a great deal better, and so he is a great 'knocker' of eminent people unless, as in the case of his sporting heroes, they are distinguished by physical prowess. He is a fiercely independent person who hates officiousness and authority especially when these qualities are embodied in military officers and policemen. Yet he is very hospitable and, above all, would stick to his mates through thick and thin, even if he thinks they may be in the wrong.

(RUSSELL WARD, 1966, pp. 1–2)

Australian colonies also developed stronger stereotypical masculine identities than the imperialist British who founded them (Moore, 1998). This was due to the lack of white women in rural Australia, the absence of Britain's complex social hierarchy and exposure to numerous different cultural norms where male-to-male intimacy was class-structured and quite usual. By the end of the 1830s the authorities grudgingly acknowledged that mateship often found its expression in homosexuality (Hughes, 1988; Jones, 1973; Moore, 1998). In the second half of the nineteenth century same-sex behaviour was identified as a distinct disease and the legal system declared male-to-male sexual behaviour an offence that was not decriminalised until 1997 in Tasmania.

By the 1840s the transplanted gentry and middle classes reclaimed their flagging physical prowess through leisure activities. In rural Australia there was less time or need for recreation, although race meetings, cricket and football matches were regular community events (Moore, 1998). Hard rural labour preserved 'manhood' right into the early twentieth century. However, pair bonding and reliance on one's mate lies forever at the heart of masculine social behaviour in Australia (Hughes, 1988). And Australian manliness became closely identified with mateship.

This mateship ethos was bolstered and perpetuated throughout the 20th century by the two world wars, the Anzac legend, sporting activities and such films as *Crocodile Dundee* and *Breaker Morant*. These Australian legends have similar essential characteristics to those of their predecessors. They are firmly heterosexual, generally working class, honest, hardworking, egalitarian, competitive, independent, antiauthoritarian and larrikins who are true to their mates, to whom they always give 'a fair go'. The key difference is that, in the past, bushmen and 'the bush' stood for the 'real Australia' and mateship and mates stood for the 'real Australian' (Haltof, 1993).

Today real Australians, while still male, are now more traditionally seen on big city football fields and cricket pitches and on big city surf beaches than riding on a sheep's back. Does this mean that the typical Australian stereotype – the rural male – is being replaced by more urban perceptions of Australian-ness? If so, where does this leave the bush in the 21st century? These become important factors when we look at how rural men, in particular, view their health.

PAUSE AND THINK

Rural men are known to view health services as 'illness services' rather than preventative services; and they often present late in onset of a disease. What aspects of this history have impacted on these health beliefs and values?

RURAL AUSTRALIA: 1900–2000s

The second century of 'settling' rural Australia had a significant impact on the development of the values and priorities that rural people hold dear. These are reflected in the way they differ from city people in how they view themselves and their health.

The new federal government in 1901 passed the *Immigration Restriction Act*, which ended the employment of Pacific Islanders, placed certain restrictions on immigration and provided for the removal of prohibited immigrants from the Commonwealth (Department Immigration and Border Protection, 2012). At this time sugar farmers were offered a subsidy for replacing non-white workers with white labour.

Several historical circumstances played a critical role in changing the population of rural Australia, none more so than the two world wars. In 1917, as the First World War (1914–18) drew to a close, the government introduced the *Returned Soldier Settlement Act*, which made land of between 70 and 320 acres available to returned soldiers on a perpetual lease (Jones, 1973). However, during the Great Depression that followed, many walked off their farms as they were inexperienced farmers with little capital on farms too small to make a family living, or in climates unsuited to the type of farming they chose. Many of the farmers 'went broke and joined the ranks of the unemployed "humping their blueys*"' around Australia' (Nalson, 1977, p. 315).

The Depression also affected the rural women – the wives. Wives were seen by the military to be the responsibility of their husbands. As a result they became shadows passing over the pages of the official records, as 'there was usually no need to comment on them unless they died or caused trouble' (James, 1989, p. 16). Their roles included not only caring for the home and family, but also cooking for the seasonal herds of men, working on the farm and, often, watching their babies die in the harsh environmental conditions. Some rural women also played active, leadership roles in farming, breeding cattle, butter manufacturing and even wine making, which were never documented until recently (Doran, 1992; James, 1989; Larkins & Howard, 1976; Martinuzzi-O'Brien, 1988). Hence, most rural women's histories died with them.

Saving the country souls

An overview of the history of the people who make up rural Australia would not be complete without noting the important impact that the various churches, unions, voluntary organisations, political organisations and service organisations played in the formation of the rural Australia that we know today.

In 1912 the Presbyterian Church of Australia formed the Australian Inland Mission and the Reverend John Flynn was appointed superintendent. Flynn, who was also a doctor, founded the Royal Flying Doctor Service (RFDS) in 1928 in Cloncurry, Queensland, as a 'mantle of safety' for the people of the outback. The RFDS today is a strong and robust national organisation that provides clinical, primary health care and emergency aero-medical services to people in remote areas (Royal Flying Doctor Service, 2015).

---

*'Humping a bluey' refers to a swagman carrying his swag and belongings as he moves on foot from one place to the next, often along the wallaby track – the writers of Henry Lawson or Banjo Paterson.

The active role that the churches played in their 'Christianising of the outback' through the establishment of missions was significant. This Christianising of the outback and the establishment of missions involved many denominations, including Catholics, Lutherans, Methodists and Presbyterians, who predominated in certain areas of Australia. These missionaries were sent forth into new lands to proclaim to the Indigenous peoples an alternative message of universal salvation in Jesus Christ, hereby evangelising entire populations and cultures (Tatamai, 2000). Many rural and remote Australians are still feeling the impact of what was no doubt considered 'fine work' within the government's protection and segregation policies of the day. A National Human Rights Commission of Inquiry in 1997 found that, between 1910 and 1970, one in three to one in ten Indigenous children were forcibly removed from their families. Of these estimated 100 000 children, 63 per cent who were taken to missions were physically abused, 28 per cent were brutally abused and one in six reported sexual exploitation and abuse (Human Rights and Equal Opportunity Commission, 1997a). Most white Australians would probably assume that those who were taken as children and reared as white would now be better off. However, the opposite is true. A three-year study undertaken in the mid-1980s revealed those taken were much less likely to have undertaken post-secondary education, three times more likely to have been in jail, twice as likely to use illicit substances and much less likely to live in stable conditions than were other Aboriginal children (Human Rights and Equal Opportunity Commission, 1997a). The *Bringing Them Home* report recommended an apology be made accompanied by appropriate reparations (Human Rights and Equal Opportunity Commission, 1997b). It was not until 13 February 2008 that the then Prime Minister, The Honourable Kevin Rudd, made the historic apology, in particular to the stolen generations, which has had a significant positive impact on Aboriginal Australians and their levels of trust of government (National Sorry Day Committee, 2015).

PAUSE AND THINK

How would the history of the stolen generation impact on the levels of trust Aboriginal people might have on those in authority today – such as police or health professionals?

What would this change about how you might consult with Aboriginal peoples?

Volunteering rural women

One key role that women played, which was critical to the establishment and sustainability of rural Australia, was volunteering. Volunteering is important in building social capital in small communities and is often a critical factor for their sustainability. The first rural women's group in the world, the Agricultural Women's Organisation, was founded in Finland as early as 1797, and a decade later the first Women's Institute was founded in Canada (Doran, 1992). This was followed by international networks of rural women's organisations. In Australia, the Country Women's Association (CWA) was formed in New South Wales in 1922, with various state branches opening over the next few years. In 1945 the states federated to form the Country Women's Association of Australia (Country Women's Association of Australia, 2015). While many may think that the main role of the CWA, as we know it today, is in making lamingtons, running street stalls and knitting toilet roll dolls, nothing could be less true. The CWA today has a strong political voice for women, children and their families in rural Australia. It remains a strong symbol of country-mindedness with its sense of social distinctiveness and perception of special rural needs (Doran, 1992). The same political ideology was being developed in many rural organisations at that time.

Migration

After the Second World War (1939–45) the migration from Italy to the wheat belt of Western Australia was the beginning of a considerable change that was to occur in many rural areas of Australia (Nalson, 1977). Between the wars, and as a result of Country Party activities, areas of intensive irrigated agriculture were created in New South Wales, Queensland, South Australia and Victoria. This irrigated agriculture was labour intensive and produced low-return crops. The work attracted few Australians but migrants, mostly from Italy, Yugoslavia and other southern and eastern European countries, many from a peasant background, were willing to do the work.

By 1947, one-quarter of all overseas-born people lived in rural areas. Often coming straight from immigrant ships and speaking no English, they started to develop intensive agriculture in rural areas and on the outskirts of major cities. In Western Australia they often travelled the thousand kilometres north to Carnarvon during winter to grow out-of-season vegetables on shares of land for the Australian owners of irrigated banana plantations. This chain migration also occurred in the tobacco growing areas in Victoria and Western Australia and the sugar cane growing areas of North Queensland and New South Wales. By 1963, 50 per cent of these thrifty, hardworking migrants had saved enough to buy out their Australian bosses (Nalson, 1977). As a result, some rural areas now have extremely high concentrations of particular ethnic groups brought out by chain migration from villages overseas.

Since the Second World War the migration from small country towns to cities, consisting mostly of young people looking for work or educational opportunities, has become a significant feature of rural Australia (Rolley & Humphreys, 1993). Postwar recovery also occurred much faster in cities than in rural areas. By 1947 Australians still saw themselves as rural pioneering people though they mostly lived in cities. They were mostly of British or Irish descent and were overwhelmingly Australian born, only 10 per cent having been born overseas (Jupp, 1990). They generally had little knowledge or interest in Aboriginal life, as they saw the Aboriginal people as a dying race. There was a hierarchy of desirable immigrants: British, Scandinavians and Germans were placed above the 'coloured races', and 'the major cultural distinction was between Catholics and Protestants' (Jupp, 1990, p. 14). Despite this, Australians still considered themselves 'egalitarian and very superior to other nationalities in sport, open-air life, material well-being and lack of class distinctions' (Jupp, 1990, p. 14). Although not all Australians held these views, they were widespread.

Rural decline

The next 40 years after the Second World War saw a continual economic rural decline that changed the face of rural Australia. There was a push for technology, free trade and globalisation, and agriculture, which in the 1950s contributed 25 per cent to the gross domestic product (GDP), 'plummeted to only 2.6 per cent of the GDP' (Rolley & Humphreys, 1993, p. 244).

By the 1970s, better technology meant that fewer people were directly involved in agricultural production, farms were amalgamating and the one-way drift of sons and daughters to the city continued. These generations, who had been taught that Australia rode to prosperity on the sheep's back, found their children moving to the bright city lights and new, sophisticated city ways of thinking and doing.

'Country-mindedness'

Rural people see themselves as different from city people. It is from this perceived difference that rural people have developed what is termed a 'sense of country-mindedness', or their ideology or 'truth' about being rural people.

Country-mindedness came into being during the economic boom years of the 1860s to 1890s, which were founded on rural growth. At the time there was a high demand for wool and wheat and, later, for exported dairy products and meat (Aitkin, 1985). The majority of people lived in large, stable rural populations. In 1901, the year of Federation, the issue of free trade was pushed, and farmers and graziers found themselves in a cost–price squeeze. At the same time the arbitration system was introduced, which seemed to protect the wages of city people at the expense of those who lived in the country (Aitkin, 1985). This contributed to the self-perception among rural Australians that they were both different and vulnerable (Lockie, 2000).

Following the First World War there was a slower rural recovery. Rural areas had failed to expand in population and wealth after more than a generation of steady growth, and country people looked to their political economy for an explanation of their predicament (Aitkin, 1985). After the Great Depression that followed, growth began again, but it did not take place to any great extent in country areas (Aitkin, 1985, p. 36). This slower post-war recovery resulted in the setting up of a variety of sectional pressure groups, including farmers' and graziers' associations, in an effort to raise the rural profile and provide a voice for rural Australia.

It was as a result of this activity that several regional and state rural organisations coalesced in 1920 to form the Australian Country Party (now known as The Nationals who have coalesced with the Liberal Party). The Australian Country Party espoused elements of country-mindedness that seemed to set the stereotypical image of rural Australians for the next 80 years. It was based, above all, on the belief that farming was an ennobling experience that commanded respect, not just for the necessities it provided but because it involved hard work, perseverance and family values (Gray & Lawrence, 2001). Country-mindedness raised the profile of the role of farming and promoted the Australian image of the real Australian male – the wealthy white grazier. Country-mindedness included common beliefs such as the following:

- Australia depends on its primary producers for its high standard of living, for only those who produce a physical good add to the country's wealth.
- Therefore, all Australians, from city and country alike, should in their own interests support policies aimed at improving the position of the primary industries.
- Farming and grazing, and rural pursuits generally, are virtuous, ennobling and cooperative; they bring out the best in people.
- In contrast, city life is competitive and nasty, as well as parasitical.
- The characteristic Australian is a country man, and the core elements of the national character come from the struggles of country people to tame their environment and make it productive. City people are much the same the world over.
- For all these reasons, and others such as defence, people should be encouraged to settle in the country and not in the city.
- But power resides in the city, where politics is trapped in a sterile debate about classes. There has to be a separate political party for country people to articulate the true voice of the nation (Aitkin, 1985, p. 35).

As a result, until the 1970s rural policy was equated with agricultural policy. The stereotypical male rural family farmer was 'the embodiment of country-mindedness, and "his" interests were represented as the interests of all rural people – indeed, as the interests of all Australians' (Lockie, 2000, p. 18; Moore, 1998).

PAUSE AND THINK

Does this stereotypical view of rural people exist today?

Is this the perception that urban people hold about rural people today? If so, what impact would that have on their relationships?

Leaving the country

By the 1970s the Country Party, founded as it was on a sense of country-mindedness, had shrunk. It repositioned itself as the National Party, basing its policies on economic rationalism and managerialism (Lockie, 2000). It has since joined with the Liberal party to form the Coalition and bases its regional policies (it has no rural or remote policies) on supporting communities, using the very strength that rural people espouse – self-reliance. By 2015 The Nationals occupied only 15 of the 150 available seats in Federal Parliament (The Nationals, 2015). Like their party name, their numbers and rural policies are decreasing, and now seem to greatly reflect those espoused by their coalition partners – the Liberal Party.

In 1985 Aitkin (p. 40) wrote that, in his judgement, '"country-mindedness" has finished as an ideology as the group lost its cohesion and size'. There were fewer rural people with rural ways of thinking … and increasing numbers being born in cities. 'Like other aspects of Australia's history, the ideology may have a future as part of a romantic past, but it has ceased to have power in the practical present. Yet it did have a great run'.

Rural political forces: enter Hansonism

Is Aitkin right? Let us take a brief look at the 1998 federal election in Australia to examine this further. A new party emerged in the second half of the 1990s: Pauline Hanson's One Nation Party. The party stood up for the underdog, or the 'little Aussie battler', which was easily interpreted as the rural farmer during the drought years. It strongly opposed Aboriginal affairs, Native Title legislation* and immigration with what were seen by much of the Australian community as redneck, racist policies (Lockie, 2000). Despite this, 11 members were voted into State Parliament at the 1998 Queensland election. Their success was seen as 'a counterpunch from an angry and ailing rural and regional Queensland', from whence One Nation grew (Lockie, 2000, p. 20). Further research that year by Davis and Stimson, however, indicates that those who voted for the One Nation Party were from urban fringes and hinterlands with weak support in town and city centres (McManus & Pritchard, 2000). The party found variable support in rural areas except around the rural–urban interface of Brisbane and Queensland's major regional cities. Socioeconomically, the researchers concluded that there were few Indigenous or overseas-born supporters, and that those who voted for One Nation were largely unskilled and blue-collar workers, living on the urban fringes and dreaming the Australian dream of home ownership (Davis & Stimson, 1998, cited in McManus & Pritchard, 2000). These findings indicate that the values espoused by One Nation continue to exist in Australian society.

By 2003 the One Nation Party had self-destructed and was involved in lengthy legal battles that culminated in the jailing of Pauline Hanson and her party co-founder for electoral fraud. By 2006 there was only one elected member of One Nation in Federal Parliament. Pauline Hanson unsuccessfully ran again in the 2015 Queensland state election with 11 candidates. This leaves a handful of Nationals and independents to speak for rural Australia.

---

*Native Title legislation is legislation passed in 1993 that acknowledges the right of Indigenous Australians to own their traditional land (*Australian Concise Oxford Dictionary*, 2000).

RURAL AUSTRALIA TODAY

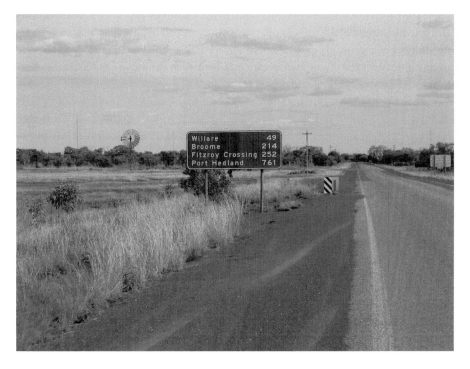

Source: Janie Dade Smith.

The face of rural communities looks considerably different these days. Services have been moved into larger regional hubs that provide better air services and more accessible roads that often bypass small towns. Greater technology, telephone banking, tele-health and internet services are provided instead of personal service, thereby reducing the number of local jobs for local youth. The privatisation of companies continues with large institutions, such as Telstra and Australia Post, reducing their services. Banks began using electronic rather than personal services, as the provision of shareholder profits became more important than the provision of basic services. There has also been a rationalisation of some of the essential health services through the use of tele-health. This includes services provided by the Royal Flying Doctor Service which, as a result of better roads and transport, has reduced clinical services to some stations and properties and replaced them with emergency and health promotion services (Royal Flying Doctor Service, 2015).

The number of farmers has decreased by 40 per cent in the past 30 years (Australian Bureau of Statistics, 2012a). They remain a strongly male population with a declining proportion of women who make up approximately 28 per cent of the farming workforce (Australian Bureau of Statistics, 2012a). In the past decade there has also been significant climate change and two major weather events that have greatly impacted upon farmers – the worst drought in 100 years and, in 2011, the most notorious flood in Australian history. Rural farmers have had to become more innovative and now produce for niche markets, for example taking up ostrich farming and growing exotic fruits, canola oil, rice, cotton and olives. There is also an increasing number of organically grown fruits and vegetables as major supermarkets respond to consumer demand. Many farmers are now leaders in the use of modern technology through the use of robotics and digital technology to manage their business, and they have the capacity for technology to resolve communication issues between the city and the bush. Mining has become the biggest rural industry with its fly-in fly-out teams of city-based professionals who add little to local economies. We also now live in an environment where sport adds more to GDP than wool or wheat (Government of South Australia, 2011).

With advanced technology and transport systems and a new economic rationalist regime, governments and big business found it less cost-effective to continue to provide their services to more isolated communities. This resulted in the closures of banks, post offices, supermarkets, hospitals and schools, and a continual economic decline that has affected farmers, pastoralists, small businesses and rural people who now find themselves adding to the rising unemployment and suicide statistics.

The overseas-born populations in rural areas account for about 12 per cent, showing a preference for city life (Australian Bureau of Statistics, 2013a). In 2013 major growth continued to be in cities with Perth being the fastest growing capital city as a result of the mining boom, where miners fly-in fly-out leaving their families in the city (Australian Bureau of Statistics, 2014a). They are now splattered in their orange vests all over outback Australia. Those people who had moved from Australian cities were mostly baby boomer retirees, who continued to prefer coastal areas and larger regional towns to inland rural areas. Today, overseas-born populations account for 26 per cent of the total Australian population. They are concentrated in the five mainland capitals with the top two groups being from England and India (Australian Bureau of Statistics, 2013a). Many of these population groups are also highly urbanised by culture with migrants born in Somalia, Lebanon, China, Greece and Asian countries being 95 per cent more likely to live in cities than Australians (Australian Bureau of Statistics, 2014b), whereas migrants from New Zealand, the United Kingdom and Germany are approximately 75 per cent more likely to live in urban areas than Australians (Australian Bureau of Statistics, 2014b).

While rural life can be challenging many find the country to be a great place to live and bring up families. There are also many newcomers with the expansion of regional government initiatives and university campuses. They attract professionals, administrators and students of all ethnicities who bring with them their own culture and families as they seek a new way of life and good coffee. Many towns are seeing an expansion of tourism as the grey nomads travel through, and some farmers are moving to farm-stay in an effort to find revenue. These innovations are slowly changing the culture of these rural towns and the values they hold dear.

CONCLUSION

Rural Australia was founded on a predominantly male base. Rural populations are culturally diverse and were made up of a combination of Indigenous people, ex-convicts and immigrants from almost every nation. Consequently, initial rural structures and previous state policies were based on male ways of doing and thinking, and on class and race structures that were often both sexist and racist.

Rural people and their forebears have endured considerable hardship, extreme isolation and tough geographical conditions to produce some of Australia's greatest economic resources. They have done this through hard work, resourcefulness, self-reliance, mateship and stoicism. These factors have given them a sense of rural community and a unique rural culture. As a result, they see themselves as different from their urban counterparts and this has been supported by government policy. Yet rural Australia is continually reported to be in crisis, with many support networks being established to address financial, social and family issues.

The rural crisis is not a single-cause issue but the result of some long-term trends, the cumulative effects of droughts and floods and some deliberate policy decisions (Jensen, 1997). There are other important matters to consider as a nation, such as the environment, climate change, the health status of Indigenous Australians, the incidence of family violence in our community and the reduction of rural services. At the same time, we are living in an environment where the 'war on terror' and international issues have demanded more attention than national and, certainly, rural issues at home. This leaves policies for rural and remote Australia being made by the large urban populations in the south east corner, who now prefer to refer to us as 'regional'.

The face of rural Australia has changed; as a consequence, it is important to start looking at the problems differently. As Jensen reminds us, 'the past does not contain the solution for the future.' There is a need to walk away from the tired and unsuccessful methods of the past and to force a cultural change on politicians and other leaders, to force a change in a mindset that has lost the war to a mindset that is determined to bring about results, and to force a commitment to genuine change and major initiatives (Jensen, 1997, p. 9).

It is up to all of us who live in rural Australia and love it – not just politicians and leaders – to find a way forward. This includes women, children and men,

Indigenous people, professionals, country people and ordinary Australians. It is time for us to change our everyday country-minded ways of thinking and doing. When we describe rural Australia, we need to exchange negative words such as deprivation, disadvantage, rural crisis, hardship, struggle and economic decline with words like technologically rich, multicultural, innovative, environmentally fascinating, resource-rich, challenging, unique and equitable. This is the 'lucky country', not the 'unlucky country'.

While there has certainly been enormous discontent, there is also enormous energy, creativity, vibrancy and commitment to a future for rural Australia. As the 2000 Human Rights Commissioner reminded us: 'this is one country as a whole, with the middle part included. The rest of the country has to remain connected so that we feel whole as a nation' (Sidoti, 2000, p. viii). It therefore seems time we reframed the national relationship that the country has with the city and celebrate our diversity.

Discussion Points

1   What impact has this history of rural Australia had on the formation of the values and beliefs that rural people have about themselves? Discuss how these values and beliefs impact upon their health beliefs.

2   Discuss the way in which this history of how Australia was settled may affect the attitudes of men in accessing health care services.

3   Is Ward's description of the typical Australian (p. 9) appropriate for today? Discuss how the history of rural Australia formed the thinking behind this statement.

4   What mental health services are available to those in rural Australia who have suffered the impact of drought and flood?

5   Do rural people today see themselves as different from their city counterparts? In what way? Discuss.

References

Aitkin, D. (1985). Countrymindedness: the spread of an idea. *Australian Cultural History*, 4, 34–40.

Australian Bureau of Statistics (ABS). (2012a). *Australian farmers and farming. Australian Social Trends.* 4102.0. Canberra: ABS. <http://www.abs.gov.au/AUSSTATS/abs@.nsf/Lookup /4102.0Main+Features10Dec+2012> Accessed 10.07.15.

Australian Bureau of Statistics. (2012b). *Unity and diversity: The history and culture of Aboriginal Australia.* Canberra: ABS. <http://www.abs.gov.au/Ausstats/abs@.nsf/0 /75258e92a5903e75ca2569de0025c188> Accessed 03.03.15.

Australian Bureau of Statistics. (2012c). *State and Territory statistical indicators, 2012.* Canberra: ABS. <http://www.abs.gov.au/ausstats/abs@.nsf/mf/1367.0> Accessed 10.07.15.

Australian Bureau of Statistics. (2013a). *Aboriginal and Torres Strait Islander peoples' labour force outcomes. Australian Social Trends*. Nov 2013. Canberra: ABS. <http://www.abs.gov.au/ausstats/abs@.nsf/Lookup/4102.0Main+Features20Nov+2013#CDEP> Accessed 10.07.15.

Australian Bureau of Statistics. (2013b). *Estimates of Aboriginal and Torres Strait Islander Australians, June 2011*. Canberra: ABS. <http://www.abs.gov.au/ausstats/abs@.nsf/mf/3238.0.55.001> Accessed 10.07.15.

Australian Bureau of Statistics. (2014a). *Regional population growth, Australia 2012–13*. Canberra: ABS. <http://www.abs.gov.au/ausstats/abs@.nsf/Products/3218.0~2012-13~Main+Features~Main+Features?OpenDocument#PARALINK2> Accessed 10.06.15.

Australian Bureau of Statistics. (2014b). *Where do migrants live? Australian Social Trends*. 2014. 4102.0. Canberra: ABS. <http://www.abs.gov.au/ausstats/abs@.nsf/Lookup/4102.0main+features102014> Accessed 10.06.15.

Australian Bureau of Statistics. (2014c). *Aboriginal and Torres Strait Islander population may exceed 900,000 by 2026*. Canberra: ABS. <http://www.abs.gov.au/ausstats/abs@.nsf/Latestproducts/3238.0Media%20Release02001%20to%202026?opendocument&tabname=Summary&prodno=3238.0&issue=2001%20to%202026&num=&view=> Accessed 03.03.15.

Australian Concise Oxford Dictionary. (2000). *Australian Concise Oxford Dictionary*. Melbourne: Oxford University Press.

Australian Pocket Oxford Dictionary. (1982). *Australian Pocket Oxford Dictionary*. Melbourne: Oxford University Press.

Country Women's Association of Australia (CWAA). (2015). *History*. CWAA. <http://www.cwaa.org.au/about-us/history/> Accessed 10.07.15.

Dempsey, K. (1990). *Smalltown – A study of social inequality, cohesion and belonging*. Melbourne: Oxford University Press.

Department of Immigration and Border Protection. (2012). *Fact sheet 8. Abolition of the White Australia Policy*. Canberra: Department of Immigration and Border Protection. <https://www.immi.gov.au/media/fact-sheets/08abolition.htm> Accessed 10.07.15.

Doran, C. (1992). *Women in isolation: A history of the Country Women's Association in the Northern Territory 1933–1990*. Darwin: Country Women's Association of the Northern Territory.

Government of South Australia. (2011). *Trends in recreation and sport*. Adelaide: Government of South Australia.

Gray, I., & Lawrence, G. (2001). *A future for regional Australia*. Cambridge, UK: Cambridge University Press.

Haltof, M. (1993). Gallipolis, mateship and the construction of Australian national identity. *Journal of Popular Film and Television*, 21(1, Spring), 27–38.

Human Rights and Equal Opportunity Commission (HREOC). (1997a). *Bringing them home report: Report of the national inquiry into the separation of Aboriginal and Torres Strait Islander children from their families*. Canberra: HREOC.

Human Rights and Equal Opportunity Commission. (1997b). *Bringing them home: A guide to the findings and recommendations of the national inquiry into the separation of Aboriginal and Torres Strait Islander children from their families*. Canberra: HREOC.

Human Rights and Equal Opportunity Commission. (2001b). *'I want respect and equality': A summary of consultations with civil society on racism in Australia*. Canberra: HREOC.

Hughes, R. (1988). *The fatal shore: A history of the transportation of convicts to Australia 1787–1868*. London: Pan Books Ltd.

James, B. (1989). *No man's land: Women of the Northern Territory*. Sydney: Collins Publishers Australia.

Jensen, R. (1997). Rural Australia: past, present and future. Rural Australia: Towards 2000 Conference, July, NSW, Charles Sturt University.

Jones, D. (1973). *Hurricane lamps and blue umbrellas: A history of the shire of Johnstone to 1973*. Innisfail: Johnstone Shire Council.

Jupp, J. (1990). Two hundred years of immigration. In J. Reid & P. Trompf (Eds.), *The health of immigrant Australia* (pp. 1–35). Sydney: Harcourt Brace Jovanovich.

Kidd, R. (1997). *The way we civilise*. St Lucia, Qld: University of Queensland Press.

Larkins, J., & Howard, B. (1976). *Sheilas: A tribute to Australian women*. Adelaide: Rigby Ltd.

Lockie, S. (2000). Crisis and conflict: shifting discourses of rural and regional Australia. In B. Pritchard & P. McManus (Eds.), *Land of discontent: The dynamics of change in rural and regional Australia* (pp. 14–32). Sydney: University of New South Wales Press.

Martinuzzi-O'Brien, I. (1988). *Australia's Italians 1788–1988*. Carlton, Vic: Italian Historical Society.

McManus, P., & Pritchard, B. (2000). Introduction. In B. Pritchard & P. McManus (Eds.), *Land of discontent: The dynamics of change in rural and regional Australia* (pp. 1–13). Sydney: University of New South Wales Press.

Moore, C. (1998). Colonial manhood and masculinities (Australian masculinities). *Journal of Australian Studies*, 56, 35–53.

Nalson, J. (1977). Rural Australia. In A. F. Davies, S. Engel, & M. Berry (Eds.), *Australian society: A sociological introduction* (pp. 304–325). Melbourne: Longman Cheshire Pty Ltd.

National Farmers Federation. (2012). *NFF Farm Facts 2012*. Canberra: National Farmers Federation. <http://www.nff.org.au/farm-facts.html> Accessed 10.07.15.

National Sorry Day Committee. (2015). *Apology anniversary*. National Sorry Day Committee. <http://www.nsdc.org.au/our-history/> Accessed 05.03.15.

Royal Flying Doctor Service. (2015). *Royal Flying Doctor Service*. <http://www.flyingdoctor.org.au/> Accessed 04.03.15.

Rolley, F., & Humphreys, J. (1993). Rural welfare: the human face of Australia's countryside. In T. Sorensen & R. Epps (Eds.), *Prospects and policies for rural Australia* (pp. 241–257). Melbourne: Longman Cheshire.

Sidoti, C. (2000). Foreword. In B. Pritchard & P. McManus (Eds.), *Land of discontent: The dynamics of change in rural and regional Australia* (pp. vii–viii). Sydney: University of New South Wales Press.

Tatamai, R. (2000). *The Catholic Church in Papua New Guinea*. <http://www.rtapng.com.pg/faith/history.html> Accessed 23.02.06.

The Nationals. (2015). *Nationals for regional Australia*. <http://www.nationals.org.au/> Accessed 05.03.15.

Ward, R. (1966). *The Australian legend* (2nd ed.). Melbourne: Oxford University Press.

Webster's Dictionary. (2010). *Webster's New World College Dictionary*. Cleveland, Ohio USA: Wiley Publishing.

CHAPTER 2

DEFINING RURAL AND REMOTE AUSTRALIA

Janie Dade Smith

Where is it that makes us most happy? One would imagine that it would be where most people choose to live, such as Sydney with its golden beaches and beautiful harbour, but nothing could be less true. The happiest people in Australia have been found to live in small rural towns with a population of less than 40 000, where they feel well connected to their communities (Cummins, 2010). The happiest electorates are the Riverina, Gippsland and Murray regions in Victoria, Ryan in Queensland and Mayo in South Australia, with Victoria being the happiest overall state (Cummins, 2010). Ironically, the most dissatisfied electorates were also the two richest and most expensive cities in Australia – Sydney and Perth (Cummins, 2010). So perhaps money doesn't make us happy after all?

Rural Australia, however, is not just a retirement place where baby boomers' dreams come true. It is a place of enormous diversity: geographically, climatically, economically, sociologically and culturally. It is the sunburnt country of extremes, from the magnificent snow-capped mountains in the south to the dense rainforest of the tropical north, to the ochre-coloured desert of the centre and beyond. It is the place where mateship, a 'fair go', resourcefulness, the Anzac legend and a hard day's work for an honest day's pay are held in high regard. It is the place where thousands of tourists come to visit each year, going home with stories of our wonderful countryside, vast distances, friendly people and fascinating fauna. But rural and remote Australia is not just the home of kangaroos, kelpies and koalas. It is also the home of some of the greatest health inequalities in the world, which increase with geographical remoteness as we will find.

This chapter explores the concepts and classifications that are used to provide health services to those who live in regional, rural and remote Australia. It then examines the inequities that exist, by comparing a very remote Indigenous community and a very remote non-Indigenous community.

URBAN AUSTRALIA

Australia is the world's largest island, with a land area of about 7 692 030 square kilometres. It is almost as large as the United States of America, 50 per cent larger than Europe and 32 times greater than the United Kingdom (Australian Government, 2015). Unlike the United Kingdom, which looks like a chess piece, or Italy, which looks like a boot, Australia, according to popular journalist Phillip Adams, looks 'more like a bum, the biggest bum on earth with Sydney and Perth at the hips and Adelaide approximating the sphincter. Which didn't do much for Tasmania' (Adams, 2003, p. 11).

Although it is the sixth largest country in terms of area, Australia is also one of the most highly urbanised and sparsely populated nations on earth, with only two people per square kilometre.

In March 2015 Australia had a population of over 23.8 million people (Australian Bureau of Statistics, 2015b). Of this population 86 per cent lived in urban areas with almost two-thirds residing in one of the nine capital cities, a proportion that is increasing annually (Australian Bureau of Statistics, 2014a). Perth was the fastest growing capital city in the country, with almost 1298 people flocking there each week, as they follow the riches of the mining boom, followed by the outer suburbs of Darwin (Australian Bureau of Statistics, 2014a). The other main areas of regional growth are the Gold Coast, Sunshine Coast and Townsville in Queensland and Newcastle, the Central Coast and Wollongong in New South Wales – all coastal areas (Australian Bureau of Statistics, 2014b).

Australia also is characterised by significant maldistribution of its population, which is concentrated in two widely separated coastal regions. The larger of these, in terms of area and population, lies in what is known as the south-east corner – the beautiful coastal regions of South Australia through to Victoria, New South Wales and south-eastern Queensland. The smaller coastal region is in the wine-growing areas of the south-west of the continent around Perth and Albany in Western Australia. In both coastal regions the population is concentrated in urban centres and surrounding areas. This means more than 80 per cent of all Australians live within 50 kilometres of the beach (Working in Australia, 2015).

There is a social trend for this maldistribution to increase within three particular population groups. The first group consists of sons and daughters as they move from smaller rural towns to go to university or to find work in the city. The second group comprises the baby boomers and retirees as they move from the cities to the more attractive coastal towns for a perceived better lifestyle. The third group is the miners and their families who are placed in cities while their parent or partners fly-in fly-out of remote mining sites. Since 2000 employment in the mining industry has more than tripled and nearly 22 per cent of Australia's mining workforce resides in Perth (Australian Bureau of Statistics, 2013). Their orange fluorescent vests are now speckled across Australian airports and they are changing the remote Australian landscape. This inflow of miners has had a huge impact on infrastructure, water supply, health care and housing, with towns like Karratha and Port Hedland in Western Australia in 2011 reporting the median weekly rent for a house being $1300 (Australian Bureau of Statistics, 2013). This movement also has important implications for health and education providers and planners, as we shall see.

PAUSE AND THINK

What impact has the mining boom had on remote communities, their services and the cost of living for long-term residents?

What do you think would be the main health concerns for miners and their families due to the fly-in fly-out nature of the work?

What are the implications for health and education providers and planners?

NON-URBAN AUSTRALIA

Australia is a highly urbanised country. In June 2013, 15.3 million Australians lived in greater capital cities, which consisted of 71 per cent of the population. The remaining 29 per cent lived in regional, remote or very remote communities (Australian Bureau of Statistics, 2014a). In the past decade there has been a shift by governments, politicians and city-based bureaucrats, who often administer rural and remote programs, to use the term 'regional' – onto which they sometimes tag 'rural'. Every time they use the term regional they are referring to anywhere in that state outside the metropolitan area, where urban ways of thinking often exist. They then occasionally tag on 'remote' as an afterthought – the forgotten population. Classification systems then divide regional areas into 'inner regional' and 'outer regional'. While differentiating between urban and non-urban is a useful beginning point, it has been difficult to achieve consensus about how best to differentiate between the different types of non-urban communities.

The focus of this book is on the health of the 29 per cent of Australians who live outside urban areas – in the parts of the country labelled rural, outer regional, rural and remote, very remote, isolated or non-metropolitan. There has been a lack of clarity in the terminology used, with many terms used interchangeably or in different ways.

Clearly, it is not possible to have one rural or non-urban lifestyle that extends across a continent as large as Australia. This simple dichotomy fails to capture the diversity of people, landscapes and towns outside the cities, including:

- the variation in climates
- the types of industry and agriculture
- the levels of infrastructure
- the economic activities and viabilities
- employment and labour patterns
- people and cultures
- health status
- demographics
- population size
- dispersal and density
- cultural groupings
- access to services.

To be able to determine the split between 'those who live in cities' and 'those who don't', the Australian Bureau of Statistics in 1999 relied on a simple split between urban and rural by classifying all parts of Australia as one or the other. However, this did not differentiate a rural town on the outskirts of Sydney from one in the middle of Australia. These classification systems have changed during this time, and I discuss the relevant systems for health professionals in this chapter.

Today, the Australian Bureau of Statistics geographically classifies Australia into six areas according to their relative remoteness (see Figure 2.1). These are important to understand as they inform policy development and the distribution of resources to people and services based on remoteness. The six remoteness areas are:

1   major cities of Australia
2   inner regional Australia
3   outer regional Australia

FIGURE 2.1 Map of remoteness areas of Australia. This map of Australia demonstrates the six classes of the remoteness structure, excluding migratory, used by the Australian Bureau of Statistics and the Australian Institute of Health and Welfare.

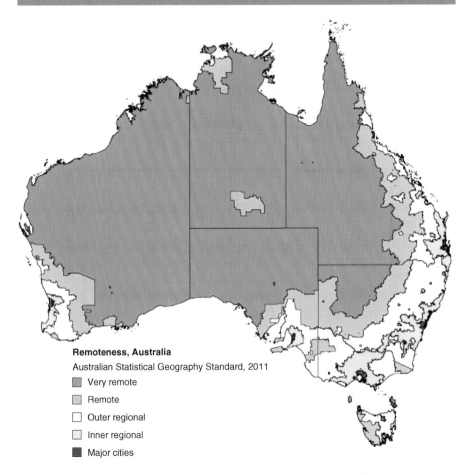

Remoteness, Australia
Australian Statistical Geography Standard, 2011

- Very remote
- Remote
- Outer regional
- Inner regional
- Major cities

Reproduced with permission from: The Australian Statistical Geography Standard, 2011. In: Australian Institute of Health and Welfare. (2014). *Access to primary health care relative to need for Indigenous Australians* (p. 6). Canberra: AIHW. <http://www.aihw.gov.au/WorkArea/DownloadAsset.aspx?id =60129547982>.

4   remote Australia

5   very remote Australia

6   migratory (Australian Bureau of Statistics, 2011).

What does inner regional Australia look like?

You can see from the map in Figure 2.1 that inner regional areas are mostly found in the south-east corner of Australia around capital cities, with the exception of those areas around Perth. One inner regional area that provides us with an example is Ballarat in Victoria.

The leafy City of **Ballarat** had a population of approximately 99 000 people in 2015, of whom nine per cent were born overseas. It is 110 kilometres west of Melbourne, an hour's drive, and it is well known for its gold rush history. It encompasses a total land area of just under 740 square kilometres with four main highways radiating from it (City of Ballarat, 2015). Ballarat has most of the facilities found in a city – traffic lights, good shopping, an airport, a large regional hospital and a large university campus. You can see that the words city and regional are used in the same sentence. This is because many regional towns have been gazetted as cities based on government criteria. Ballarat is also the place that many students undertake rural placements, and some actually make the one-hour drive to and from the city every day so that they can still live in metropolitan Melbourne.

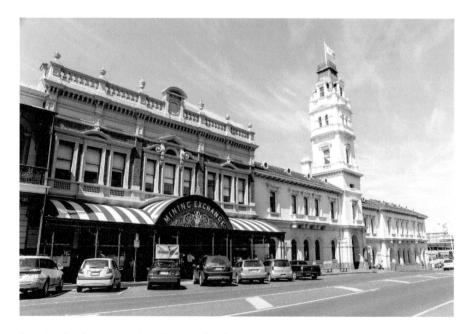

Reproduced with permission from: Shutterstock/Nils Versemann.

What does outer regional or rural Australia look like?

When we think of the term 'rural' we often think of pastoral or agricultural pursuits and 'the country', which is often characterised by simplicity and being uncomplicated. People often use the term interchangeably with 'the outback', 'the bush' and 'the country'. However, country can also mean the land of a person's birth, their mother-land, or the land where they are considered to be a native. Indigenous Australians often refer to 'my country' in this way. There are also state variations. For example, a doctor who works in the Northern Territory would describe herself as a rural doctor who works in the outback, while a doctor who works in rural Victoria would probably describe himself as a 'country doctor' who works in the country.

The term rural is now being used less often by governments and bureaucrats and is being replaced with the term 'outer regional'. This reflects the continued urbanising of Australia and takes with it some of the charm that these words bring, along with images of the Country Women's Association of Australia, the swaggie and the Royal Flying Doctor Service.

The physical distinctions typically used to describe outer regional areas in Australia are large distances, inaccessibility to services and lower population numbers, factors that can constrain the activities of the people and their levels of wellbeing.

An example is found in **Mount Isa**, an outer regional town in north-west Queensland in which copper, silver, lead and zinc are mined. It has a falling population of

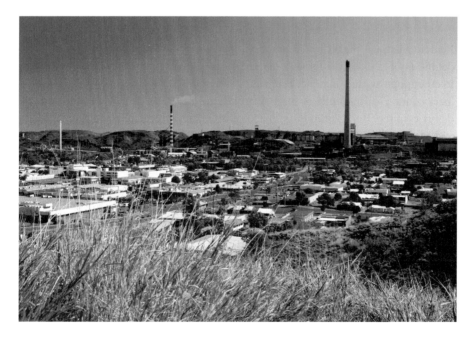

Reproduced with permission from: iStockphoto/James Bowyer.

approximately 23 000, of whom about 15 per cent are Indigenous Australians, which is five times the national average (Australian Bureau of Statistics, 2015a). Mt Isa Health Services District covers an area of over 380 000 square kilometres. There are air services in and out of Mount Isa daily. To drive to Townsville, the nearest large regional centre, 883 kilometres away, takes about 10 hours. To continue the drive to the nearest metropolitan city, Brisbane, takes a further two days or between 18 and 20 hours. During the wet season the road sometimes floods, making it inaccessible.

PAUSE AND THINK

List the issues that a patient who required radiation services for 8 weeks in a larger regional town like Townsville would have to consider. What support systems are in place to support them?

What issues would health professionals need to consider in the safe transport of a critically ill patient from Mt Isa to a larger regional or metropolitan hospital?

These factors – long distances, inaccessibility to services and lower population numbers – distinguish outer regional from urban areas and they all increase with remoteness.

REMOTE AUSTRALIA

Remote Australia makes up 78 per cent of the landmass of this great country. The definition of 'remote' is a faraway place: distant in place, space, time and connection to other populations (dictionary.com, 2015). Remote Australia is also often called the 'back country' or the 'outback', particularly in the Northern Territory and the central desert country. The term implies that very little happens there in the human sense, and that what does happen can be slow and undramatic. But as Thomas Keneally (1983) tells us, nothing could be less true. Just like the temperature, everything in the remote context is multiplied including the flies, the distances one has to travel to get anywhere and the lack of resources.

Remote areas are characterised by small and highly dispersed populations, higher proportions of Indigenous people and less access to all services. Roads are usually long, dusty and unsealed, with wandering stock and wildlife – typically sheep, cattle, kangaroos, emus and, in Central Australia, the odd camel. Under these conditions, a 100-kilometre road trip can take several hours.

Remote communities include railway sidings, mining towns, cattle stations, pastoral leases, discrete Indigenous communities, outback towns, tourist resorts, shipping and Australia's surrounding oceans, islands and Antarctica. All are remote, and all are different from one another and function in diverse ways.

There is an old saying in remote areas that 'if you've seen one remote community, then you've seen one remote community'. This saying emphasises the uniqueness and different characteristics found in each community. It also alerts remote health professionals to the issues they might need to consider when they move from one community to another, which could mean unlearning what they think they already know – especially if state boundaries are crossed. These issues may involve learning:

- a different language
- different cultural norms and practices
- about differing health status
- practical issues, such as dealing with water supply, travelling in certain weather conditions, knowing who to approach and other local oddities.

What does remote look like?

Remote is enormously diverse, from the huge central desert to the ski slopes in the south, the ochre mountains of the west and the crocodile-infested rivers of the north. The further you travel from the cities, past the networks of small rural towns, as the paved roads become longer and straighter or turn to gravel or dirt, as the climate becomes more extreme and the landscape more intimidating and more beautiful, when hours of travel are required to get from one town to the next, most of us would have a sense that we have left rural Australia and entered remote Australia. One becomes acutely aware that, not only is the city far away, but everyone else is too.

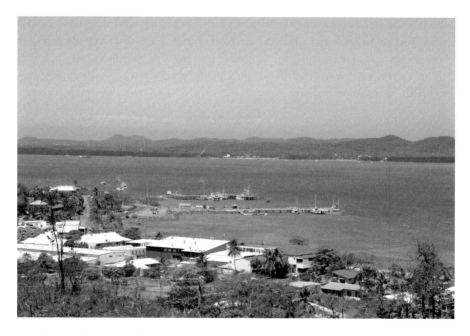

Reproduced with permission from: Flickr/John Benwell.

Only those who have never been to a remote area could imagine that it is difficult or confusing to differentiate between remote and rural areas (Kelly & Smith, 2007).

As an example of the sheer geographical and access issues associated with being remote, take **Thursday Island** in the Torres Strait, which is increasingly becoming a tourist attraction. Thursday Island, off the tip of far north Queensland, is very small. It is too small to have an airstrip, yet it has several air services a day. These aeroplanes land, after their two-hour trip from Cairns, on Horn Island, a larger island next to Thursday Island. Passengers then travel by bus to the wharf and by ferry to Thursday Island. The whole trip takes about four to five hours depending on the weather. Therefore, a trip to Thursday Island for the first time can offer a few surprises for the uninitiated. To transport a seriously ill patient from Thursday Island, or from one of the smaller outer islands, to a major regional centre also offers unique challenges. It can involve all manner of transport including a helicopter, boat, ferry, truck, ambulance and aircraft. Frequently, emergency air services are prevented from travelling or landing by animals on the airstrip or by climatic conditions such as fog, cyclones or torrential rain. So, while Thursday Island may not be considered as remote as many small, remote towns, it presents its own unique challenges.

Isolated

Another word often used interchangeably with remote is 'isolated'. Isolated can refer to being isolated from our family and traditions; from our social, cultural, gender or professional group; or physically by geographical distance or climatic conditions. People living in cities can feel isolated if they have few friends or are poor, homeless, unemployed or sick. Urban fringe doctors working in the western suburbs of Sydney, who provide services to culturally diverse groups, could be considered as isolated if cultural access to services is denied. Therefore, social factors that impede access to those things that make people feel connected in some way with their culture, health and socioeconomics also need to be considered, especially when we examine geographical classification systems.

WHY DEFINE REGIONAL, RURAL AND REMOTE?

It is important to be able to define what is regional, what is remote and what is neither, for a number of reasons. First, definitions enable us to establish the populations of towns and where particular groups of people, who may have special needs, live. For example, 21 per cent of Indigenous Australians live in remote or very remote areas compared with 1.7 per cent of the non-indigenous population (Australian Institute of Health and Welfare, 2014b). We know that the health status of Indigenous Australians is far below that of other Australians, as is their housing and access to education, and that this becomes worse with geographical remoteness. Therefore, knowing the distribution of Indigenous Australians (see Figure 2.2) assists in planning health care, education and housing services.

Second, definitions assist governments in allocating resources and services. This includes determining the number of schools, banks and health care facilities required

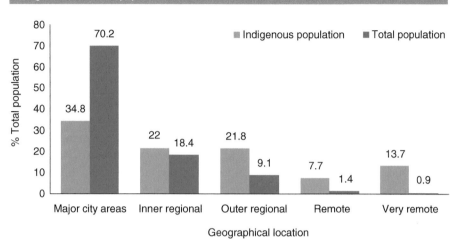

FIGURE 2.2 The geographical distribution of the total Australian population and the total Indigenous Australian population.

Adapted from: Australian Bureau of Statistics (2011). Aboriginal and Torres Strait Islander and non-Indigenous population 30 June 2011. 3238.0.55.001 – *Estimates of Aboriginal and Torres Strait Islander Australians, June 2011.* <http://www.abs.gov.au/ausstats/abs@.nsf/mf/3238.0.55.001>.

to meet the population's needs and funding programs and projects to support rural and remote initiatives.

Third, definitions assist in ensuring that the services provided are affordable, and that those who suffer socioeconomic disadvantage are not further disadvantaged by where they live.

Classifying for urban, regional and remote regions

There are three main classification systems that have been developed, which allow us to collect and examine information about a range of factors, including:

- the structure and nature of the population being serviced
- patterns of morbidity and mortality within the population
- the special needs of particular population groups
- the distribution and availability of the health workforce
- information about infrastructure – the number and type of health services provided and the patterns of utilisation.

To be useful, any such geographical classificatory system should allow us to distinguish any differences *within* the non-urban sector, as well as allowing comparison *between* urban and non-urban Australia. However, terms to differentiate between rural or remote Australia have not been precisely defined, and it has remained unclear when remote rather than rural should be used.

The three main classification systems used in health

There have been three main attempts to develop a geographical classification system over the past two decades that are important for health professionals to understand. These classification systems enable the government to coarsely divide the national population into groups that live in similar types of geographical areas, based upon which they allocate resources and the workforce (Australian Institute of Health and Welfare, 2015).

1   The first system, The **Rural, Remote and Metropolitan Areas** (RRMA), developed in 1999, relates directly to the medical profession to measure and manage the distribution of the national general practitioner (GP) workforce, and the range of incentive and training programs. RRMA measures remoteness in a straight-line distance between goods and services to the nearest urban centre. Three zones – metropolitan, rural and remote – are subdivided into seven categories that are built on the Index of Remoteness (see Table 2.1). The Department of Health ceased using RRMA for new programs from 2009, but it is still being used with some programs and will be reviewed as to whether the Modified Monash Model will better assist them to meet their policy objectives (Australian Institute of Health and Welfare, 2015).

2   The **Modified Monash Model,** introduced in early 2015, is based on research conducted by Monash University as to how geographical locations relate to key general practice workforce indicators (Table 2.2). The Monash research showed that the degree of remoteness and population size of a town provide a reliable, accurate measure to determine how attractive it would be for a medical practitioner to want to work and live there. This new system will assist with the distribution of incentives to the General Practice Rural Incentives Program and target

TABLE 2.1   RRMA classification system

ZONE		CATEGORY
Metropolitan zone	M1	Capital cities
	M2	Other metropolitan centres (urban centre population > 100 000)
Rural zone	R1	Large rural centres (urban centre population 25 000–99 999)
	R2	Small rural centres (urban centre population 10 000–24 999)
	R3	Other rural areas (urban centre population < 10 000)
Remote zone	Rem1	Remote centres (urban centre population > 4999)
	Rem2	Other remote areas (urban centre population < 5000)

Adapted with permission from: Australian Institute of Health and Welfare. (2015). *Rural, Remote and Metropolitan (RRMA) classification.* Canberra: AIHW. <http://www.aihw.gov.au/rural-health-rrma-classification/>.

MODIFIED MONASH CATEGORY	INCLUSIONS – ALL AREAS CATEGORISED BY AUSTRALIAN STATISTICAL GEOGRAPHY STANDARD (ASGS)
MM 1	RA1 – e.g. capital cities
MM 2	RA2 and RA3 that are in, or within 20 km road distance of, a town with a population greater than 50 000 – e.g. Hobart, Ballarat (Vic), Bundaberg, Cairns, Townsville, Darwin
MM 3	RA2 and RA3 that are not in MM2 and are in, or within 15 km road distance of, a town with a population 15 000 to 50 000 – e.g. Coffs Harbour (NSW), Maryborough (Qld), Warrnambool (Vic), Kalgoorlie (WA)
MM 4	RA2 and RA3 that are not in MM2 or MM3, and are in, or within 10 km road distance of, a town with a population 5000 to 15 000 – e.g. Lithgow (NSW); Sale (Vic); Margaret River (WA); Charters Towers (Qld)
MM 5	All other areas in ASGS RA2 and RA3 – e.g. Gundagai (NSW); York (WA); Port Fairy (Vic); Hay, Bega (NSW); Mossman (Qld)
MM 6	All areas categorised ASGS RA4 that are not on a populated island that is separated from the mainland in the Australian Bureau of Statistics (ABS) geography and is more than 5 km offshore
MM 7	RA5 (very remote) – all other areas – that being ASGS RA5 and areas on a populated island that is separated from the mainland in the ABS geography and is more than 5 km offshore – discrete remote Indigenous communities, islands and migratory

TABLE 2.2 **Modified Monash Model***

*The DoctorConnect website provides an interactive map to determine all towns in Australia and their MMM classification: <http://www.doctorconnect.gov.au/internet/otd/publishing.nsf/Content/MMM_locator>.

Adapted from: Australian Government. (2015). *Rural Classification Reform: Frequently asked questions.* Canberra: Department of Health. <http://www.doctorconnect.gov.au/internet/otd/publishing.nsf/Content/Classification -changes>.

doctors to areas most in need (Department of Health, Australian Government, 2015).

3 **Accessibility Remoteness Index of Australia plus (ARIA+)** was redeveloped from ARIA in 2001. It was designed to be an unambiguous geographical approach to defining remoteness based on road distances between populated localities and service centres (Australian Population and Migration Research Centre, 2015). The road distances are then used to generate a remoteness score for any Australian location (see Figure 2.3). ARIA+ calculates numerical values for anywhere in Australia that range from 0 to 12, where 0 equals major metropolitan areas and 12 equals very remote areas. It then divides locations into five categories (see Table 2.3) based on natural breaks in the 0–12 continuum (Australian Population and

FIGURE 2.3 Accessibility/Remoteness Index Australia (ARIA+). This map clearly indicates the six areas, excluding migratory, and the names of some of the communities in each category.

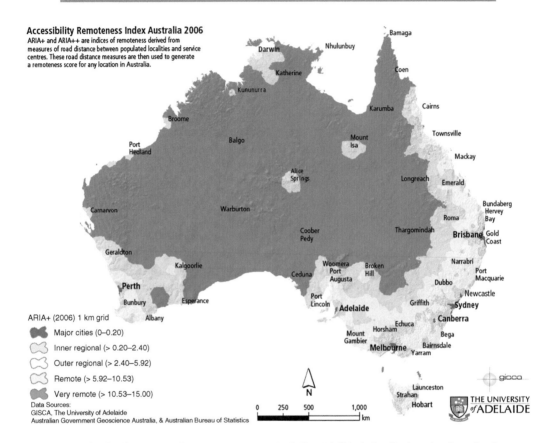

Reproduced with permission from: Baxter, J., Hayes, A., & Gray, M. (2011). *Families in regional, rural and remote Australia* (Facts sheet). Melbourne: Australian Institute of Family Studies.

TABLE 2.3 ARIA+ classification system

SERVICE CENTRE CATEGORY	URBAN CENTRE POPULATION
A	250 000 persons or more
B	48 000–249 999 persons
C	18 000–47 999 persons
D	5000–17 999 persons
E	1000–4999 persons
F (ARIA++ only)	200–999 persons

Adapted with permission from: Australian Population and Migration Research Centre. (2015). *ARIA+ (Accessibility/Remoteness Index of Australia).* <https://www.adelaide.edu.au/apmrc/research/projects/category/about_aria.html>.

Migration Research Centre, 2015). Since it is a measure of increasing 'remoteness', the term 'rural' is not defined, nor definable, in ARIA values. Geographical remoteness was seen to be a better indicator of disadvantage than subjective labels such as rural. Its advantages over other methods of measuring remoteness are that it is a purely geographical measure of remoteness and it is flexible, clear, precise and relatively stable over time (Australian Population and Migration Research Centre, 2015). There have been a number of adaptations of the ARIA+ system relevant to specific health professional groups such as pharmacists, who have a PhARIA that is based on road distance to the five closest pharmacies.

Although we have these two main measures of geographical remoteness they do not, however, measure the morbidity or mortality of the population, the cultural grouping or the socioeconomic status of the population being serviced – all factors that impact upon health status.

It should be remembered that it is data collected on the geographical classification that should inform decision making, not the classification itself. Any geographical classification only provides the framework upon which to classify and compare a range of data (Glover & Tennant, 2003). This is particularly important when funds are allocated using only these classifications, as remoteness may only be one factor affecting health issues.

PAUSE AND THINK

Using the DoctorConnect and the ARIA+ classification systems identify your town or one that you have been to in rural or remote Australia and see where they are classified.

Compare the health, education and social services provided in that town to those in a more urban area.

APPLYING THE CLASSIFICATION TO PRACTICE IN VERY REMOTE AUSTRALIA

Seventy-eight per cent of the landmass of this great country is considered to be remote or very remote. As you move further away from the eight capital cities, the more disperse the population becomes. Towns are infrequent and far apart, and the accessibility, safety and quality of health services can become progressively compromised. Remoteness is identified with a lack of accessibility to services, especially those regarded as 'normal' in urban areas, such as food supply and health care services (Kelly & Smith, 2007). This lack of accessibility becomes more pronounced in those communities described as 'very remote'.

When you enter very remote Australia, as classified by ARIA+, you are truly heading 'off the beaten track'. You usually do not end up in one of these places by accident – they are usually not on the way to anywhere else, they are not usually on a map and it often takes hours of travel along dusty, corrugated dirt roads to get there. You are, in effect, entering outback Australia. It is possible to perish in this sort of country. You would usually need a four-wheel drive vehicle, a reserve fuel tank, a couple of spare tyres, several litres of water and a satellite phone or two-way radio if you wish to keep in touch while you are on the road. You often need a permit in advance to visit a discrete Indigenous community in very remote Australia. Roads can be impassable at times – depending on weather conditions like flooding – and they are not always fenced, so wandering livestock, kangaroos, camels and other animals might be a problem (Kelly & Smith, 2007). More than 25 ARIA+ classified very remote communities are located on islands that are only accessible via air or sea travel. Some communities on the mainland are only accessible by air. This helps to conceptualise the context of very remote health service provision, where accessibility holds real challenges.

What is also noticeable when travelling in very remote Australia is the much higher proportion of Indigenous people. Indigenous people make up 45 per cent of the very remote population (Australian Institute of Health and Welfare, 2014b). They largely live in the 1187 discrete Aboriginal and Torres Strait Islander communities and, although they share the same geographical space as non-Indigenous people, they rarely mix as they live in towns located far away from one another. Most of the health services in these very remote, discrete Aboriginal communities are found in just three states – Western Australia, Queensland and the Northern Territory.

To interpret remote health data, we require a basic understanding of conditions on the ground. To illustrate this, we need to examine the structure and distribution of health services in *very remote Australia*. All ARIA+ very remote towns and communities have populations of less than 1000 (Australian Institute of Health and Welfare, 2014b). Let us now explore what this means for health services in these areas.

Providing health services in very remote areas

Table 2.4 demonstrates the differences between the two types of very remote communities and the inequities that exist. One community is a discrete very remote *Indigenous* community and the other is a very remote *non-Indigenous* community. Yet they are classified as the same under the ARIA+ classification scheme – as very remote.

Table 2.4 contains a combination of information from the Australian Bureau of Statistics and the Australian Institute of Health and Welfare (Australian Bureau of Statistics & Australian Institute of Health and Welfare, 2008; Australian Bureau of Statistics, 2009; Australian Institute of Health and Welfare, 2014b, 2014d), plus local knowledge based on the experience of the authors (Ellis & Kelly, 2005; Kelly & Smith, 2007).

TABLE 2.4 Comparing two very remote communities that are both based on the same ARIA+ category		
FEATURE	INDIGENOUS COMMUNITY	NON-INDIGENOUS COMMUNITY
Town	Not on most maps	Included on most maps
	Permit required to enter the community	Some mining communities are closed
Roads	Dirt road off the highway	Sealed roads on the highway
Economic base	Usually no industry	Usually mining or pastoral industry
Population	200–1000 people	200–1000 people
	80% Indigenous	80% non-Indigenous
	78% speak an Indigenous language at home (Australian Bureau of Statistics [ABS] & Australian Institute of Health and Welfare [AIHW], 2008)	82% speak English at home (ABS & AIHW, 2008)
Income	Median income is $394 per week (Erny-Albrecht, Raven & Blywood, 2014)	Median income is $869 per week – higher than any other region (Erny-Albrecht et al., 2014)
Houses	39% overcrowded (AIHW, 2014d)	Houses usually in good repair and uncrowded
	40% of houses require major repairs (ABS, 2009)	
Water supply	Is tested irregularly	Town supply is usually tested regularly and is safe to drink
Sewerage	Problems and overflows are extremely common	Sewerage usually works and does not overflow
Health services	Usually a single Aboriginal and Torres Strait Islander primary health care service without inpatient facilities, providing 24-hour emergency care and visiting services to outlying communities	Usually a hospital with acute and 24-hour inpatient care, as well as visiting specialists and allied health. Of the 68 very remote hospitals in Australia, 59 are located in non-Indigenous communities
Emergency care	Provided by a registered nurse or Indigenous health worker with telephone advice from a doctor. The Royal Flying Doctor Service (RFDS) transfers patients to a regional hospital	Provided by ambulance, then a doctor and registered nurse – in the accident and emergency department. RFDS transfers stabilised patients to a regional hospital if necessary
Health services employer	Usually the state or territory government; about half of all Indigenous primary health care services are Aboriginal community controlled	Usually the state or territory government supplemented by private GP services and a pharmacy

Continued

TABLE 2.4 **Comparing two very remote communities that are both based on the same ARIA+ category–cont'd**		
FEATURE	INDIGENOUS COMMUNITY	NON-INDIGENOUS COMMUNITY
X-rays	A registered nurse or Indigenous health worker takes X-Rays	There is usually access to an appointed radiographer
Scope of practice for registered nurses	Registered nurse roles are 'extended' and include prescribing, diagnosing and managing patients based on clinical guidelines (CARPA Clinical Procedures Manual for example)	While broader and deeper, the scope of practice for registered nurses is similar to advanced urban registered nurses
Private health services	There are usually no private health services – e.g. pharmacy, pathology, allied health	There may be private health services such as a pharmacy or other allied health services
Non-emergency transport – road travel	Usually takes more than a day's road travel on dirt roads, which can be impassable at times. Very few Indigenous households have access to a vehicle	Road travel is more likely to be on paved roads. Most own or have access to a vehicle

Notes:

1   Indigenous primary health care service is the most common health service provided in discrete very remote communities. Fifty-six per cent of Indigenous people in discrete communities lived 100 kilometres or more from the nearest hospital (ABS & AIHW, 2008).

2   This is a profile of the most common type of health service provided in non-Indigenous towns in very remote Australia. Some health services will be exceptions.

Classifying for disadvantage

Table 2.4 clearly demonstrates the inequities in getting to and from two very remote communities. It also compares provision of the two very different health services: the haves and the have-nots. Non-indigenous towns and services tend to resemble smaller versions of outer regional Australia. They also attract the lion's share of 'hard-to-find' doctors. In contrast, the absence of on-site doctors in remote Indigenous communities has led to a 'different' model of health service – Indigenous primary health care services, which differ between states and regions. For example, in Queensland primary health care services are classified as 'hospitals', which means they are operated in the hospital 'acute medical care' paradigm. Therefore, resources are largely allocated based on the work of doctors through the Medicare system. So, when there are no doctors located in these communities, this impacts on both the resourcing mechanisms and the scope of practice of largely government-employed staff. This results in registered nurses and Indigenous health workers performing roles and undertaking procedures usually restricted to doctors – prescribing, diagnosing and managing (CRANAplus, 2015). These factors influence a person's access to the service due to cultural and other issues. Additionally, issues of continuity of care are affected as there are often very high turnover rates of remote nursing staff.

Clearly, there is more going on than disadvantage due to geography and classifications alone. There appear to be twin key factors at play – remoteness and the cultural grouping of the population being serviced. When combined, both factors appear to have a strong influence on the type and level of service being provided to a very remote community. These factors will undoubtedly influence the health outcomes of the population, which are already compromised especially for the remote Indigenous population. However, the effects may be insignificant while Indigenous people continue to live in crowded houses in communities with unreliable water supplies, broken sewerage systems, poor food supplies and open garbage dumps (Australian Institute of Health and Welfare, 2014c). These are just a few of the factors that need to be taken into account when interpreting data that deal with remoteness and disadvantage in very remote Australia.

CONCLUSION

Australia appears to be the 'land of plenty', or 'enough', apart from discrete Indigenous communities in remote and very remote areas, which remain pockets of significant need. It seems that, if people are unwell, they will generally receive appropriate levels of care across urban, regional and remote Australia unless they live in very remote Indigenous communities and inland Australia.

A major problem in understanding the health of people in regional and remote Australia is the limited availability, representativeness and quality of data. Very few data sources are complete, accurate, regionally representative and unambiguous enough to allow meaningful comparisons between populations from different areas. This applies particularly to remote and very remote areas where there are low population numbers but high numbers of Indigenous Australians. While some remote communities have been found to report better Indigenous health data than cities, the data usually only represent three or four states and often the data sources are incomplete. What is consistent between groups is the poorer health status for all Australians who live remotely.

The extra challenge is one of Indigenous health, not necessarily the health of those living in remote areas. Further work is required to tease out the differences in morbidity and mortality *between* Indigenous and non-Indigenous populations in very remote Australia. Remoteness can explain some of the disadvantage, but it does not explain the disparities that exist between equally remote Indigenous and non-Indigenous communities.

When the data regarding rural and remote health service delivery using the ARIA+ classification were published, it had the effect of pulling aside a veil on very remote health service provision. An ever-widening gap in health and wellbeing evident *within* geographical classificatory systems was exposed. Also exposed were discriminatory practices that favour one subgroup at the expense of another, and population statistics on racial and ethnic composition that can be used by policy makers to identify selected subgroups in need of support to allocate the required social resources. Ratios of health care practitioners to population in a particular area are often used to judge accessibility. But such ratios are crude at best. They do not tell the whole story, since people in areas with ratios comparable to others of similar size may still be disadvantaged (Kelly & Smith, 2007). With this come thoughts about institutional racism. Although new classification systems are being implemented, in reality they only focus on the medical workforce and incentives rather than the socio-economic realities of many of these very remote communities.

Discussion points

1 Using the RRMA or ARIA+ classification system, find three towns in each category that you have been to, lived in or know quite well. Discuss the health and other services provided in each of the towns. What gaps, inequities and inconsistencies have you found between the services in each town?

2 If you were responsible for allocating rural and remote health resources, would you do so equally on the basis of the information that you found in discussion point 1? If not, why not? Discuss.

3 Refer to Table 2.4. Discuss the inequities between the two very remote communities. What surprised you in this table?

4 Why would remote and very remote areas be better at collecting Indigenous identification data than city areas? Discuss.

5 Where would you look for information about how many doctors work in very remote Australia?

6 What health indicators would you use to demonstrate that remote Australians are disadvantaged when compared to those living in major cities? Discuss.

References

Adams, P. (2003). Brains, brains, brains; oi, oi, oi. *The Weekend Australian Magazine*, 1–2 March, 11.

Australian Bureau of Statistics (ABS) (2009). *National Aboriginal and Torres Strait Islander Social Survey, 2008*. Canberra: ABS. <http://www.abs.gov.au/ausstats/abs@.nsf/Latest products/4714.0Main%20Features102008?opendocument&tabname=Summary&prodno=471 4.0&issue=2008&num=&view=> Accessed 12.07.15.

Australian Bureau of Statistics (2011). *Remoteness structure*. Canberra: ABS. <http://www.abs.gov.au/websitedbs/D3310114.nsf/home/remoteness+structure>Accessed 12.07.15.

Australian Bureau of Statistics (2013). 4102.0 – *Towns of the mining boom. Australian Social Trends*, April 2013. Canberra: ABS. <http://www.abs.gov.au/AUSSTATS/abs@.nsf/Lookup/4102.0Main+Features10April+2013> Accessed 12.07.15.

Australian Bureau of Statistics (2014a). *Estimates and projections, Aboriginal and Torres Strait Islander Australians, 2001 to 2026*. Canberra: ABS. <http://www.abs.gov.au/AUSSTATS/abs@.nsf/DetailsPage/3238.02001%20to%202026> Accessed 03.03.15.

Australian Bureau of Statistics (2014b). 4102.0 – *The average Australian. Australian Social Trends*, April 2013. Canberra: ABS. <http://www.abs.gov.au/AUSSTATS/abs@.nsf/Lookup/4102.0Main+Features30April+2013#back7> Accessed 12.07.15.

Australian Bureau of Statistics (2015a). *Mt Isa LGA*. Canberra: ABS. <http://stat.abs.gov.au/itt/r.jsp?RegionSummary&region=35300&geoconcept=REGION&dataset=ABS_NRP9_LGA&datasetLGA=ABS_NRP9_LGA&datasetASGS=ABS_NRP9_ASGS&regionLGA=REGION&regionASGS=REGION> Accessed 12.07.15.

Australian Bureau of Statistics (2015b). *Population clock*. Canberra: ABS. <http://www.abs.gov.au/ausstats/abs@.nsf/0/1647509ef7e25faaca2568a900154b63> Accessed 08.03.15.

Australian Bureau of Statistics & Australian Institute of Health and Welfare (AIHW) (2008). 4704.0 – *Health and welfare of Australia's Aboriginal and Torres Strait Islander peoples*. Canberra: ABS and AIHW.

Australian Government (2015). *The Australian continent*. <http://www.australia.gov.au/about-australia/our-country/the-australian-continent> Accessed 09.03.15.

Australian Institute of Health and Welfare (2014a). *Access to primary health care relative to need for Indigenous Australians*. Canberra: AIHW. <http://www.aihw.gov.au/WorkArea/DownloadAsset.aspx?id=60129547982> Accessed 11.03.15.

Australian Institute of Health and Welfare (2014b). Chapter 7, Indigenous health. In *Australia's health 2014*. Canberra: AIHW.

Australian Institute of Health and Welfare (2014c). *Australia's health 2014*. Canberra: AIHW. <http://www.aihw.gov.au/australias-health/2014/indigenous-health/> Accessed 12.09.15.

Australian Institute of Health and Welfare (2014d). *Housing circumstances of Indigenous households: Tenure and overcrowding*. Canberra: AIHW. <http://www.aihw.gov.au/WorkArea/DownloadAsset.aspx?id=60129548056> Accessed 12.09.15.

Australian Institute of Health and Welfare (2015). *Rural, Remote and Metropolitan (RRMA) classification*. Canberra: AIHW. <http://www.aihw.gov.au/rural-health-rrma-classification/> Accessed 12.09.15.

Australian Population and Migration Research Centre (2015). *ARIA+ (Accessibility / Remoteness Index of Australia)*. <https://www.adelaide.edu.au/apmrc/research/projects/category/about_aria.html> Accessed 13.03.15.

City of Ballarat (2015). *City of Ballarat Profile*. <http://www.ballarat.vic.gov.au/> Accessed 12.03.15.

CRANAplus (2015). *Framework for remote practice*. Cairns: CRANAplus. <https://crana.org.au/files/pdfs/Framework_Remote_Practice_FINAL.pdf> Accessed 14.03.15.

Cummins, R. (2010). *What makes us happy? Ten years of the Australian Unity Wellbeing Index*. Melbourne: Australian Unity and Deakin University.

Department of Health, Australian Government (2015). *Rural classification reform: Frequently asked questions.* Canberra: Department of Health. <http://www.doctorconnect.gov.au/internet/otd/publishing.nsf/Content/Classification-changes> Accessed 12.09.15.

dictionary.com (2015). British dictionary definitions for remote dictionary.com. <http://dictionary.reference.com/browse/remote> Accessed 12.07.15.

Ellis, I., & Kelly, K. (2005). Health infrastructure in very remote areas: an analysis of the CRANA bush crisis line database. *The Australian Journal of Rural Health, 13*(1), 1–2.

Erny-Albrecht, K. B. L., Raven, M., & Bywood, P. (2014). *PHCRIS policy issue review: Fly-in fly-out/drive-in drive-out practices and health service delivery in rural areas of Australia.* Canberra: Primary Health Care Research & Information Service. <http://www.phcris.org.au/publications/policyreviews/report.php?id=8425> Accessed 17.07.15.

Glover, J., & Tennant, S. (2003). *Remote areas statistical geography in Australia: Notes on the Accessibility/Remoteness Index for Australia (ARIA+ version)*; working paper no 9. Adelaide: Public Health Statistical Information Unit, University of Adelaide.

Kelly, K., & Smith, J. D. (2007). Chapter 5. What and where is rural and remote Australia? In J. D. Smith (Ed.), *Australia's rural and remote health: A social justice perspective.* Melbourne: Tertiary Press.

Keneally, T. (1983). *Outback.* Lane Cove, NSW: Hodder & Stoughton (Australia) Pty Ltd.

Working in Australia (2015). *Australia's beach lifestyle.* <http://www.workingin-australia.com/live-and-settle/life-in-australia/beach-lifestyle#.VaI47U0w-Uk> Accessed 11.03.15.

CHAPTER 3

CULTURE AND HEALTH

Robyn Williams | Janie Dade Smith | Regan Jane Sharp

A people without the knowledge of their past history, origin
and culture is like a tree without roots.

(MARCUS GARVEY)

Imagine the perfect world where our children play in the sunshine with their multi-cultural friends, where everyone is treated equally, where we all understand and respect each other for our strengths and our differences. To live in such a peaceful multicultural society it is important to understand why we 'think what we think' and why different cultural groups 'think what they think'. This understanding is particu-larly important for health professionals who will all at various times work in cross-cultural contexts. Working as a 'culturally safe' practitioner is just as important as being a 'clinically safe' practitioner. A crucial part of being culturally safe is being able to define our own culture, to know how our own cultural identity influences and shapes our work practice and being able to negotiate shared meaning and relation-ships of trust with *all* people receiving our care.

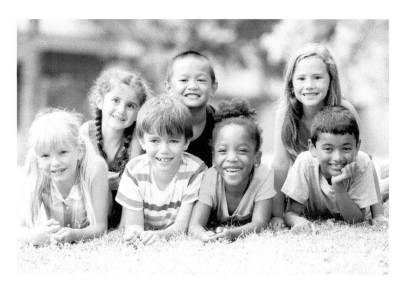

Reproduced with permission from: iStockphoto/Christopher Futcher.

Learning about our own cultural identity, particularly for those from the dominant or largest cultural group, is an interesting process that can be confronting and extremely challenging. This is because we commonly think that our way of doing or seeing things is the most obvious and logical way. This chapter aims to challenge those beliefs so that you, as a health professional, can provide the most appropriate services to all who make up our very culturally diverse population.

This chapter also examines the issue of culture from international, national and rural perspectives. It explores how to turn one's gaze from 'the other' and how to look at one's self, that is, what goes into making up our professional and personal identity and how this impacts on work practice. It then explores in detail three key concepts, racism, social justice and cultural safety, and applies these principles through the use of a case study.

WHAT IS CULTURE?

Culture describes the particular way of life of a group of people, as they are living today. It is like a group's own particular pattern or template for living. It includes what they *think* – their beliefs, values and philosophies; what they *say* – their stories, myths, languages, symbols and traditions; what they *do* – their lifestyles, customs and behaviours; what they *believe* – their ambitions, traditions and expectations; and what they *make* – their buildings, technology and food.

Culture is learned. It evolves, adapts and is passed down from generation to generation. It is based on shared perceptions about the cultural group's beliefs, values, philosophies and norms (Tidwell, 2003). It is these shared perceptions that define the culture and bind the group together. It tells them what is 'pretty' and what is 'ugly'; what is 'right' and what is 'wrong'. It influences their preferred way of thinking, of behaving and of making decisions (Eckermann et al., 2012).

Culture is constantly changing; it has to in order to survive. Our culture changes slowly and constantly as we find new ways of doing things and through our exposure to other cultures. Discoveries and innovations, such as television and the internet, and social and political movements, such as the women's movement, help bring about these changes. We borrow and discard from other cultures, such as worldwide fast food chains like McDonald's where we now find Australians asking for fries instead of chips. Our long-term contact with other cultures also brings about change in how we view the world (Tidwell, 2003). These subtle influences affect our culture and slowly and constantly change our own template for living as a group as we accept, respect and take on these beliefs and practices as our own. This means that we always have a culture. It is not something we can lose; it is what we are living now (Cadet-James, 2003).

Different cultures often have difficulty in understanding one another. This is not just due to differences in language and lifestyle, but also to the different processes they use to interpret the world and consequently make their decisions. These decisions are based on their own set of principles, values and philosophies and their different ways of knowing and doing (Eckermann et al., 2012). It is often easier to see 'differences' in other people than in ourselves; often we cannot recognise our own culture because it is so much a part of us. This can then raise a 'fear of difference' between two groups, which is based on the insecurity that arises from unfamiliarity. Consequently, most of us think that what we see and believe is the 'right or only' way. This often leads us to make judgements or disapprove of others who think or behave differently from ourselves. This is particularly prevalent for those who belong to the largest and dominant group, largely because this is the section of society that has the most influence on how people behave.

There are a variety of different subcultures within every culture (Dreachslin, Gilbert, & Malone, 2012). These include the practices of a school group – 'school culture'; or the values of a workforce – 'corporate culture'; or the perceptions of a gendered group – 'male culture'; or the actions of a particular group – 'the culture of violence'. The women's movement of the 1970s created one such subgroup and substantially changed the way in which women are now viewed by, and socially integrated into, society. There may also be subcultures between mainstream groups, such as gays, lesbians, bisexuals, transgenders, queer and intersex people, the elderly, single parents, intravenous drug users, teenagers, football players and different professional groups. One culture that dominates all health professionals is 'medical culture', which is based on the scientific rationalist and biomedical model of health care. For centuries it has provided the lens through which we understand the scientific basis of illness; it has provided society with one 'worldview' of health and illness.

What is worldview?

The concept of worldview provides a lens for understanding culture. It refers to how different people or groups of people perceive and relate to the world in different ways. Worldviews influence how we 'understand the world' and all aspects of life. It affects how we experience health and illness, what it means to be well, what we do when we are sick, who we talk to and how we understand the causes and treatments of our conditions.

Worldview is also tied to the concept of different 'knowledge'... how we 'know' the world, which will influence understandings of all aspects of life, including health. If we only know one way of seeing the world, or one way of understanding it, we will take this to be the 'true' way of seeing the world – it becomes our 'reality'. However, we then may be more likely to disregard others' worldviews, or to not see them as legitimate ways of knowing about the world.

We all make assumptions about what is true and these assumptions are embedded within our knowledge systems. All knowledge is also political, in that it is constructed by relationships of power based on domination and subordination. The objectivist, scientific view of knowledge is dominant in Western society and particularly in areas such as health.

These concepts of knowledge and worldview are very important to understand, as they are fundamental to what we understand about culture. It is important to remember that it is not just other cultures whose worldviews we need to recognise. MacLachlan (1997, p. 59) said that we need to 'think through' our own culture, which means being aware of our own worldviews and understandings to help us explain

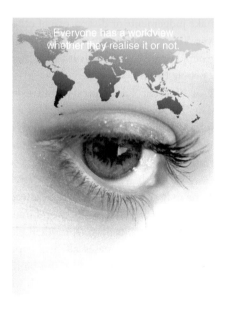

Everyone has a worldview whether they realise it or not.

Reproduced with permission from: Shutterstock/ARENA Creative.

why we think and act the way we do. In doing so, we can understand that our way of experiencing the world is just one way, rather than the only or the right way.

To be an effective health professional, it is important to be aware that not all groups think like you do, particularly if you are part of the dominant group. When one culture tries to convert another culture to its way of thinking or doing, it often results in 'culture conflict'. This can occur when one cultural group has power over another, and where it tries to impose its systems and organisations, beliefs and values on the less powerful – usually by violence or legislative sanctions (Eckermann et al., 2012).

Understanding health culture

The concept of health differs between individuals, both within and across different cultures, and this difference has important implications for health systems and services. The word 'health' carries considerable cultural, social and professional baggage and it is a key to our culture. It is a word that involves important ideas and strongly held values (Baum, 2008). Using it in different ways gives rise to particular ways of seeing the world and behaving.

In many Western countries such as Australia, the dominant health systems operate using a **biomedical model of health** (Baum, Bégin, Houweling, & Taylor, 2009). When a biomedical approach is used, the body is essentially viewed as a machine with a set of interrelated parts. The malfunctioning or 'sick' part is isolated, causes are sought and treatment is instigated. From this description, it can be seen that this biomedical model is derived from a typically Western scientific framework of knowledge and understanding, based on objectivity and scientific rationalism. This means breaking something down into its smallest components for analysis, rather than seeing something as a whole (Crotty, 1998).

As with many other cultures, Indigenous Australians tend to see health from a holistic perspective, where it is not just the physical wellbeing of the individual but includes the social, environmental, cultural and spiritual wellbeing of the whole community (NAHS Working Party, 1989).

Therefore, as health professionals it is important to question one's own understandings of health, to begin to understand how health can differ across cultures. Differing and often competing worldviews, language barriers and misunderstandings can inhibit effective service delivery. A major factor that influences access to and equity in a service is the appropriateness of the service to all of its users and the previous experiences of the client, both within wider society and within the service industry.

PAUSE AND THINK

Think about your own worldview of health. How do you define it?

What factors have you brought to this worldview from your own family?

Recognising difference

People who look physically different from the mainstream group cannot hide their identity or choose not to disclose it. Every day they come in contact with mainstream groups or belief systems where they are aware of their differences. These experiences, many of which begin in childhood, will strongly contribute to the identity and sense of self held by marginalised individuals and groups. These experiences will interact and be simultaneously influenced by cultural differences, family and worldview.

In some cases individuals can choose when to declare their 'differentness'. For example, they can decide not to tell the GP that they use recreational drugs or have hepatitis C – for fear of being labelled a drug user; they might not tell their next door neighbour that they are gay or lesbian – for fear of being judged or subjected to homophobia; they might not tell their workmates that they are a devout Christian – for fear of being discriminated against for their religious beliefs; or a teenager might not tell their midwife that they have had an abortion – for fear of being judged as promiscuous or stupid. These people still suffer marginalisation and discrimination from mainstream (or other minority) groups, but it is less constant because physically they can 'blend in with the crowd'.

INTERNATIONAL PERSPECTIVES

A number of new Australians, in particular health professionals, are being moved to rural and remote areas as they come through our borders from war-torn countries, where many have been victims of terror, displacement and violence. We no longer live in an insular world where we can choose to ignore the activities of other countries. As our nation becomes more multicultural, it is important that we have some insight into some of the rites and rituals that other cultures practise so that we can understand the thinking behind what they do, and their beliefs and value systems. Once we can see the thinking behind the action, it becomes easier to tolerate or respect these cultural groups for thinking what they think, and to suspend judgement about those things that we do not understand (Eckermann et al., 2012). This may then provide us with some insight into why they think that. It is really a matter of tolerance and respect.

Rites and rituals

First, let us look at the number of ways in which we all learn our value systems throughout our lives. This occurs through traditions that are passed on from parent to child, and family to family; through rituals that we hold dear such as christenings, marriages and funerals; through those rites of passage that acknowledge a new phase of development, such as bar mitzvahs and school graduation ceremonies; and through our religious, cultural and political beliefs.

There are key rituals that we accept in all cultures at the most important times in our lives, such as at birth, when we become adults, on marriage and at death. These are the occasions when we take time to acknowledge, recognise, respect and honour the new, the maturing process and the dear departed. In Australia we honour our fallen soldiers – 'lest we forget'; our 'lovable larrikins' such as Ned Kelly; and of course our sporting, music and activist heroes, on whom we bestow awards such as 'Australian of the Year'. Each culture does these things differently, and the traditions are passed down from generation to generation, from cultural group to cultural group and from religion to religion. Honour, therefore, forms part of the value system upon which cultures base their philosophies.

Not all countries have the freedoms, guaranteed human rights and value systems that Western cultures take for granted. In other cultures, what Australians proudly consider their cultural norms could be seen as crimes of the state or acts that would bring great dishonour and disrespect on the family. Some cultures can have overtly defined roles for men and women. For example, women may not be considered equal to men; the institution of marriage and the concept of 'marriageability' may be held in the highest regard; women may be 'protected' by men; and there may be strong traditional family or caste* systems. Examples of acts that might be considered disrespectful or a social crime could include females wearing revealing clothes or travelling without a male companion in many Muslim countries or females marrying into another caste system in India.

Likewise, there are numerous cultural practices that many Australians may consider wrong, ridiculous or even barbaric in the context of their own cultural template for living. These include: praying three times a day; requiring women to wear veils; paying dowries so that daughters can marry; arranging marriages; and circumcising or killing daughters. For example, in Pakistan the United Nations estimates that there are over 5000 honour killings every year (cited: Chesler, 2010). These women are killed at the hands of their fathers, brothers and husbands in the name of honour and tradition. The value and belief system behind these killings is based on strong patriarchal and tribal traditions that regard the male as the sole protector and controller of the female, and her 'right to life' as conditional on her obeying social norms and traditions (Morgan, 2003). If the male's protection is violated he is viewed as losing his honour, which in turn brings dishonour to his family. The thinking behind this is that he either failed to protect her, or failed to bring her up correctly (Jones, 2008).

In our Western cultural value system we treat honour killings as murder and as a violation of our most basic human right: our right to life. In Western cultural value systems our right to life and the rights of women to be equal to men, to be protected from violence and abuse and to marry whom they want are taken for granted. They are assumed to be basic human rights; but of course not everyone adheres to these

*Caste system is a system of social hierarchy particularly used in Hindu society, where members have no social contact with other classes but are socially equal to one another and often follow the same occupations (*Australian Concise Oxford Dictionary*, 2000).

beliefs, which is evident in our high rates of domestic violence across all levels of society.

The cultural conflict here lies in the ways in which these two value systems see the role, value and 'humanness' of women compared with men. The value systems are supported by learned traditions that are passed down from one century to the next.

Now let us examine our own Australian culture and the values, beliefs and philosophies that characterise our template, and the way in which we live as a group.

AUSTRALIAN CULTURE

Australian culture consists of a diverse combination of cultural groups. Walking down some of the city streets in metropolitan Melbourne or Sydney, you could be forgiven for thinking you were in Tokyo, Saigon, Rome or Athens.

Most Australians see Australia as a relatively young country because they calculate its age in terms of European settlement. However, there were ancient Indigenous cultures and traditions in existence for at least 45 000 years before the arrival of Europeans (Human Rights and Equal Opportunity Commission, 1997). Yet Australia's now dominant cultural group has taken on few of these traditions, apart from a growing appreciation of Indigenous art, dance and bush tucker. Due to colonisation, the very essence of Australian culture has become that of the dominant English and Europeans, and more recently the United States. It includes those characteristics and icons that we now hold dear as a nation such as our obsession with 'football, meat pies and Holden cars'.

In Australia today there are more Italians, South Africans and Greeks than there are Indigenous Australians, and there are many sixth and seventh generation Australians who think of nowhere else as home. It is our borrowing from different cultures that has given this great country of ours its diversity and richness and makes us one of the more successful multicultural societies in the world.

Typical Aussies

What underpins the worldview, values, philosophies, belief systems and ways of doing that make Australian culture different from other cultures? On what have we forged our national identity?

First, we have the values that we as a nation hold dear, and upon which Australian culture is based. As Australians we take great pride in what we see as uniquely Australian values, such as 'our sense of fairness, that is, giving and getting "a fair go"; our camaraderie – "mateship"; our sense of optimism – "she'll be right"; and our sense of equality and egalitarianism' (Sidoti, 1996, p. 1).

Second, there is our philosophy for living, which is based on a sense of our basic human rights supported by our values of equity – fairness, equality and sameness. As Australians we now take for granted our right to work, vote, travel and speak freely; our freedom of religion and from arbitrary arrest; and the right of ethnic and racial minorities and those with disabilities to protection (Human Rights and Equal

Opportunity Commission, 2015b). Generally, we believe that women should be treated as equal to men, able to work for the same pay as men and to wear whatever clothing they choose. We believe all adult people should be free to marry, or not to marry, have their own sexual preferences and choose their own partners. Most Australians see these beliefs as their right, without question. In fact these human rights, which we take for granted, provide us with a strong core national value system that is based on justice, equality and a 'fair go' for all. They form our national identity and they are the reason why so many people want to live in our wonderful country. This philosophy is right for us as a group of people. Today, if we did not hold these values and philosophies, we would probably be labelled 'un-Australian'.

The third factor, our belief system, is based on our concept of human rights plus our value system. Generally speaking, we have a value system that tells us what is 'beautiful' – being thin and young; what is 'ugly' – being fat and old; what is 'right' – getting ahead and having a nice house, a good job and lots of money; and what is 'wrong' – breaking the law or abusing children. As Australians generally, we make our decisions accordingly.

This has not always been the case in Australian life. Australian culture, like all other cultures, is forever changing. For example, the discovery of the contraceptive pill in the 1960s and the 1970s push by the women's movement for equal rights produced many innovations, including a change in government policy that brought about supporting parents' benefits and abortion legislation. This enabled women, for the first time, to choose whether or not to keep their babies rather than have them adopted out, and to escape from violent and unhappy relationships. These changes brought with them new freedoms, belief systems, lifestyles, expectations and values, new ways of behaving and making decisions, new government policies and new perceptions of male and female roles. This has consequently changed our cultural template for living as a group.

In 2015 the push for 'marriage equality' will have another long-term impact on our belief systems, values and expectations, and will change not only our policies but our template for living as a group – one that is inclusive of those with sexual preferences different from the dominant group.

RURAL CULTURE

There are many subcultures within the overall Australian culture. Rural culture is one, which is important for health professionals to understand. As we have already noted, rural people see themselves as different from city-dwelling Australians, and they have different perceptions of health. This worldview is probably due to the different experiences of rural people that resulted from historical perceptions of the 'strong, rugged, male' foundations laid in rural history. Hence, the values and beliefs illustrated in such expressions as 'a hard day's work for an honest day's pay', 'sticking by your mates through thick or thin' and 'not big-noting yourself' continue to be held strongly by rural people. Although this ethos is also held by other Australians, it is far more pronounced among the people of the bush, who believe in the superiority of their way of life (Dempsey, 1990) and who are renowned for their independence, resourcefulness, capacity for hard work and stoicism in the face of adversity (Rolley & Humphreys, 1993).

These distinctive sets of values, beliefs and priorities form Australia's rural culture – its template for living as a group. These values and beliefs were perpetuated in the 1920s by political attitudes that fostered a sense of 'country-mindedness' and the ideology or 'truth' of being rural people. Farming was seen as an ennobling experience that commanded respect because it involved hard work, perseverance and strong family structures (Gray & Lawrence, 2001). The image of a 'real' Australian that was promoted to the world was one of a countryman, able to tame his environment and make it productive through hard work (Aiken, 1985). City life was decried as competitive and nasty, and city people as being much the same the world over (Aiken, 1985). In more recent times, movies like *Crocodile Dundee* and television series like *McLeod's Daughters* have perpetuated this rural belief system. While many of the values of the time were both sexist and racist, the values behind them were largely based on the concept of a 'fair go', a belief in the productivity of hard work and the optimism and stoicism expressed in 'she'll be right, mate'. This is where rural people's characteristic perceptions about their own health may have originated.

Rural communities are made up of long-term residents: tradespeople, general workers, farmers, teachers and professional people. While it is generally understood that rural people tend to be very friendly, hospitable and loyal, Ken Dempsey (1990) in his study *Smalltown* found that there are also some other unique characteristics that differentiate the archetypal rural person from the city-dwelling Australian. He found that there are often very clear divisions between certain groups in small towns, and he places them into four categories: the 'no-hopers' – long-term residents who are usually the drinkers, unemployed and unkempt; the 'blockies' – hippie types who build a shelter on a block to get away from the city but end up on the dole and are not welcome in the community; 'deviant women' – women without local kinship who visit bars and are often judged on their performance as mothers; and 'transients' – 'two-bob blow ins' who owe no loyalty to the town, such as professionals and especially teachers (Dempsey, 1990, p. 48). It is from these kinds of perceptions that worldviews of rural culture have been formed.

Rural communities also possess systems of social status that can be distinguished by wealth, longevity in the community, perceived gender roles, religion, class, social standing and reputation for service (Stehlik, 2001). Rural people can also marginalise 'newcomers': those who may have different politics, religion, class or cultural background (Dempsey, 1990). There is often distrust and suspicion of newcomers, who can be defined as those who were not born in the town, or who do not have their family name on a plot at the cemetery. There is a potential for marginalising particular people who may be labelled 'fly-by-nighters' and 'no-hopers' by the locals (Dempsey, 1990). These can include short-term professionals on rotation or miners who fly in and fly out. Many newcomers have been sanctioned and sometimes driven from the community if they have failed to conform to the community's standards.

This process is called **stereotyping** and is about attributing certain characteristics to a group based on some common factor the group has – such as being from a rural town and therefore not being as bright as someone from the city.

As health professionals it is important to understand how these values and belief systems affect how people from different cultures and different cultural groups form their worldview, as well as their concept of health and illness.

Medical culture

Our medical system is derived from Western worldviews, our understandings of health, the body and our scientific rationalist thinking. On this basis it is not surprising that significant issues can arise when a person of a different worldview or cultural background interacts with such a system. This can impact on how a patient or client accesses a system, how they are diagnosed and how they are treated, as well as how compliant they are with the treatment recommended. As has also been seen, culture can be viewed from a number of perspectives when talking about interactions with the medical system. One of the most powerful examples comes from Indigenous experiences with a non-Indigenous medical system. Many Indigenous people report difficulties with mainstream medical services and many cases result in avoidance. Some culturally related examples include the physical environment for healing, family, communication and compliance. These issues can cause harm for clients who may not be receiving care in a culturally safe way.

CULTURAL SAFETY

The concept of cultural safety first came to prominence in New Zealand in the late 1980s from work spearheaded by Māori nurses including Papps and Ramsden (1996) and some of their Pakeha (white) colleagues. They identified issues relating to the interactions between Māori, the New Zealand health system and the institutions who educate health professionals for their roles. These issues included students' ongoing experiences of institutional racism, especially in the education system, and lack of appropriate tertiary education opportunities for Māori.

According to Woods (2010), the construct of cultural safety was originally inspired by the principles of *protection, participation* and *partnership* that were derived from the 1840 Treaty of Waitangi in New Zealand. This treaty, although not always fully honoured, was the foundational agreement between the Māori, the Indigenous people of the land, and the Pakeha, or British colonists. Cultural safety has subsequently been perceived as a guide for responding to the health problems of many of the world's most vulnerable or marginalised ethnic groups, that is, where similar experiences of colonisation have frequently led to significant health disparities between the Indigenous peoples and more recently arrived colonists in New Zealand, Australia and Canada.

So what does cultural safety mean? Cultural safety has its antecedents as a philosophy of health care that aimed to improve the health of all Indigenous peoples in First World colonised countries by providing culturally appropriate health care services. It is framed as a social justice approach to health care, aiming to address the health status of Indigenous peoples through continuous improvement in their health communication and interactions with health service providers (Kowal & Paradies, 2005; Ramsden, 2002). It needs to be said, though, that the concept of cultural safety has grown much more in recent years and has been broadened to include working cross-culturally in diverse contexts – not only in Indigenous health.

Cultural safety requires health professionals to undertake a process of personal reflection of their own cultural identity to be able to recognise the impact that their own culture has upon their health care practice. An acceptance and respect of cultural and individual difference is a critical factor in culturally safe practice.

Williams (1999, p. 1) tells us that cultural safety is about having a 'shared respect, shared meaning, shared knowledge and experience, of learning, living and working together with dignity, and truly listening'. Cultural safety can therefore be 'as simple as "having manners" and treating others with dignity and respect', and it can be 'as complex as having a discussion on culture and power' (Williams, 1999). 'Unsafe cultural practice would therefore comprise any action that diminishes, demeans or disempowers the cultural identity and well-being' of the person whose health is being acted upon (Nursing Council of New Zealand, 2011, p. 9). Cultural safety also extends beyond ethnic groups and includes 'age or generation; gender, sexual orientation, occupation, socioeconomic status, ethnic origin or migrant experience, religious or spiritual beliefs and disability'(Nursing Council of New Zealand, 2011, p. 6).

Principles of cultural safety

Ramsden (2002) describes three key principles that underlie the concept of cultural safety:

1 **p**artnership
2 **p**articipation
3 **p**rotection.

These 'three Ps' provided the building blocks for developing culturally safe professional health practice. When put into action these principles require:

- commitment from all involved to embrace cultural safety in a meaningful and transformative way
- developing all resources in partnership and using participatory models of appropriate health care
- protection against individual, structural and institutional racism
- acknowledgement that feelings of isolation and culture shock are common
- acknowledgement of language and cultural barriers that prevent meaningful exchanges

- recognition that concepts of health and wellness vary between cultures
- recognition of a client's past negative experiences with the system, both direct and observed (Ramsden, 2002).

How do you achieve cultural safety?

The following model has been adapted from Ramsden's work (cited Eckermann et al., 2012, p. 187) and is used to describe the three interrelated domains of culturally safe practice (see Figure 3.1). These three domains can be concurrent, and will vary with individual experience depending on the context and over time. The domains can begin initially by being aware that there is 'difference', such as differences in language, culture, appearance, gender, upbringing and socioeconomic status. They can then flow onto being sensitive and finally move to safe practice – as experienced by both the practitioner and the person whose health is being acted upon.

Cultural awareness domain – cultural awareness is a beginning step toward understanding that there is difference. It acknowledges the different social, economic and political contexts in which people exist. It is much more than information about formal cultural rituals and practices. For example, it could include sitting down with someone from another culture and talking about being parents of teenagers, thereby building relationships through establishing common ground and celebrating differences.

FIGURE 3.1 Culturally safe practice.

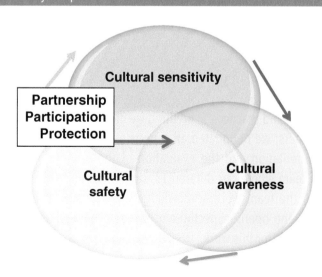

Cultural sensitivity domain – this is more than cultural awareness; it is about acting upon and legitimising difference through understanding, accepting, respecting and validating cultural difference. This domain involves a process of self-reflection and introspection where a person can begin to understand the formation of their beliefs and values (Bird-Rose, 2005; Ramsden, 2002). For example:

> I returned to Bali for the fifth time and was greeted by our Balinese driver whom we knew quite well. I was very pleased to see him and I went to kiss his cheek and suddenly realised that perhaps it was culturally inappropriate. He looked relieved and shook my hand enthusiastically to convey his pleasure.
>
> (WILLIAMS, 2015)

This quote demonstrates a process of self-reflection when two different sets of beliefs and traditions were in play.

Cultural safety domain – cultural safety means an environment that is spiritually, socially and emotionally safe, as well as physically safe for people; where there is no assault, challenge or denial of their identity, of who they are and what they need. It is about shared respect, shared meaning, shared knowledge and experience, of learning together with dignity and truly listening. Unsafe cultural practice is any action that diminishes, demeans or disempowers the cultural identity and wellbeing of an individual or group (Williams, 1999).

Culturally safe practice requires openness, honesty, acceptance, reflection, commitment and respect. It is important to recognise that actions often speak louder than words – the way we move, our approach, the expressions on our face and the look in our eyes are all signs that make any words, actions or reactions truthful. It is also crucial to recognise people can only speak with authority about their *own* experiences. As such, cultural safety enables individuals to retain their right to determine if the process or outcome of experience (past and present) is culturally appropriate (Ramsden, 2002). For example:

> We developed a cultural immersion program for medical students. We were a diverse and international cross-cultural team of nine with different beliefs, values and practices. Everything we did was in partnership with all team members; we negotiated all aspects – the program, the resources, the implementation and the evaluation of the program. It was a very respectful team where our differences, similarities and what each person brought to the team were acknowledged. We all learnt more than we taught by being open, respectful and standing back when required. We won two awards for this work.
>
> (SMITH et al., 2015)

Cultural safety in Australia

My story as an educator

A few years ago, I ran a remote health workshop on working cross-culturally with two Aboriginal facilitators. There was a mixed bunch of participants – ranging from 'newbies' to 'cynical old hands' with varying degrees of clinical as well as cultural competence. Mr R was a young man fresh off the plane from Tasmania who was heading out to a remote community in Arnhem Land with his family. During the introduction, he stated that he had (not knowingly) 'met an Aboriginal person, but he was feeling fairly confident clinically and wasn't afraid of asking questions'. About a third of the way into the first session on engaging in effective and respectful communication with Indigenous peoples in the delivery of health services, Mr R said: 'No offence, but this cultural safety stuff is bullshit and I can't see what it has to do with my job'. I commended him on feeling comfortable enough to speak his mind and then the group proceeded to have quite a robust discussion.

Eighteen months later, Mr R turned up at another workshop I was facilitating. He sought me out at the first break, thanked me and told me that he had been thinking about what I said in the previous workshop and that now it was making sense. This got me thinking and wondering how to create opportunities for people to get the importance of this concept and take on board that working in a culturally safe way is equally as important as being clinically safe.

What does a culturally safe health care environment look like?

A culturally safe environment is one that accepts the legitimacy of difference and diversity in human values, beliefs, behaviours and social structures. It exists in an environment where people feel spiritually, socially, emotionally and physically safe. In essence, its practice is based upon trust and genuine partnerships.

Critically, it does not require the examination of any culture other than our own – so as to be open-minded and flexible in attitudes towards people from cultures other than our own. Identifying what makes others different is simple – understanding our own culture and its influence on how we think, feel and behave is much more complex and a lifetime journey.

The occurrence or success of cultural safety is determined by the experience of the person whose health is being acted upon – the recipient – as well as the staff involved.

Culturally safe care is met when:

- one's actions include **recognising, respecting and nurturing** the unique cultural identity of an individual

- one's actions support the **positive health, wellbeing and empowerment** of those with whom you live, work and interact
- it involves revealing, understanding and responding to the **power relationships** between a service provider and the people who use the service
- it challenges service providers to **examine their own practices** (encompassing their own culture, history, attitudes and life experiences).

To provide a culturally safe and quality service, providers must **engage in self-reflection** so that any service is provided knowing that the clients or users of the service have cultural values and norms that are different from their own. (This means looking at preconceived ideas and stereotypes.)

In a relationship where one has institutional power, it is the '**moment of trust**' where the client or patient does not feel the need to hide or protect their difference.

Terminology

There are many words that are used interchangeably with cultural safety, including cultural competence, cultural security, cultural respect and cultural responsiveness. Many of these terms have been adapted from other countries with a similar history of colonisation of Indigenous populations, such as New Zealand and Canada (Sherwood & Edwards, 2006). Let us briefly unpack these terms and what they are taken to mean.

Cultural security is built from the acknowledgement that 'awareness' of culturally appropriate service provision is not enough. It shifts the emphasis from attitudes to behaviour, focusing directly on practice, skills and efficacy. This includes workforce development, workforce reform, purchasing of health services, monitoring and accountability, and public engagement (Human Rights and Equal Opportunity Commission, 2010). This means ensuring all voices are heard and respected, in relation to our community challenges, aspirations and identities, and that this is done in such a way that the community have ownership over themselves (Human Rights and Equal Opportunity Commission, 2010).

Cultural competence is a term that has risen to prominence in nursing education over the last 10 years and, more recently, in medical education (Australian Medical Council, 2013; Committee of Deans of Australian Medical Schools, 2004). It has been defined as a 'set of congruent behaviours, attitudes, and policies that come together in a system, agency, or amongst professionals that enables them to work effectively in cross-cultural situations' (Cross, Bazron, Dennis, & Isaacs, 1989, p. 4).

Cultural responsiveness is defined as an extension of patient centred-care. It includes paying particular attention to social and cultural factors in managing

Terminology—cont'd

therapeutic encounters with patients who are from different cultural and social backgrounds. This is viewed as a cyclical and ongoing process, requiring health professionals to continuously self-reflect and proactively respond to the person, family or community with whom they interact (Indigenous Allied Health Australia, 2013).

Cultural respect aims to uphold the rights of Indigenous peoples to maintain, protect and develop their culture and achieve equitable outcomes (Australian Health Ministers' Advisory Council, 2004). It includes a commitment that health services will not compromise the legitimate cultural rights, practices, values and expectations of Indigenous peoples.

Cultural diversity is not only focused on ethnicity but also on gender, age, disability and sexual orientation.

Culture conflict occurs when one culture tries to convert another culture to its way of thinking or doing. This can occur when one cultural group has power over another, and where it tries to impose its systems and organisations, beliefs and values on the less powerful, usually by violence or legislative sanctions (Eckermann et al., 2012).

Culture shock is that feeling of uneasiness or disorientation that a person experiences when in unfamiliar surroundings or with a dominant culture that is different from their own. This often happens when visiting another country or when cultural practices and language are different from their own.

POWER, AUTHORITY AND HEALTH CARE OUTCOMES

It is important to discuss the issue of power when we discuss culture and health care as they are intrinsically related. The medical profession is a useful area to begin to explore the notion of power and authority. The general public can easily recognise the authority that doctors, who reputedly hold the highest level of specialist medical skills and knowledge, have in the health system. So does power automatically come with authority and status? And how are this power and authority maintained?

There are many symbols in the health system linked to power and authority. Traditionally, the white jacket, complete with the stethoscope, was part of the 'image of the doctor' perpetuated by the media.

Uniforms are another powerful symbol in health. Nurses and midwives have longstanding traditions of wearing uniforms that have transformed over the years from the white starched uniform and cap to coloured corporate style dress and more recently 'scrubs'. The argument for the continued use of uniforms includes easy identification, professionalism and infection control. But how does the presence of the uniform influence the relationship between professional and client?

PAUSE AND THINK

Why is it that doctors, acute care nurses and midwives have always worn uniforms but social workers, mental health nurses and other allied health workers do not?

Is it because of the need to protect and be protected for those professions involved in 'hands on' care?

Nurse managers, community nurses and midwives are rarely exposed to bodily fluids, other than in labour and birth settings. So why do they continue to wear uniforms?

Health professionals' source of knowledge and power confers authority over clients. It is important to be aware that power can be understood in many ways and takes many forms. Some are obvious; others are very subtle but no less powerful.

Some of the types of power commonly encountered include: *authority* – a soldier obeying an order; *force* – a court order removing a child from its carer, *coercion* – the threat of physical violence with actual violence being used, or *inducement* or *manipulation* (Chenoweth & McAuliffe, 2005, p. 36).

Communication has an important influence on the dynamics of power between groups and individuals in the health care environment. The ability to communicate clearly and assertively has been recognised as an essential skill in the management of workplace demands and stress for health professionals. Assertive communication helps to reduce conflict with others and therefore serves as a useful skill to maintain long-term wellbeing for everyone.

When dealing with people from other cultural groups, it is crucial to ask who provides care and who is responsible for making decisions within the client and family context. For many cultural groups, this means taking into consideration the kinship and family structure and what determines acceptable social behaviour. For example, an Aunty may have the authority to speak on a child's behalf.

When any health professional is working in a cross-cultural context it is critical to work in a culturally safe and effective way that includes:

- respect for each other's culture, knowledge, experience and obligations
- not assaulting a person's identity
- treating each person with dignity.

When people interact in a health setting, the symbols and language used directly influence each person, for example by using medical terminology instead of plain English. Outcomes are dependent on these communications, and so are trust and respect.

Symbols such as uniforms, stethoscopes and even the system of appointments (show up and wait) can result in confusion, fear, intimidation and disorientation, even before the professional encounter begins. When these factors combine with

---

PAUSE AND THINK

It is now time to think about power and privilege in the context of culture. Consider:

1   What do you think it means to have control over your own health?

2   Have you ever been to the doctor and felt put down, not listened to or not taken seriously?

3   When someone asks you for advice about their health, how do you go about answering their questions?

---

cultural differences the outcomes and processes of health care can be haphazard and less than ideal. It is almost like a triple whammy when you combine these three factors together – the client, the health professional and the cross-cultural interaction.

For example, when a health professional talks about someone going to the doctor or the hospital, they usually say that the client 'presents', as in 'the patient presented with the following symptoms'. Some argue that the use of this kind of language takes something away from an individual's identity whereby they are regarded as an object to be operated upon. Perhaps this is one of the central points of cultural safety: each person is a member of a group and is also an individual with their own priorities and identity. To assume otherwise is disempowering as it fails treat the person with respect, dignity or validate their identity as a human being.

Lupton (2012) describes the health encounter as a voluntary agreement between the patient and the provider, where they agree to participate on the grounds that they think it will be of benefit, but not necessarily because they agree that the provider is intrinsically more worthy (Lupton, 2012). Therefore, the practitioner needs to acknowledge an unequal power relationship exists in the health encounter and there is a potential impact on the client and their health outcomes.

Power, influence and a reputation for 'getting it right' or 'being the expert' can change the way people respond to health advice, and that response is often critical to health outcomes. If a client tries to access a health service but feels disrespected, they are less likely to trust it or follow advice given. Similarly, if the health professional is only interested in the presenting disease rather than the person it may result in non-compliance.

These skills applied well can make significant differences to your practice and effectiveness, and will increase the chance that your professional performance improves your clients' lives.

Willis and Elmer (2011, p. 257) argue that 'the medical encounter must be understood as a social interaction and not simply as a clinical encounter'. It is also important to remember that power imbalances and their effects in these situations may not always be intentional. They can arise from patterns of work such as time management, from appearance and a sense of 'otherness' developed over time or from assumptions

PAUSE AND THINK

What are the likely outcomes when a health professional:

- does not make assumptions about who you are
- speaks with respect and understanding
- shows interest in your priorities (e.g. family and work obligations)?

Ask yourself:

- Are you paying attention to the person in front of you? Or are you operating from assumptions that do not apply to them?
- What did you learn from them?
- How did you become better at your job as a result of meeting that person?
- How can you build your knowledge of culture and people from this interaction?

about which behaviours are acceptable and which ones are derided within the dominant group.

Control over health information also plays a disempowering role in health care. This is even more unhelpful for people who are already disenfranchised or marginalised, for example refugees or people with disabilities. The effect often can be so great that health care and its benefits are systematically denied to some people.

CASE STUDY

The following case study provides an opportunity for you to explore your own values and cultural understandings by applying them to health professional practice. Using the principles and the three domains for achieving cultural safety, reflect on the practice of this allied health professional working in a remote Indigenous setting. Discuss how recognition of differences and power imbalances between patients and health professionals helps to improve the safe delivery of health services.

Note: This case study can be used as a teaching and learning resource in tutorials or to generate discussion in a small group setting.

Case study 1: Cultural safety – Kelly White

Kelly White is a 32-year-old clinical psychologist. She has worked as part of the assessment team at Metropolis Hospital's Secure Mental Health Unit for the past nine years. She also spends time at Metropolis University marking papers and occasionally guest lecturing. Having succumbed to her desire for a sea change, Kelly accepts a position in the small remote community of Littleton. She works for the local Aboriginal Community Development Corporation (ACDC) at their primary health care centre. Her role is to participate in the development of their Youth Suicide Strategy as part of the ACDC Taskforce. Kelly is very enthusiastic about this new position, and she hopes this will be an opportunity for her to apply her years of experience in a different cultural setting.

Kelly's first week in Littleton is a very eye-opening experience and she encounters many issues that she has never faced before. Most of her clients are Aboriginal. Though they are there by choice, many of her clients will not look her in the eye and seem very reluctant to talk. While many of the women appear introverted and say very little in Kelly's presence, she later sees them talking, laughing and behaving in extroverted ways outside the clinic. Many of the men talk to Kelly as though she is a child, and they seem determined to talk only about their physical health and their family members – not about themselves personally. Kelly is also confronted by a subtle sense of segregation within the community between the Aboriginal people and the non-Aboriginal people who live there. She is unsure about how she fits into this environment.

After six weeks of consulting on the Youth Suicide Strategy, Kelly feels out of her depth. She has found her work with ACDC to be more challenging than she expected. Kelly is confused about the apparent gender hierarchy in the taskforce – many of her contributions are ignored and she is frequently told suicide is different for 'Blackfellas'. She feels that, although she is very skilled as a professional, her skills do not seem relevant to many of her clients' problems. Kelly begins to question her own professional competence and how she applies her knowledge and skills when treating her new clients.

In the past week Kelly has become quite angry on occasions and is feeling very isolated. She decides to discuss her concerns with Daisy, one of her colleagues. Daisy is an Aboriginal Health Practitioner at the health centre and sits in on many of the Youth Suicide Strategy development meetings. She seems to be very close to many of the locals. Daisy agrees to mentor Kelly and begins by discussing cultural safety.

Case study questions

1   Discuss which domain of cultural safety you believe Kelly is in. Is she working in a culturally safe manner?

2   Discuss the signs and symptoms of culture shock. Is Kelly suffering from culture shock? Explain your answer.

3   Using the three Ps of cultural safety (partnership, participation and protection), discuss the issues that you think Kelly has accepted and those that she needs to understand and work on.

4   What should Kelly do to get the women to engage in a partnership with her?

5   Why do the men wish to only discuss their health problems?

6   Why do the men dismiss Kelly's contributions?

7   What issues within the community does Kelly have to address in order for her to be sufficiently informed and able to work in a participatory way?

8   What would be the most suitable way for Kelly to discuss her concerns with Daisy?

RACISM

What is racism?

Racism, like sexism and classism, is about power. The *Oxford Dictionary* (2015) defines racism as the 'belief that all members of each race possess characteristics, abilities, or qualities specific to that race, especially so as to distinguish it as inferior or superior to another race or races' and the expression of such prejudice.

It is the approach by which one dominant racial group has, and maintains, power over another racial group and subordinates it. This subordination is often based upon a belief that some races are genetically superior and that races differ decisively from one another. Racism is then often coupled with *ethnocentrism* – the notion that one race is absolutely superior to other racial groups. Racism then becomes an institutionalised system of power and subordination, created and perpetuated by the dominant racial group.

This system of power is openly entrenched within our institutions. It includes the way in which the institution is organised in all aspects of its workings – economically, politically, socially and culturally. It ensures that the dominant racial group has, and maintains, power and privilege over all others in all aspects of life (Derman-Sparks & Brunson, 1997). It is something we learn as we grow up, just as we learn about our own cultural norms, values and beliefs. We are socialised into it from probably two years of age, and most certainly by three to four years (Derman-Sparks & Brunson, 1997). One could therefore argue that, essentially, we are all racist; it is something we need to unlearn throughout our lives.

However, Derman-Sparks and Brunson (1997) argue that it is the outcome of individual, cultural and institutional policies and actions, rather than the intent behind them, that determines the presence of racism. As a result, it is more about 'what you do' than about 'what you think' – it is about your actions. One may therefore act in a racist manner without knowing it, and without thinking of oneself as racist. One of the challenges in discussing racism is that few people would label themselves as racist. Yet often in the media we hear reports about racist acts in sports, on public transport and by individual members of the public. The truth is that hatred and intolerance underlie all societies. They simmer closely below the surface of all our dealings in this country (Hall, 1998).

Often the terms **ethnicity** and **race** are used interchangeably; while they are related, they are not the same. The concept of *ethnicity* is based on the idea of a social grouping marked especially by shared nationality, tribal affiliation, shared genealogy or kinship and descent, religious identification, language use or specific cultural and traditional origins. However, the concept of *race* is premised on biological classification – genetic similarities, familial traits and heredity (e.g. blue eyes, a big nose or brown hair).

Racism can present itself in several ways through stereotyping, prejudice and discrimination. It is important for all health professionals to understand and take responsibility for how racism manifests itself because it can affect both health care delivery and health outcomes.

Stereotyping is about placing all people with certain characteristics in a group based on some commonalities that the group has – such as 'all blondes are dumb', 'all Muslims are terrorists'. Making assumptions to predict behaviours in individuals or groups who are different from ourselves can lead us to stereotype. Stereotyping does not tend to allow for individual differences within cultures and commonly victimises groups by blaming their cultures for perceived and negatively valued practices.

Prejudice is the process of making a judgement about an individual or group on the basis of their social, physical or cultural characteristics. It is usually based on a stereotype rather than on actual evidence. Prejudice is usually negative but it can also be positive such as 'one can be prejudiced favourably towards Thai cooking or the Wilderness Society' (Hollinsworth, 1998, p. 48). All of us carry around erroneous or unsubstantiated beliefs about the world, or at least others in it. In most cases, however, when confronted with new information or experiences that contradict or question such errors, we can change our mind without too much difficulty or trauma. Just like over-generalisations, prejudices are usually highly resistant to change.

Discrimination is the unjust or prejudicial treatment of different categories of people, based especially on the grounds of race, age or sex (Oxford Dictionary, 2015). The Human Rights and Equal Opportunity Commission (2015a, p. 1) states that: 'Racism, racial discrimination, xenophobia and all kinds of related intolerance have not gone away' in Australia. Their 'persistence is rooted in fear: fear of what is different, fear of the other, fear of the loss of personal security. And while we recognize that human fear is in itself ineradicable, we maintain that its consequences are not...'

Understanding one's own prejudices, and taking responsibility for how these feelings can affect health care, is one of the most significant things an individual can do to improve health outcomes. Most people do not intend to be racist in their attitudes but every time a negative feeling towards someone based on their culture, language, behaviour or beliefs is assigned, this is a form of racism. Working with groups or clients who are from a dissimilar culture does not require an overemphasis on the differences that could impede relationships between the provider and the client. It is more important to focus on similarities and what we have in common.

Types of racism

There are three key forms of racism. They all interact with one another:

Institutional racism 'refers to the ways in which racist beliefs or values have been built into the operations of social institutions in such a way as to discriminate against, control and oppress various minority groups' (Henry, Houston, & Mooney, 2004). This includes all those structures, systems and services that are automatically built into an organisation or institution, such as its mission, policies, organisational structures and economic system, as well as its corporate culture, which reflects and perpetuates its beliefs and behaviours (Derman-Sparks & Brunson, 1997). It is the thinking behind 'this is how we do it here' and 'we have always done it like this'. In Australia these institutional structures are essentially built upon Western ways of doing and knowing; priorities are set according to this thinking. A good example is found in the inequitable way in which Aboriginal Community Controlled Health Organisations (ACCHO) receive 'body part' funding, when Indigenous people tend to have a holistic view of health. Yet the funding is based on body parts and separate funding streams for conditions such as diabetes and heart disease. This means that one ACCHO had 26 different sources of funding upon which they had to report (Henry et al., 2004).

Cultural racism or ethnocentrism is the set of cultural beliefs, values, symbols and underlying rules of behaviour that teach and endorse notions of the dominant culture's superiority (Derman-Sparks & Brunson, 1997). It reflects the ideology of the dominant group with identifiable structures and practices and plays a critical role in socialising people to participate in, and maintain, institutional racism (Derman-Sparks & Brunson, 1997). A good example can be found in the Australian education system, which is based on non-Indigenous ways of teaching and learning. Despite the fact that we now know Indigenous children often respond and engage in different ways from non-Indigenous children (Human Rights and Equal Opportunity Commission, 2001), the system continues to be unresponsive to cultural differences in learning and teaching contexts.

Individual racism constitutes more than mere prejudice, or stereotyping of specific groups of people. It also includes the attitudes and behaviours that enable, and maintain, the power relationships of racism (Derman-Sparks & Brunson, 1997). Although acts of racism may appear to be specific to the person carrying them out, they are often fuelled by, and reflect, institutional and cultural dimensions of racism (Derman-Sparks & Brunson, 1997). Examples include name-calling during sporting activities or in the schoolyard that is ignored by those whom the institution places in authority. Racism is therefore a result of racial prejudice plus institutional power.

Overt and covert racism

Racism can operate overtly; that is, through policies and practices that openly maintain the right of the dominant group to the exclusion of others. Australian examples are the White Australia Policy, which persisted for more than 100 years in Australia, and the Queensland *Aboriginal Preservation and Protection Act* from 1939–1966, which excluded Indigenous children from attending school or from enjoying the usual liberties of other Australians (Kidd, 2007).

Racism also operates covertly through hidden practices that consistently perpetuate inequitable relationships (Derman-Sparks & Brunson, 1997). This occurs in many of our systems, including in our prisons, where mainstream intelligence testing and other research tools are used, even though a quarter of inmates are Indigenous, many have literacy problems and English is often their second or third language. Sometimes covert racism becomes overt. A good example is found in the furore of 'Ban the Burqa' in the Federal Parliament House in 2015, which was based on fear arising from the different values and beliefs systems and tensions that simmer below the surface in the Australian population.

Dealing with racism – building resilience

Racism can be very confronting and damaging. Racism is more than just words or actions. It includes invisible barriers, big and small, that can prevent people from doing well in life and can affect health outcomes. How do we deal with this? One way of looking at this is that, in every act of racism, there are three actors – the *perpetrator*, the *victim* and the *bystander*(s) – and each one plays a role and each has a responsibility to do something about it. Beyond Blue (2015) offer three main actions:

1 Report it.
2 Stand up for it.
3 Stop it.

The Human Rights and Equal Opportunity Commission (Human Rights and Equal Opportunity Commission, 2015c) recommends the actions outlined in Figure 3.2.

PAUSE AND THINK

Think about an act of racism that you have witnessed, or that has happened to you. Identify the perpetrator, the victim and the observer. How was it managed and how could that management have been improved? How do you feel as a result of this incident?

SOCIAL JUSTICE

Australians generally have a strong sense of social justice and belief in the freedom to live in a fair society. So what does social justice mean? 'Justice' means 'fairness' and is based on a human right. 'Social' refers to 'society', which is made up of human beings. Therefore, social justice refers to 'a fair society'. It essentially means giving people a fair chance, a share or a choice based on their human rights as determined by the United Nations Universal Declaration of Human Rights (United Nations, 1948). These include our rights to life, free speech and a vote; our freedom to choose our religion and to travel, to marry or not, to work; to protection from arbitrary arrest and the right of ethnic and racial minorities, and those with disabilities, to protection. Most importantly, these human rights include our right to health (Human Rights and Equal Opportunity Commission, 2015b).

FIGURE 3.2 What to do about racism.

If you see racist behaviour in public, you could....

 Say something if it feels safe to do so. It doesn't have to be aggressive, in fact it's often more effective if it's not. It could be as simple as saying "Why don't you just leave him/her alone?"

If it doesn't feel safe to say something, you could....

 Tell someone responsible such as the driver if it's happening on a bus or tram or a security guard if it's happening at a club or venue.

 Call the police on 000 if you think that you or somebody else may be in danger.

 Think about how you can support the target of the abuse.
– for example, you could go and sit or stand next to them and check if they're ok.

If you see racist material online, you could....

 Report it.
Most social networking sites have policies for dealing with offensive content and enable users to report this material. More information is usually available on these sites under "guidelines", "standards" or "terms of use".

 Say something. Go to the Anti-Hate website to check out messages you can post in response to "haters" online.

If you see racism directed towards a classmate, colleague or team-mate, you could....

 Say something. Check out the Speak UP! Handbook for ideas of things to say to counter prejudice in any situation.

 Let them know they can complain. The Australian Human Rights Commission can investigate and resolve complaints of race discrimination in areas including employment, education, sport, accommodation and the provision of goods and services. The complaints process is free and confidential. For more information go to the Complaints page.

 Suggest they talk to someone. Most schools, workplaces and sports clubs will have a policy for dealing with bullying and harassment, including racism. You might like to suggest to the person experiencing the racist behaviour that they seek advice from the contact person named in the policy such as the student welfare officer at school, human resources in the workplace or manager or club official in a sports club.

 Click on the image to check out Play By the Rules 'Racism In Sport' toolkit.

Adapted with permission from: Play by the Rules. <www.playbytherules.net.au>.

A way to describe social justice and how it applies to real life is best conveyed by this story by Frank Brennan, a Jesuit priest and lawyer and well-known spokesperson on Indigenous land rights (Brennan, 1989, cited in Smith, 1995). Brennan describes how, as a young boy, he went to boarding school. While he was very bright academically, he was never very good at sport and was therefore a member of the D grade football team. The A grade team were always allowed to play on the level field, which was protected from the wind, but the D grade team had to play on the hill slope. He tried to convince his teachers that, if they were allowed to play on the flat oval, the D grade team's game would greatly improve and the A grade team would be challenged, as they would have to try to play better on the hill slope. However, this was never allowed. The A grade team were the fittest and best, so they should have the best oval, and the D grade team were the worst, so they were given the worst oval. They would never have the opportunity to access the resources of the best team because they would never equal them, in skill or in status.

Hence, social justice is also about fair and equal access to services and resources and to freedom and choice to decide how we as Australians want to live our lives, irrespective of where we live or our culture (Human Rights and Equal Opportunity Commission, 2015b).

CONCLUSION – IT'S A MATTER OF RESPECT

As Australians we largely define our national character in terms of values such as fairness, acceptance, equality, human rights and social justice.

> However, if we looked a little more closely at ourselves we would see that things could be fairer than they are. We could be more accepting than we are, and our participation in the economic, social and cultural life this country has to offer could be more equitable and inclusive than it is.

> (SIDOTI, 1999, p. 1)

Our current inequitable and non-inclusive attitudes and policies are going to be exacerbated by an influx of new Australians, who have come from unjust and extremely inequitable societies – their very reason for coming to the 'lucky country' in the first place. Many are moving to rural and remote Australia as they pass though the immigration system. They are often survivors of trauma and torture. They will hold different values, beliefs and practices, which does not make them any less human, just different. To be able to be fair, we need to appreciate this difference and treat all cases equally, and different cases differently (Brennan, 1989). This may mean that we need to unlearn what we think we know, question our own values and cultural norms and be open to doing so in an environment of tolerance and respect, since countries can no longer be insular in today's global environment.

Tolerance is not just about understanding or accepting; it is more about tolerating other cultures, and people as human beings, as a mark of respect for their values, philosophies, belief systems and ways of doing. Wilson (1998), however, argues that, while tolerance is essential for a peaceful and united community, it is not enough. He states that to develop a multicultural community spirit we need to 'express a rich and lively interest in one another', really celebrate our diversity and 'have an instinct for compassionate sharing and sensitivity to another's needs' (Wilson, 1998, p. xiv). This does not mean that we necessarily agree with what other cultures do; in fact, we can vehemently disagree, especially over issues that violate others' basic human rights. What is important is that we do not view people as being any less human than ourselves, and that we can respect their rights as human beings to participate in our society as equals.

Hence, to be able to respect other cultures, it is vital to understand our own culture. It is not so much to understand 'what we do', such as drinking beer, having barbecues and 'taking the mickey out of each other' (teasing), but the 'thinking behind what we do' – our belief systems and our philosophy about what is important in our lives. It is the lack of understanding that different cultures have about 'why we do what we do' that creates conflict.

Eckermann et al. (2012) tell us that an acceptance of different cultures does not mean that we have to abandon our own traditions and philosophies. Rather, we need to suspend judgement about those things that we do not understand, make a conscious effort not to determine what is 'good' and 'bad' for others and constantly question our predisposition to seek security in those things that we feel we 'know' about other groups (Eckermann et al., 2012). For health professionals, acceptance also means that we need to provide health services in a culturally safe manner.

Discussion points

1. Describe your own culture – what are your beliefs, values and traditions that make up your own template for living as a group?
2. Review current newspapers that reflect the common beliefs found in mainstream Australian culture. Discuss.
3. What social trends have changed during your lifetime that are affecting Australian lives now?
4. What international practices have been borrowed by Australian culture?
5. Discuss three key ways of preventing culture conflict. How does it occur?
6. Think of three examples of covert and overt racism that you have observed. Discuss.
7. Think of the government departments and institutional systems that you have worked in, and examine whether their systems or policies could fit into the definition of institutional racism. Discuss some systems that do not. How do they work?
8. Discuss how rural and remote health practitioners could work in a more culturally safe way.

References

Aiken, D. (1985). Country-mindedness: the spread of an idea. *Australian Cultural History*, 4, 34–40.

Australian Concise Oxford Dictionary (2000). *The Australian concise oxford dictionary* (3rd ed.). Melbourne: Oxford University Press.

Australian Health Ministers' Advisory Council (AHMAC). (2004). *Cultural respect framework for Aboriginal and Torres Strait Islander health 2004–2009*. Adelaide: Department of Health, South Australia, Australian Health Ministers' Advisory Council – Standing Committee for Aboriginal and Torres Strait Islander Health Working Party.

Australian Medical Council (AMC). (2013). *Standards for assessment and accreditation of primary medical programs by the Australian Medical Council 2012*. Canberra: AMC.

Baum, F. (2008). *The new public health* (3rd ed.). Melbourne: Oxford University Press.

Baum, F. E., Bégin, M., Houweling, T. A. J., & Taylor, S. (2009). Changes not for the fainthearted: reorienting health care systems toward health equity through action on the social determinants of health. *American Journal of Public Health*, *99*(11), 1967–1974.

Beyond Blue. (2015). *The invisible discriminator*. Melbourne: Beyond Blue. <https://www .beyondblue.org.au/resources/for-me/stop-think-respect-home/the-invisible -discriminator?utm_source=bing&utm_medium=cpc&utm_campaign=NonGeo -RaceDiscrim-OtherKW&utm_term=beyond%20blue%20racism&sekw=34629437575> Accessed 26.10.15.

Bird-Rose, D. (2005). *Reports from a wild country: Ethics for decolonisation*. Sydney: University of New South Wales Press Ltd.

Brennan, F. (1989). Social justice, human and civil rights: how do they affect the delivery of health care in remote areas? Paper presented at the 2nd Council of Remote Area Nurses of Australia National Conference, Canberra.

Cadet-James, Y. (2003, May 2003). [Personal communication].

Chenoweth, L., & McAuliffe, D. (2005). *The road to social work and human service practice: An introductory text*. Melbourne: Thomson.

Chesler, P. (2010). Worldwide trends in honor killings. *Middle East Quarterly, Spring*, 3–11.

Committee of Deans of Australian Medical Schools (CDAMS) (2004). *CDAMS Indigenous health curriculum framework*. Melbourne: CDAMS.

Cross, T., Bazron, B., Dennis, K., & Isaacs, M. (1989). *Towards a culturally competent system of care* (Vol. 1). Washington D.C.: Georgetown University Child Development Center, CASSP Technical Assistance Center.

Crotty, M. (1998). *The foundations of social research: Meaning and perspective in the research process*. St Leonards NSW: Allen & Unwin.

Dempsey, K. (1990). *Smalltown: A study of social inequality, cohesion and belonging*. Melbourne: Oxford University Press.

Derman-Sparks, L., & Brunson, C. (1997). *Teaching/learning anti-racism: A developmental approach*. New York: Teachers College Press, Columbia University.

Dreachslin, J. L., Gilbert, M. J., & Malone, B. (2012). *Diversity and cultural competence in health care: A systems approach*. Hoboken: Jossey-Bass.

Eckermann, A. K., Dowd, T., Chong, E., Nixon, L., Gray, R., & Johnson, S. (2012). *Binan Goonj: Bridging cultures in Aboriginal health*. Chatswood NSW: Elsevier International.

Gray, I., & Lawrence, G. (2001). *A future for regional Australia*. Cambridge, UK: Cambridge University Press.

Hall, R. (1998). *Black armband days* (1st ed.). Milsons Point NSW: Vintage Publishers.

Henry, B., Houston, S., & Mooney, G. H. (2004). Institutional racism in Australian health care: a plea for decency. *Medical Journal of Australia*, *180*, 517–520.

Hollinsworth, D. (1998). *Race and racism in Australia* (3rd ed.). Katoomba NSW: Social Science Press.

Human Rights and Equal Opportunity Commission (HREOC) (1997). *Bringing them home report: Report of the national inquiry into the separation of Aboriginal and Torres Strait Islander children from their families*. Canberra: HREOC.

Human Rights and Equal Opportunity Commission (2001). *Social justice report 2001.* Canberra: HREOC.

Human Rights and Equal Opportunity Commission (2010). *Aboriginal and Torres Strait Islander Social Justice Commissioner social justice report 2010.* Report No. 1/2011. Canberra: HREOC.

Human Rights and Equal Opportunity Commission (2015a). Extract from the *Vision Declaration for the World Conference Against Racism.* Canberra: HREOC. <https:// www.humanrights.gov.au/hreoc-website-racial-discrimination-national-consultations -racism-and> Accessed 22.07.15.

Human Rights and Equal Opportunity Commission (2015b). *Human rights explained.* Canberra: HREOC. <https://www.humanrights.gov.au/education/human-rights-explained -index> Accessed 22.07.15.

Human Rights and Equal Opportunity Commission (2015c). *Racism stops with me: Tips for bystanders.* Canberra: HREOC. <http://itstopswithme.humanrights.gov.au/what-can-you-do/ speak/bystanders> Accessed 25.06.15.

Indigenous Allied Health Australia (IAHA) (2013). *Culturally responsive health care.* Canberra: IAHA. <http://iaha.com.au/wp-content/uploads/2013/09/Position_Paper _Culturally_Responsive_Health_Care.pdf> Accessed 22.07.15.

Jones, A. (2008). Case study: Honour killings and bloody feuds. <http://www.gendercide.org/ case_honour.html> Accessed 20.07.15.

Kidd, R. (2007). *Hard labour – stolen wages, national report on stolen wages.* <www.austlii.edu.au/au/journals/AILRev/2007/85.pdf> Accessed 08.04.15.

Kowal, E., & Paradies, Y. (2005). Ambivalent helpers and unhealthy choices: public health practitioners' narratives of Indigenous ill-health. *Social Science & Medicine, 60,* 1347–1357.

Lupton, D. (2012). *Medicine as culture: Illness, disease and the body* (3rd ed.). London: Sage.

MacLachlan, M. (1997). *Culture and health.* San Francisco: Wiley.

Morgan, D. (2003). *Kurdish women take action against honour killings.* <http:// www.kurdmedia.com/kwahk/r_dm_kurdishwomenaction.htm> Accessed 22.07.15.

National Aboriginal Health Strategy Working Party (1989). *National Aboriginal health strategy.* Canberra: Commonwealth of Australia, Australian Government Printing Service.

Nursing Council of New Zealand. (2011). *Guidelines for cultural safety, the Treaty of Waitangi and Māori health in nursing and midwifery education and practice.* <www .nursingcouncil.org.nz> Accessed 25.07.15.

Oxford dictionary. (2015) *Online Oxford dictionary: language matters.* <http:// www.oxforddictionaries.com/definition/english/discrimination>.

Papps, E., & Ramsden, I. (1996). Cultural safety in nursing: the New Zealand experience. *International Journal for Quality in Health Care, Oct 1996,* 491–497.

Ramsden, I. (2002). *Cultural safety and nursing education in Aotearoa and Te Waipounamu [thesis].* Wellington: Victoria University.

Rolley, F., & Humphreys, J. (1993). Rural welfare – The human face of Australia's countryside. In R. Epps (Ed.), *Prospects and policies for rural Australia* (pp. 241–257). Melbourne: Longman Cheshire.

Sherwood, J., & Edwards, T. (2006). Decolonisation: A critical step for improving Aboriginal health. Special issue: Advances in Indigenous health care. *Contemporary Nurse, 22(2),* 178–190.

Sidoti, C. (1996). *The human rights of rural Australians, First occasional paper of the Human Rights and Equal Opportunity Commissioner.* <www.hreoc.gov.au> Accessed 08.12.02.

Sidoti, C. (1999). Rural health: a human right. *Australian Journal of Rural Health, 7*(4), 202–205.

Smith, J. D. (1995). *Suicide sacrifice or success: Nursing on another path.* Inaugural community health nursing conference, Cairns, FNQ Community Health Nurses Association.

Smith, J. D., Wolfe, C., Springer, S., Martin, M., Togno, J., Sargeant, S., et al. (2015). Using cultural immersion as part of teaching Aboriginal and Torres Strait Islander health in an undergraduate medical curriculum. *Rural and Remote Health, 15*(3), 3144.

Stehlik, D. (2001). Out there: spaces, places and border crossings. In L. Bourke (Ed.), *Rurality bites* (pp. 30–42). Altona, Vic: Pluto Press Australia Pty Ltd.

Tidwell, C. (2003). *Culture definitions and traits.* <http://www2.andrews.edu/~tidwell/bsad560/Culture.html> Accessed 20.07.15.

United Nations. (1948). *All human rights for all – Fiftieth anniversary of the universal declaration of human rights 1948–1998*, Universal declaration of human rights, resolution 217 A(111), 10th December. <www.un.org/Overview/rights.html> Accessed 20.07.15.

Williams, R. (1999). Cultural safety: what does it mean for our work practice? *Australian and New Zealand Journal of Public Health, 23*(2), 213.

Williams, R. (2015). Personal communication.

Willis, K., & Elmer, S. (2011). *Society, culture and health: An introduction to sociology for nurses.* South Melbourne, Vic: Oxford University Press.

Wilson, R. (1998). Foreword. In D. Hollinsworth (Ed.), *Race and racism in Australia* (2nd ed., pp. xii–xv). Katoomba NSW: Social Science Press.

Woods, M. (2010). Cultural safety and the socioethical nurse. *Nursing Ethics, 17*(6), 715–725.

CHAPTER 4

INDIGENOUS AUSTRALIA

Jacinta Elston | Janie Dade Smith

Indigenous Australia is diverse. Most Indigenous Australians live in city suburbs or large regional areas; many run their own businesses, go to university, work for the public service, raise healthy children, play sport and contribute to society. Some are world-renowned for their political, artistic, academic and written work, and many are prominent in public life as sporting heroes or ceremonial performers. Yet they rarely make positive headlines in the media. Indigenous society today is known to many Australians only through mostly negative media images that were implanted into our brains by the media as a result of the Northern Territory Emergency Response to child abuse in remote Northern Territory communities in 2007 (Wild & Anderson, 2007). It conjured up images of great ochre deserts in remote Australia with thousands of sickly children, intoxicated men and women and ungodly acts, but nothing could be less true. Indigenous Australians drink less than non-Indigenous Australians, many remote communities are dry, and only 24 per cent of the population live in remote Australia. Indigenous Australians are unique in their aspirations and values. However, their problems are not unique; they are shared by other indigenes in Fourth World countries* around the world. The most striking difference for Indigenous Australians is their health status, which compares poorly with that of indigenes in other countries (Freemantle, Officer, McAullay, & Anderson, 2007).

*The Fourth World is comprised of countries that are characterised by their experience of being colonised by a dominant group. Many Fourth World people have been forced to assimilate and have lost their land, their economic base and their autonomy (O'Donoghue, 2001).

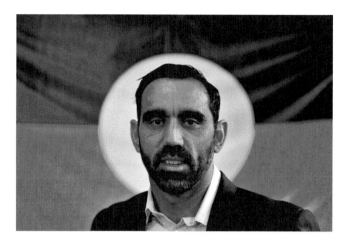

Reproduced with permission from: AAP Image/Paul Miller.

There are many issues one can discuss at the great Aussie barbecue but, like politics and religion, the 'Aboriginal problem' is an issue that everyone has an opinion on. Many Australians also exhibit a fear of difference in colour, race, language and lifestyle. This leaves a multicultural Australia whose issues of cultural diversity, racism and national identity are among the most hotly contested, emotionally charged and important challenges confronting us (Hollinsworth, 2010). The 2015 furore over the crowd behaviour towards Aboriginal footballer Adam Goodes provides a good example of how racism continues to simmer slowly under the surface in all of our dealings in this country. It also proves that Australians have generally been poorly educated about Aboriginal and Torres Strait Islander peoples. It is almost as if they have learnt about two parallel histories, where the lives of the two groups have no common meeting points.

Many stories have been told, mostly from a white, male perspective. Many of these stories have perpetuated stereotypes of Indigenous Australians that are based on outdated policies, theories and beliefs. In this chapter we will pull from this parallel history two key issues using the writing of predominantly Indigenous authors and respected historians. The first is the thinking behind the colonising process from which the stereotyping about Indigenous Australians was often first formed. The second is an examination of the policies that impact upon the lives and health of Indigenous Australians today and especially those who live in remote Australia.

SETTING THE SCENE

Who are Indigenous Australians?

When we talk about the Indigenous peoples of Australia, we refer to both Aboriginal and Torres Strait Islander peoples. Ethnically and culturally, Aboriginal people and Torres Strait Islanders are distinct cultural groups with different histories, different languages and different cultural norms. In the 2011 census there were 669 881 Australians who identified as being Aboriginal and/or Torres Strait Islander, an increase of over 30 per cent from the previous census in 2006, making up about 3 per cent of the total Australian population (Australian Institute of Health and Welfare, 2014). Of these, 6 per cent identified as being Torres Strait Islander and 4 per cent as both Aboriginal and Torres Strait Islander. It should be noted that the 2011 data could be considered an undercount as the identification question was not answered by over one million people at that time (Australian Institute of Health and Welfare, 2014).

Historically, Aboriginal people lived in up to 600 different clan groups on mainland Australia, each with its own tribal land, language, law and culture (Australian Government, 2015a). Torres Strait Islanders come from 14 inhabited islands in the Torres Strait, which lie between the tip of Cape York Peninsula in Queensland and the south of Papua New Guinea.

Prior to the settlement of Australia, Broome (1982) suggests that Aboriginal peoples were largely coastal people who gradually moved down the coastline and over the years travelled via the lakes and rivers into the hinterland. Leading traditional lifestyles for thousands of years, they were extremely efficient hunters and gatherers and they employed considerable levels of resource management. Aboriginal people lived for over 2000 generations in small societies where everyone knew everyone else (Broome, 1982). Strong kinship ties provided security and intimacy and bound together the community.

The traditional Aboriginal web of life was closely knit with spirituality, Aboriginal lore and kinship systems, underpinning traditional beliefs and practices. The land was considered not only to give life: it was life (Broome, 1982). Each Aboriginal clan group had a significant relationship of connectedness and being with the land within their 'own country'. Dudgeon, Oxenham and Grogan (1996, p. 32) tell us that:

> … people belonged to the land: people, animals, flora and the land were one. The people's power and sense of being came from the land. Pride and esteem emanated from celebrating the land, which included the cosmos and intricate interaction of spiritual beings, whose continuing action gave meaning, purpose, and strength to all living and non-living things.

Special significance was given to ancestors and their resting places. The lives of Aboriginal people were shaped by their Dreamtime stories, which were 'both an explanation of how the world came into being, and how people must conduct their behaviour and social relations' (Broome, 1982, p. 15). These are important points – the connection to land, spirituality, roles and relationships – that are continually represented in Aboriginal stories and artworks.

The Aboriginal kinship system encompassed the nuclear and extended family as a whole group. There were specific codes of behaviour for every kinship relationship: for instance, 'a mother-in-law and a son-in-law did not speak to each other and an uncle's role was to teach his nephews the art of hunting' (Broome, 1982, p. 16). This system enabled Aboriginal people to work out exactly where they stood in relation to any other members of the tribe, even outsiders. Economic activity was based on immediate use, not on the creation of surplus for exchange, and a generous system of sharing existed with reciprocity as the centre of social organisation (Reynolds, 1982). Reciprocity was so fundamental to Aboriginal society that, as Thompson noted in the 1940s, there was no tra-

Kinship system from Reconciliation Australia. Video access through Student Consult.

ditional word meaning 'thank you' in the clans that they knew, as life was a shared existence (cited in Reynolds, 1982). So what belonged to one, belonged to everyone. This concept continues to exist in Indigenous Australian society today.

When British colonisers came into this intelligently balanced material and spiritual world Aboriginal people at first thought they were 'resuscitated natives', or spirits of black men who had 'returned to life in a different colour' (Eyre, Buckley, cited in Reynolds, 1982, p. 30).

Colonising the world

In the 1700s around the world colonies were being established: in Canada by the French, South Africa by the Dutch, Australia by the English. The process of colonisation worldwide was based on a set of principles that influenced European attitudes, scientific beliefs and theories.

The theories and principles formed the set of values, beliefs and philosophies and the cultural template that was used for living at that time. They also provided the context within which the governments and colonies dealt with the Indigenous inhabitants of the countries that were being colonised. In Australia, they allowed the dispossession of Aboriginal land, the institutionalisation of racism and, as historian Henry Reynolds argues, the process of attempted genocide (Reynolds, 2001).

In the mid-1700s, as explorers started travelling the world, they met people who looked 'different' from themselves and they began speculating about the reasons for this difference. It was from this time that two predominant scientific theories prevailed in Europe that were based on speculation about the nature of humanness (Eckermann et al., 2012).

PAUSE AND THINK

What was the thinking behind these British colonisers' actions?

What was their cultural belief and value system?

Why did they 'think what they thought'? And what was their reasoning behind it?

What was the cultural template upon which they based their actions? Refer to Chapter 3 for more information on cultural perspectives.

The **Great Chain of Being Theory** arranged all living matter in a hierarchy, from the simplest organisms at the bottom to man at the top (Eckermann et al., 2012). Human beings were also arranged in this hierarchical order. Like a staircase, it started with the simplest creatures, the primates (monkeys), on the bottom step. On the next step up were the 'noble savages' – the Australian and Northern American natives, then the Negroes, then the brown and yellow-skinned peoples and, finally, the white-skinned peoples at the top, along with God. This theory was scientifically supported by phrenology, a study of the shape, volume, weight, size and configuration of skulls (Reynolds, 1989), which was used to 'prove' European superiority over other cultural groups and thereby justify the dispossession of Aboriginal peoples (Broome, 1982).

The Great Chain of Being theory had widespread support until well after the 1850s. By then almost half the southern continent was held by European invaders, who were driven on by dreams of mining and pastoral wealth supported by research reports (Broome, 1982). The publishing of Charles Darwin's *The Origin of Species* in 1859 further supported the current ideas about race.

The second theory was **Social Darwinism,** which is an adaptation by other scholars of Charles Darwin's influential theory of evolution, applied to the physical, cultural and intellectual evolution of non-Europeans. It was based on notions about 'survival of the fittest and natural selection', 'by which favourable variations survived and developed to form a new species' (Broome, 1982). It was argued that weaker races would die out through a process of natural selection, sanctioned racial violence, endorsed feelings of superiority and, in Australia, it left the Aboriginal people to bear the blame for their own extinction (Ober, Peeters, Archer, & Kelly, 2000; Reynolds, 1987).

Broome (1982) argues that these scientific theories, which have since been discredited, supported European Australians in their racist views of Aboriginal Australians, which were based on ignorance, lack of sympathy and a need to rationalise their seizure of Aboriginal land. The vestiges of this form of thinking still live on today in the minds of many people as they are passed on from one generation to the next in the form of racism.

Colonisation was based on three main beliefs:

1 **basic ethnocentrism,** where Europeans saw their culture as being absolutely superior to all others

2 **xenophobia,** whereby the Europeans had a morbid fear of foreigners or anything that seemed unfamiliar (Eckermann et al., 2012)

3 the **Protestant work ethic**, which stressed the importance of achievement, of materialism and of wealth as an indicator of God's grace. With increasing industrialisation and economic expansion came the need for more resources (Eckermann et al., 2012).

BRITISH COLONISATION OF AUSTRALIA

It is estimated that there was a population of 750 000 Indigenous Australians before European settlement (Australian Bureau of Statistics, 2002). When Australia was 'discovered' by the British in 1770, it was regarded as uninhabited or empty – terra nullius* – and classified as Crown land. The Aboriginal inhabitants were seen as 'flora and fauna' and were thought to have no culture, no morality, no religion, no soul and no humanity. There were massacres and open guerrilla warfare between settlers and Aboriginal people as areas were opened up for British settlement, and rapid dehumanisation of Aboriginal groups occurred (Eckermann et al., 2012). The colonial push was different in different states of Australia, but the result was the same: dispossession of land and culture. Government policies were based on the colonisers' perceived superior values and pseudoscientific beliefs and, consequently, no treaty or agreement was made between the settlers and the Indigenous inhabitants who, it was thought, would die out. By 1947 the population was estimated to be about 300 000 Aboriginal people, a reduction of between 50 and 90 per cent depending on geographic area (Eckermann et al., 2012).

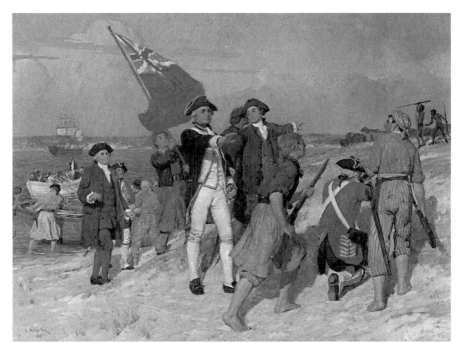

E. Phillips Fox. *Landing of Captain Cook at Botany Bay*, 1770. 1902 oil on canvas, 192.2 × 265.4 cm. National Gallery of Victoria, Melbourne. Gilbee Bequest, 1902. Reproduced with permission.

*'Terra nullius' is land belonging to no one, the ownership of which in international law can therefore be claimed by another nation (*Australian Concise Oxford Dictionary*, 2000).

> ### PAUSE AND THINK
>
> Why was no treaty negotiated with Aboriginal Australians, when treaties were signed in other countries being colonised at the same time – the United States, Canada and New Zealand?
>
> What impact has this lack of treaty had on Aboriginal Australians today?

AUSTRALIAN POLICIES OF THE DAY

Just as there were hundreds of different tribes that could almost be described as separate nations, so were there as many different policies in the colonies (now states) of Australia.

These policies were based on the theories of Social Darwinism and the Great Chain of Being and the intellectual notions of the time. Eckermann and her colleagues (2012) found that every Act of Parliament imposed on Aboriginal people between 1890 and the 1960s can be classified as an example of institutional racism. It is difficult here to state that these policies were introduced with uniformity across all Australian states and territories, as there were many jurisdictional differences. For that reason, the following is merely a thumb print of the policies of the time.

> ### PAUSE AND THINK
>
> It is important when working with local Indigenous groups to learn the relevant state and local history, as this will contribute to your understanding of the issues and, ultimately, help facilitate stronger working partnerships. This is discussed in more detail in Chapter 6, which provides the 12 principles for working cross-culturally and consultation signposts.

Ten key Australian policies are described below, based on the prevailing intellectual beliefs and pseudoscientific theories at the time.

Policy 1 – Colonisation: European settlement 1788–1880 When Australia was 'discovered' in 1770 by Captain Cook, he claimed the land as uninhabited, or terra nullius. It was therefore classified as Crown land, and Governor Phillip proclaimed British sovereignty over it in 1788 (Eckermann et al., 2012; Hollinsworth, 1998). This action was considered normal according to current European values at the time. The Indigenous inhabitants had not used the land in the ways that Europeans considered it should be used, such as for agriculture and settlement in cities, and they had created no signs of civilisation (Eckermann et al., 2012). As the land was regarded as terra nullius, any attempts Aboriginal people made at resisting were interpreted as rebellion, not war. This is how the occupation and dispossession were rationalised. The outcomes were the appropriation of Aboriginal homelands and a process of extermination or domestication, sickness and a loss of Aboriginal law, leadership, traditions and language (Eckermann et al., 2012).

Policy 2 – The White Australia Policy: 1850s–1973 This did not specifically target Aboriginal peoples. This is important because it had a lasting impact on the national and social development of Australia and contributed towards the set of white cultural values and beliefs that helped form the national self-identity of Australians. 'True blue' Australians were, of course, white; and the White Australia Policy excluded and marginalised groups based on their ethnicity and race (Human Rights and Equal Opportunity Commission, 2001). The policy therefore provided a platform upon which to build and perpetuate the stereotypes of other cultural groups, and it resulted in systemic racism and intolerance of diverse cultural groups (Human Rights and Equal Opportunity Commission, 2001). The policy also formed a set of cultural norms – white ways of thinking and doing – upon which many of Australia's government structures and public institutions are built.

Policy 3 – 'Protection' through segregation: 1890s–1950s It was thought that, due to the perceived inferiority of the Indigenous peoples (ethnocentrism), they would die out (Social Darwinism) and that an era of protection and 'smoothing the dying pillow' would follow (Protestant ethic). This process of 'protection' saw the forced segregation of Aboriginal people from their homelands onto missions and reserves, where they were provided with poor living conditions, meagre rations of sugar, tea and flour, as well as controlling substances of tobacco and opium. The state policies differed, but these missions and reserves* were run by a 'Chief Protector of Aborigines' who was appointed to be the legal guardian of all Aboriginal and 'part' Aboriginal children up to 16 years (giving them a similar status to 'wards of the state'†). They were excluded from state schools and were divided into 'full-bloods' and 'half-castes' (Great Chain of Being theory). The forcible removal of children ensued (the stolen generation). The Protector had the power to control the movement, speech, marriage, bank accounts, wages, wills, property and debts of all Aboriginal people (Kidd, 2002). Different cultural groups were forced to live together on missions and reserves, which often created great disharmony. Curfews were imposed in country towns. Perth was prohibited to Aboriginal people, and Brisbane allocated a boundary line to Aboriginal people along what is now called Boundary Road. The term 'Aborigine' was defined by an Act of Parliament and Aboriginal people were not allowed to drink, vote or receive social service benefits (Kidd, 2002; Langton, 2001). Some were given a certificate of exemption, or 'dog tag' as it was known, which allowed them to participate in mainstream society, although they were banned from visiting their families on the reserve (Council for Aboriginal Reconciliation, 1994). All rites and customs that were

*Missions and reserves were places where Indigenous Australians were sent to live as a result of government policies between the late 1800s and the 1970s. They had strict government controls, employed protectors and were often run by religious organisations.
†A ward of the state is a child admitted to government control, an institution or a hostel (Human Rights and Equal Opportunity Commission, 1997b, p. 609).

seen as injurious to the welfare of Aboriginal people on the reserves were prohibited – these included tribal language and law (Eckermann et al., 2012).

At Federation of the six colonies in 1901, the Constitution of Australia made only two references to Aborigines. Section 127 excluded them from the census (although heads of cattle were counted); and Section 51 (Part 26) gave power over Aborigines to the States rather than to the federal government. This was the situation until the referendum in 1967.

Policy 4 – Assimilation: 1950s–1960s Assimilation replaced segregation as official policy in 1951, since it was clear that the Aboriginal people were not dying out. Assimilation was based on the assumption that Aboriginal Australians would attain the same lifestyle, customs, laws and traditions as other Australians through a process of generational cultural adjustment (Broome, 1982). Nonetheless, in the hands of the administrators it became a policy 'to change Aborigines into Europeans with black skins' (Broome, 1982, p. 171). The assimilation policy was later found to be both 'systemic racial discrimination, and genocide, as defined by international law' (Human Rights and Equal Opportunity Commission, 1997b, p. 266). In Queensland the policy of segregation continued until 1965.

Policy 5 – Integration: 1967–1972 In 1967, the federal government held a constitutional referendum in which over 90 per cent of Australians voted in favour of transferring power from the States to the Commonwealth with regard to Aboriginal people, and to count Indigenous Australians in the census (Attwood, Markus, Edwards, & Schilling, 1997). Hughes tells us that 'the referendum victory was a watershed, as it gave black Australians basic human rights and laid the foundations for the land rights movement of the '70s' (cited in Attwood et al., 1997, p. ix). In 1971 Indigenous Australians were included in the census for the first time. While this new integration policy placed more emphasis on positive relations, it was really assimilation under another name.

Policy 6 – Self-determination: 1972–1975 The Federal Department of Aboriginal Affairs (DAA) was established in 1972. It was responsible for the development of national policies in consultation with Aboriginal and Torres Strait Islander people, thus restoring power to Aboriginal people and Torres Strait Islanders to make their own decisions about their own way of life. It was, however, still a bureaucracy based on a consultative process. The Queensland Government rejected this and continued with assimilation policies until 1982 (Ober et al., 2000).

Policy 7 – Self-management 1: 1975–1988 The federal government expected Indigenous Australians to be held accountable for their own decisions and financial management (Eckermann et al., 2012). With this came a strong push for land rights and separate legal, health and housing services.

Policy 8 – Self-management 2: 1988–2004 Indigenous Affairs were reorganised under an elected body – the Aboriginal and Torres Strait Islander Commission (ATSIC), which was made up of community-elected Aboriginal and Torres Strait Islander peoples – to manage some of their own affairs. There was a focus on welfare, housing, health, employment and education (Eckermann et al., 2012). The Council for Aboriginal Reconciliation was established in 1991 but was defunded in 2001. During this time there was much discussion about a treaty and extensive work was undertaken under the banner of reconciliation, though Government only implemented a few of the Council's recommendations. At the same time the World Health Organization reported that Aboriginal health was among the worst of any Indigenous group in the world. In 1995 the health portfolio was transferred from ATSIC back to the Commonwealth Government under the auspices of the Office of Aboriginal and Torres Strait Islander Health within the Health Department. Between 2002 and 2004 a whole-of-government cooperative approach was trialled in 10 communities and the role of ATSIC was reviewed under the Minister for Immigration, Multicultural and Indigenous Affairs. There was no longer a Minister specifically for Indigenous affairs. On 16 July 2004 the Federal Parliament of Australia abolished ATSIC. More than one billion dollars of former ATSIC programs were transferred to mainstream departments who were required to accept responsibility for Indigenous services and accountability for the outcomes (Human Rights and Equal Opportunity Commission, 2004).

Policy 9 – Shared responsibility: 2004–2014 The Office of Indigenous Policy Coordination (OIPC) was established within the Department of Immigration, Multicultural and Indigenous Affairs (DIMIA) to coordinate a whole-of-government approach to programs and services for Indigenous Australians. It also provided advice on Indigenous issues to the Minister and aimed to develop new ways of engaging directly with Indigenous Australians at regional and local levels. This engagement was achieved through the development of Regional Partnership Agreements (RPAs) that aimed to customise and shape Australian Government interventions in a region and develop Shared Responsibility Agreements (SRAs) at community level (Office of Indigenous Policy Coordination, 2006). SRAs spell out what communities, governments and others will contribute to achieving long-term changes in Indigenous communities and are made at a local level. Examples of SRAs include: the government providing funding to convert a building into a day-care centre; upgrading the oval and basketball courts and building swimming pools in return for the community undertaking responsibility for training and the provision of better care for children. In several communities there is a 'no pool no school' rule, whereby the pool is funded by the government while the community provides activities and care for the pool, and ensures that the children attend school (Office of Indigenous Policy Coordination, 2006). This increased level of control over communities through the SRAs could appear to be reminiscent of previous government policies, and one could be mistaken for seeing it as assimilation under another name. For example, up until the 1960s, Aboriginal children were barred from municipal pools and schools because of the colour of their skin.

Policy 10 – Indigenous Advancement Strategy 2014–current In 2014 the Office of Aboriginal and Torres Strait Islander Health was amalgamated into the mainstream Department of Health. The Australian Government's policy framework for Aboriginal and Torres Strait Islander people was set by the Department of the Prime Minister and

Cabinet, under the leadership of the Prime Minister, and the Minister for Indigenous Affairs, through the 'Indigenous Advancement Strategy' (IAS; Australian Government, 2015c). The strategy streamlines activities into five broad programs: jobs, land and economy; children and schooling; safety and wellbeing; culture and capability; and remote Australia strategies. In 2015, the Department administered funding to many Aboriginal and Torres Strait Islander and non-Indigenous organisations in an attempt to create a more streamlined and less onerous submission and reporting process reducing over 150 programs into the five streams. In addition to the IAS, two significant campaigns have been in operation for several years that have the potential to positively impact on the health and wellbeing of Aboriginal and Torres Strait Islander people, and how service providers and health care professionals approach their work in these communities: Closing the Gap and the Constitutional Recognition campaigns.

HEALTH POLICY TIMELINE: 1967–2016

The timeline in Table 4.1 describes some of the major developments in Indigenous affairs nationally and the numerous Indigenous health policies, strategies, reports and inquiries that have occurred in the 49-year period since the referendum. This timeline by no means describes all of the reports or inquiries, only many of those that impacted upon the health of Indigenous Australians. Prior to the 1967 referendum and prior to the 1950s, there was a significant lack of formal health policy relating to Aboriginal and Torres Strait Islander people. Commentaries and reports on the poor health status were only found in the documents and records of government officials, anthropologists and other officers of the colonies.

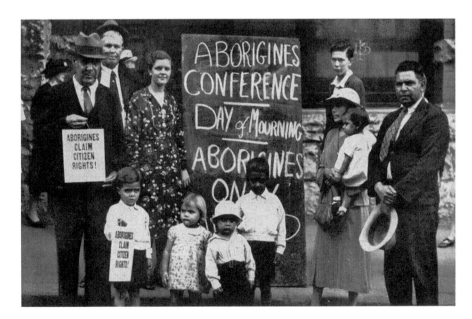

Reproduced with permission from: State Library of New South Wales.

1950–1963

POLICY – ASSIMILATION
Outcome: Aboriginal Australians would attain the same lifestyle, customs, laws and traditions as other Australians. Later defined by International law as systemic racial discrimination and genocide (Human Rights and Equal Opportunity Commission [HREOC], 1997a)

1967

CONSTITUTIONAL REFERENDUM
Outcome: The Commonwealth Government handed the power from the states to legislate for Indigenous Australians and allowed their inclusion in the census for the first time

1968

Office of Aboriginal Affairs is established
Outcome: Aboriginal health units were established in four states

1969–1972

POLICY – INTEGRATION
Except Queensland, which continued assimilation until 1982
Outcome: Placed more emphasis on positive relations, but was really assimilation under another name

1970

Report on the Health of Aboriginal Children in Queensland Settlements and Missions,1967–1969 **is presented in the Annual Report of the Queensland Institute of Medical Research**
Note: There was little data on the health status of Aboriginal and Torres Strait Islander peoples as no process to collect national Indigenous health data existed at this time
Outcome:
The report revealed:
- stillbirth rates 4.2 times higher.
- death from prematurity 3.9 times higher.
- infant mortality 6.3 times higher.
- toddler death rates 13.4 times higher.
- 47% of all deaths related to gastroenteritis and/or pneumonia.
- 85% of all children suffered from malnutrition
The report was censored before its release and a feeding program was initiated (Kidd, 1997)

1971

Aboriginal Medical Service (AMS) was established in Redfern, Sydney
Outcome: First community-controlled AMS in Australia

1972–1975

POLICY – SELF – DETERMINATION
Outcome: The Department of Aboriginal Affairs (DAA) was established. It started consulting with Indigenous peoples on national policy for the first time

1972: 26 January
Aboriginal people erected the Tent Embassy, Parliament House, Canberra
Outcome: It drew attention to their having no legal freehold title to any part of Australia (Council for Aboriginal Reconciliation, 2001)

Continued

Table 4.1 Policy timeline 1967–2015–cont'd

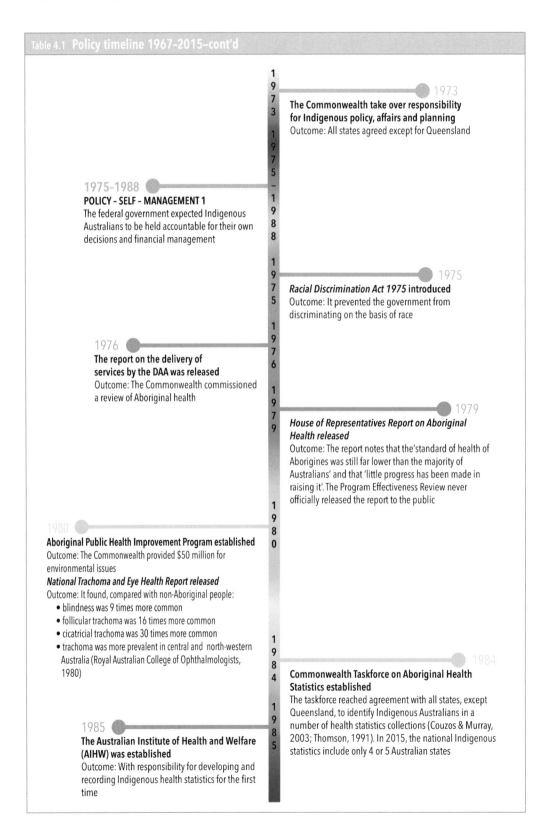

1973
The Commonwealth take over responsibility for Indigenous policy, affairs and planning
Outcome: All states agreed except for Queensland

1975–1988
POLICY – SELF – MANAGEMENT 1
The federal government expected Indigenous Australians to be held accountable for their own decisions and financial management

1975
Racial Discrimination Act 1975 **introduced**
Outcome: It prevented the government from discriminating on the basis of race

1976
The report on the delivery of services by the DAA was released
Outcome: The Commonwealth commissioned a review of Aboriginal health

1979
House of Representatives Report on Aboriginal Health **released**
Outcome: The report notes that the 'standard of health of Aborigines was still far lower than the majority of Australians' and that 'little progress has been made in raising it'. The Program Effectiveness Review never officially released the report to the public

1980
Aboriginal Public Health Improvement Program established
Outcome: The Commonwealth provided $50 million for environmental issues
National Trachoma and Eye Health Report released
Outcome: It found, compared with non-Aboriginal people:
• blindness was 9 times more common
• follicular trachoma was 16 times more common
• cicatricial trachoma was 30 times more common
• trachoma was more prevalent in central and north-western Australia (Royal Australian College of Ophthalmologists, 1980)

1984
Commonwealth Taskforce on Aboriginal Health Statistics established
The taskforce reached agreement with all states, except Queensland, to identify Indigenous Australians in a number of health statistics collections (Couzos & Murray, 2003; Thomson, 1991). In 2015, the national Indigenous statistics include only 4 or 5 Australian states

1985
The Australian Institute of Health and Welfare (AIHW) was established
Outcome: With responsibility for developing and recording Indigenous health statistics for the first time

Table 4.1 **Policy timeline 1967–2015–cont'd**

1988–2004
POLICY – SELF-MANAGEMENT 2
Outcome: Aboriginal and Torres Strait Islander representation through an elected body, Aboriginal and Torres Strait Islander Commission (ATSIC; from 1990), to manage some of their own affairs

1989
The National Aboriginal Health Strategy **(NAHS), developed by Aboriginal people, was presented by government**
Outcome: It recommended that $3 billion was required to deal with the enormous Indigenous health problems. The government allocated $232 million over five years (NAHS Working Party, 1989). It has never been fully implemented and has instead formed the basis for numerous other reports
The first National Health Survey **was conducted**
Outcome: This was the *first time* it had included identification of Indigenous people – but it did not include all states

1991
The Aboriginal and Torres Strait Islander Health Goals and Targets **was produced by ATSIC**
Outcome: It built upon the NAHS report and was seen as a means of evaluating the effectiveness of NAHS
The Royal Commission into Aboriginal Deaths in Custody **was released**
Outcome: The Commissioner made 339 recommendations, including the implementation of the NAHS report and cultural training of the health workforce. Between 2000 and 2004 imprisonment rates for Indigenous women rose by 25% and for Indigenous men by 11%. In 2006 there were more deaths in custody than in 1988 when the Inquiry was initiated (HREOC, 2006)
The Council for Aboriginal Reconciliation was established by the Prime Minister
Outcome: It was set up to build relationships for change between Indigenous and non-Indigenous Australians
National Health and Medical Research Council (NHMRC) *Guidelines on ethical matters in Aboriginal and Torres Strait Islander health research* **was released**
Outcome: It outlined the steps researchers should follow when working with communities, taking into account the cultural differences and sensitivities that have been the crux of the problems in the past (NHMRC, 1991)

1988
The Royal Commission into Aboriginal Deaths in Custody initiated
Outcome: They investigated 99 deaths in custody that had occurred over the previous 9 years, of whom half had been separated from their families (HRSCoATSIA, 1994). Aboriginal people at that time made up 14% of the total prison population and were up to 15 times more likely to be in prison than non-Aboriginal people (HREOC, 2006)

1990
Aboriginal and Torres Strait Islander Commission (ATSIC) was established, replacing DAA
Outcome: Tripartite Forums were established in the states and the Territory to provide national coordination and representation for many services for Indigenous peoples, including health

1992
The High Court of Australia handed down its *Mabo* **decision**
Outcome: It grants title of land on Murray Island to the proponents, in recognition of the special relationship that Aboriginal and Torres Strait Islander peoples have with the land (Council for Aboriginal Reconciliation, 2001). The Mabo decision effectively challenged the concept of terra nullius, recognising customary rights to land as part of common law based on traditional customs, rather than as statute law, which is legislated in parliaments (Hollinsworth, 1998). This meant that Indigenous Australians could claim native title to land as a legal right, rather than as a political gift or through welfare provision (Hollinsworth, 1998)

Continued

Table 4.1 Policy timeline 1967–2015–cont'd

1993

National Aboriginal Community Controlled Health Organisation (NACCHO) was formed
Outcome: It forms an umbrella organisation for the growing number of Aboriginal Medical Services. In 2015 there were over 150 AMSs nationally
The Native Title Act 1993 **became law**
Outcome: It recognised native title and a process for native title rights (Council for Aboriginal Reconciliation, 2001)
The Human Rights and Equal Opportunity Commission (HREOC) employed its first Aboriginal and Torres Strait Islander Social Justice Commissioner
Outcome: He stated in his 1994 report: 'There should be no mistake that the state of Indigenous health in this country is an abuse of human rights. A decent standard of health and life expectancy equivalent to other Australians is not a favour asked by our peoples. It is our right – simply because we too are human' (HREOC, 2005, p. 11)

1994

The National Aboriginal and Torres Strait Islander Health Survey **is conducted for the first time by the Australian Bureau of Statistics (ABS)**
Note: Identification of Aboriginality was reported as remaining incomplete in most areas. The findings in this report were therefore likely to be a substantial underestimate (AIHW, 1996)
Outcome: When compared with other Australians they found:
• the gap in life expectancy had widened
• diabetes death rates were 12 times higher for men and 17 times higher for women
• 15–20 years gap in life expectancy
• death rates between 25 and 54 years were 5–7 times higher.
• infant mortality rates were 3–5 times higher
• low birth weight rates were double
• maternal deaths were 10 times higher
• hospital admission rates were 50% and 60% higher for women and men, respectively (AIHW, 1996)
Evaluation of NAHS report undertaken
Outcome: Two evaluations were commissioned and found that NAHS had never been effectively implemented and that all governments had grossly under-funded initiatives, especially in remote and rural areas (NAHS Evaluation Committee, 1994)

1995

Indigenous health was transferred from ATSIC to the Commonwealth Health Department
Outcome: The Office for Aboriginal and Torres Strait Islander Health (OATSIH) was established to manage Indigenous health
Framework Agreements were established between the states and the federal government
Outcome: To provide advice on policy, planning and Indigenous health issues. Six out of eight states signed
The Ways Forward: National Aboriginal and Torres Strait Islander Mental Health Policy National Consultancy Report **was released**
Outcome: This report provided an overview of the mental health needs and problems of Indigenous people around Australia. It proposed a comprehensive national program under Aboriginal control to address years of neglect in this area

1996

The Aboriginal and Torres Strait Islander Health and Welfare Information Unit undertook a review to develop a national plan for Aboriginal and Torres Strait Islander health information
Outcome: The plan was the result of extensive consultation and included state and Territory reports and case studies of good practice in health information for Indigenous health (AIHW, 1997). 20 years later the data still only includes 4 or 5 states and often excludes large states such as Victoria
National Aboriginal and Torres Strait Islander Social and Emotional Wellbeing Action Plan **was launched**
Outcome: It built on the Bringing Them Home Report to provide a coherent approach to Aboriginal and Torres Strait Islander mental health. It resulted in $20 million being allocated for curricula development, information systems, linkages and clinical services (Office of Aboriginal and Torres Strait Islander Health, 2001)
National Aboriginal and Torres Strait Islander Hearing Strategy **was approved**
Outcome: The federal budget allocated $5.7 million to improve the delivery, detection and treatment for hearing health in the 0–5-years-old age group, and the management of services and community programs (Department of Health and Aged Care [DHAC], 1996)

Table 4.1 Policy timeline 1967–2015–cont'd

1997

Bringing Them Home Report – a national inquiry into the separation of Aboriginal and Torres Strait Islander children from their families – released by the Human Rights and Equal Opportunity Commission (HREOC, 1997a)

Annual 'Sorry Days' were convened each year thereafter to commemorate the release of this report

Outcome: Making hundreds of recommendations, the Commission concluded that an extremely gross violation of human rights had occurred during the period of the assimilation policy that was genocidal in character (HREOC, 1997a). Those taken were found to be much less likely to have undertaken post-secondary education, and were:

- three times more likely to have been in jail
- two times as likely to use illicit substances
- much less likely to live in stable conditions than Aboriginal children who were not removed (HREOC, 1997a)

ABS and Australian Institute of Health and Welfare (AIHW) launched the first *Health and Welfare of Australia's Aboriginal and Torres Strait Islander Peoples* report

It included statistics on the health and welfare of Indigenous Australians for the *first time*

Outcome: They found, compared with non-Indigenous Australians, that Indigenous Australians:

- die at a younger age from almost every type of disease or condition for which information is available
- have a life expectancy about 15–20 years lower
- have babies that are 2–3 times more likely to be of low birth weight and 2–4 times more likely to die at birth
- are 2–3 times more likely to be hospitalised
- have death rates that are higher at every age, with the largest gap in adults aged 25–54 years, who have rates that are 6 to 8 times higher
- are twice as likely to smoke
- are more likely to abstain from drinking alcohol (33% versus 45%)
- have child abuse and neglect rates that are 2–3 times higher for physical, emotional and sexual abuse, and 6 times higher for neglect
- have double the number of adults employed as community service workers
- 4 to 10 Indigenous households were estimated to have insufficient income to meet basic needs (ABS & AIHW, 1997)

The National Training and Employment Strategy for Aboriginal and Torres Strait Islander health workers and professionals working in Aboriginal and Torres Strait Islander health was released

Outcome: They recommended processes that strengthened the Aboriginal and Torres Strait Islander health workforce through training, employment initiatives, working conditions, professional development and cultural awareness training for all health professionals

House of Representatives released the first in a series of submissions in response to their inquiry into Indigenous health

Outcome: It contained 212 submissions received in response to their inquiry into Indigenous health

1997:26–28 May

Australian Reconciliation Convention was convened by the Council for Aboriginal Reconciliation

Outcome: Attended by 1800 participants, this event was a historic landmark in the reconciliation process. It stimulated a grassroots people's movement around the country (Council for Aboriginal Reconciliation, 2001)

1998

AIHW and National Centre for Epidemiology and Population Health (NCEPH) released expenditures on health services for Indigenous peoples for the first time

Tasmania and the Northern Territory sign Framework Agreements for the first time

Outcome: This is the first time that an industrialised country had estimated the health service expenditure for its Indigenous people. It showed the recurrent expenditure was about $853 million, about 8% higher than for other Australians. It also found that the median weekly income of Indigenous males was $189 compared with $415 for non-Indigenous males (AIHW & NCEPH, 1998)

1999

The National Audit Office released the *National Aboriginal Health Strategy* – delivery of housing and infrastructure to Indigenous communities

Outcome: It found that ATSIC's analysis and reporting of performance information for NAHS for 1997–1998 was inadequate and recommended targets, output and outcome measures be developed for employment and training (National Audit Office, 1999)

The Community Housing and Infrastructure Needs Survey (CHINS) was conducted by the ABS on behalf of ATSIC

Outcome: A comprehensive survey of housing and infrastructure in discrete remote Indigenous communities was undertaken to provide future policies and targeted programs in areas of identified need. It clearly showed that remote Indigenous communities did not have the infrastructure required to attain or maintain health

Continued

Table 4.1 Policy timeline 1967–2015–cont'd

 2000

House of Representatives Standing Committee into Family and Community Affairs tabled its final report, *Health is life,* following five volumes of submissions regarding the Indigenous health status inquiry

Outcome: The report made 35 recommendations, similar to those made in the 1989 NAHS report, including the supply of fresh food and water in remote areas, housing infrastructure and education to workforce training and reconciliation (House of Representatives, 2000). The government accepted six recommendations outright, a further 15 in principle, noted 13 and rejected one

 2000: 27 May

Corroboree 2000 – the Council for Aboriginal Reconciliation ceremonially presented the national reconciliation documents to national leaders and the people of Australia

Outcome: More than 250 000 people joined the People's Walk for Reconciliation across Sydney Harbour Bridge. In December the Council presented its final report and recommendations to the Prime Minister (Council for Aboriginal Reconciliation, 2001)

2001

The National Council for Aboriginal Reconciliation was closed down on 1 January

Outcome: The government rejected most of the recommendations made in the national reconciliation documents (HREOC, 2005)

Reconciliation Australia was established

Outcome: An independent, not-for-profit organisation established by the former Council for Aboriginal Reconciliation (Reconciliation Australia, 2006)

Redfern AMS celebrated 30 years of health care provision

Department of Health and Aged Care (DHAC) released the *Aboriginal and Torres Strait Islander Coordinated Care Trials National Evaluation Report 1*

Outcome: The report described the background, descriptions, experiences and outcomes of the four coordinated care trials conducted during 1997–1999

DHAC published *Better health care: Studies for the successful delivery of PHC services for Aboriginal and Torres Strait Islander Australians*

Outcome: It examined primary health care and national and international evidence of the effectiveness of this approach in improving Indigenous health outcomes

AIHW released *Expenditures on Health Services for Aboriginal and Torres Strait Islander Peoples for the Period 1998–1999*

Note: Only 50% of the expenditures could be included in the analysis due to poor data (AIHW, 2001)

Outcome: They reported similar findings to the 1995–1996 report, with total expenditures being $1245 million, equivalent to $3065 per Indigenous person, compared with $2518 per non-Indigenous person. Medicare and the Pharmaceutical Benefits Scheme (PBS) expenditures were 37% lower than for non-Indigenous people (AIHW, 2001)

2001: October

Dr Arnold 'Puggy' Hunter Memorial Scholarship Scheme commenced, named after the Aboriginal leader in health

Outcome: Three Indigenous nursing students and five medical students were awarded the first scholarships. In 2015 the scheme included all health related disciplines

2002

The Council of Australian Governments (CoAG) commissioned the Review of Commonwealth/State Services Provision to produce regular reports against key indicators of Indigenous disadvantage

Outcome: The purpose of this report was to measure the impact of policy changes on the Indigenous community

***The National Strategic Framework for Aboriginal and Torres Strait Islander Health: A Framework for Governments* was endorsed by the Australian Health Ministers Advisory Council (AHMAC)**

Outcome: The Framework was based on nine principles. It was built on the 1989 National Aboriginal Health Strategy and addressed approaches to primary health care within contemporary policy environments

The NHMRC *Road map: A strategic framework for improving Aboriginal and Torres Strait Islander health through research* was endorsed by the NHMRC

Outcome: The purpose was to identify areas of research that would underpin better policy and practice to improve Indigenous health. It committed to spending 5% of the Medical Research Endowment Account on Aboriginal and Torres Strait Islander health research, and Indigenous participation on the NHMRC Council and its principal committees (NHMRC, 2002)

The Australian National Audit Office (ANAO) concluded its follow-up to the 1998 performance audit of the Department of Health and Ageing to determine the extent that the department had implemented the recommendations

Outcome: ANAO found that eight of their 12 recommendations had been implemented, but they were impeded from meaningful reporting against the performance indicators due to the gaps and deficiencies in the reliability, or lack of, available data, which was the single most significant quality issue (ANAO, 2002)

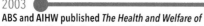
Table 4.1 Policy timeline 1967–2015–cont'd

2003

ABS and AIHW published *The Health and Welfare of Australia's Aboriginal and Torres Strait Islander Peoples 2003* **(ABS & AIHW, 2003)**

Outcome: They reported that Indigenous Australians:
- were twice as likely to live in rented accommodation
- were under-represented in child-care facilities
- had 6 times more child protection orders
- represented 43% of all 10–17-year-olds in detention
- were twice as likely to be of low birth weight
- had twice the perinatal death rate
- 17% of those assisted by SAAPs (homeless people) were Indigenous, of whom 33% were escaping from domestic violence

Hospitalisation for:
- assault was 8 times higher for males and 28 times higher for females
- respiratory disease was 3 times higher
- injury and poisoning were double in discrete remote communities, where
- over a quarter of communities failed water testing
- half reported sewerage overflow (ABS & AIHW, 2003)

In July the National Strategic Framework for Aboriginal and Torres Strait Islander Health: Framework for Action by Governments was released

Outcome: The framework built on the 1989 NAHS report and the 2000 reconciliation framework. It was based on nine principles and addressed approaches to primary health care and population health within contemporary policy environments and planning structures (National Aboriginal and Torres Strait Islander Health Council, 2003)

2003
2004
2007
2005

2004–2007

POLICY – SHARED RESPONSIBILITY

Outcome: The Office of Indigenous Policy Coordination (OIPC) was established to coordinate a whole-of-government approach to programs and services for Indigenous Australians

In November 2004 the National Indigenous Council was appointed

2005: 16 March

The Aboriginal and Torres Strait Islander Commission (ATSIC) and its service delivery arm, the Aboriginal and Torres Strait Islander Services (ATSIS), were abolished

Outcome: New arrangements as at 1 July – more than $1 billion of former ATSIC/ATSIS programs were transferred to mainstream departments. ATSIC Regional Councils ceased to exist. The Social Justice Commissioner urged Governments to work together to facilitate and fund alternative regional representative structures (HREOC, 2005)

2005

State of the Service 2003–2004 **report released**

Outcome: It reported that Indigenous Australian public service employment rates were the lowest in 10 years and were declining (HREOC, 2005)

The Community Development Employment Projects (CDEP) discussion paper, *Building on Success* **was released**

Outcome: The paper proposed reforms to the CDEP scheme with stronger focus on employment, community activities and business development (HREOC, 2005)

The United Nations Committee on the Elimination of Racial Discrimination observations on Australia were released

Outcome: The Committee acknowledged progress but noted their concerns regarding:
- the government's rejection of most of the recommendations adopted by the Council of Aboriginal Reconciliation in 2000
- the abolition of ATSIC
- the gaps in housing, employment, health and income of Indigenous peoples
- the continued existence of mandatory sentencing in Western Australia and the overrepresentation of Indigenous people in prisons, particularly the increasing numbers of Indigenous women (HREOC, 2005)

Continued

| Table 4.1 | **Policy timeline 1967–2015–cont'd** |

2005

Overcoming Indigenous Disadvantage – Key Indicators 2005 Report released by the Steering Committee for the review of Government Service Provision, Productivity Commission

Note: Like most of the above reports, the Committee noted that the data for Indigenous people remained deficient. In 2015 most data sets still only included four or five states. These estimates are conservative

Outcome: The committee found that, between 2000 and 2004:
- 49% over 18 years reported a disability
- year 12 retention rates rose by 4%
- year 9 retention rates declined by 11%
- average weekly household income rates were $374, down $20 per week
- 25% increase in female imprisonment rates
- 65% of Indigenous homicides involved alcohol

And, when compared with non-Indigenous peoples, Indigenous Australians were:
- 11 times more likely to be imprisoned
- 19 times more likely to be in juvenile detention
- 2–3 times more likely to suicide
- twice as likely to be admitted to hospital for infectious diseases
- twice as likely to smoke
- 2–3 times more likely to die in infancy
- twice as likely to be born with low or extremely low birth weight (ABS & AIHW, 2005; Steering Committee for the Review of Government Service Provision, 2005)

ABS and AIHW *released The Health and Welfare of Australia's Aboriginal and Torres Strait Islander Peoples, 2005.* **They reported improvements in the quality and quantity of Indigenous data collected (ABS & AIHW, 2005)**

Note: This may impact upon the data produced

Outcome: It contained specific and limited information on Torres Strait Islanders for the first time.

From 1994/6–2002 they reported:
- an increase in primary and secondary school enrolments
- rising employment levels of 7%
- a decline in infant mortality (though it was still double)
- 70% were living in regional and remote areas
- diabetes rates were 4 times more prevalent, and hospitalisation rates were 5 times higher
- dialysis rates were 9–17 times and mortality rates were 11 times higher than non-Indigenous Australians
- lifespan was approximately 17 years less for both males and females (ABS & AIHW, 2005)

2006

2006

Federal Budget released in May

Outcome: The government announced that Australia was debt-free and had a substantial surplus (AMA, 2006)

National Rural Health Alliance media release – budget commitment to remote Indigenous stores

A national survey found that 60% more adults in remote areas were now missing out on food than 4 years ago due to lack of money (National Rural Health Alliance, 2006). The government commits $48.1 million over 3 years to support remote Indigenous stores in the provision of fresh foods for remote communities

The Australian Medical Association (AMA) *Report Card 2006 Aboriginal and Torres Strait Islander Health* **was released**

Outcome: The AMA identified a $460 million annual shortfall in Indigenous primary health care spending. It called on the federal government to close the gaps within 5 years (jointly with NACCHO) and set provision for primary health care services and core fund them at actual cost (AMA, 2006)

Standing Committee on Aboriginal and Torres Strait Islander Health, Statistical Information Management Committee (2006) released *National Summary of the 2003 and 2004 Jurisdictional Reports Against the Aboriginal and Torres Strait Islander Health Performance Indicators*

Outcome: This report was the second national summary of 56 health performance indicators for Aboriginal and Torres Strait Islander peoples, developed to monitor whether the health of Indigenous people was improving, and to highlight problem areas and priorities. Due to the relatively poor quality of the Indigenous health data, the committee found it impossible to make comprehensive state comparisons (AIHW, 2006)

The Indigenous Summit on Child Abuse and Violence was announced in June following the Northern Territory Crown Prosecutor leaking confidential documents to the media

The summit focused on law, order and policing. Health was left off the agenda. The government responded with policies to strengthen administration, policing and mandatory reporting of child abuse and violence, citing a system of paternalism to be introduced that is based on competence rather than race

At the same time, the Weekend Australian reported states and territories under-spending the allocated $141 million for building homes for Aboriginal people. In 2003–2004 the under-spend was $55.1 million (17–18 June 2006)

Table 4.1 Policy timeline 1967–2015–cont'd

2007

The Northern Territory National Emergency Response (also referred to as 'the intervention')
Outcome: This dramatic response was developed targeting welfare provision, law enforcement, and land tenure by the Howard government as a result of the Inquiry into the Protection of Aboriginal Children from Sexual Abuse, titled *Ampe Akelyernemane Meke Mekarle: 'Little Children are Sacred'.*
(The rates of abuse were false and founded on fraudulent information given to the Hon Minister Mal Brough's office)
Launching of the *'Close the Gap Campaign'* by the Committee of Australian Governments (CoAG)
Outcome: CoAG commits to 'closing the gap' in life expectancy between Indigenous and non-Indigenous Australians in one generation and sets a strategy – *Closing the gap*

2008 13th February

Prime Minister, the Hon Kevin Rudd, apologises and says 'Sorry' to Indigenous Australians and the Stolen Generation
Outcome: The apology is on behalf of successive governments for the 'profound grief, suffering and loss' due to separation from their families. The nation stops to hear the apology, which has a significant national impact
Government funding impetus improves
Outcome: CoAG announce they will contribute $806 million (federal) and $772 million (all states) to Aboriginal and Torres Strait Islander health over the next 4 years, which is the biggest single injection of Indigenous health spending in decades (NACCHO, 2008)
Australia supports the United Nations Declaration on the Rights of Indigenous Peoples
Outcome: The Howard government had rejected the declaration previously, despite Canada, USA and New Zealand signing it, fearing a separate customary law
Prime Minister Kevin Rudd says 'Sorry' to the Forgotten Australians
Outcome: The apology includes migrants and Indigenous people who were victims of abuse in orphanages and institutions between 1930 and 1970, who suffered abuse similar to the Stolen Generations of Aboriginal peoples

2010

The UN Committee on the Elimination of Racial Discrimination reports
Outcome: The UN Committee delivers a damning report on Australia's failure to meet international commitments on eliminating discrimination (The Greens, 2010)

2011

The Australian Parliament passes with bi-partisan support the *Aboriginal and Torres Strait Islander Peoples Recognition Bill 2012*
Outcome: The bill recognises the unique and special place of Aboriginal people and sets out a review process to progress the route to a referendum

2013: 14 March

The Northern Territory Country Liberal Party elects Gamilaroi man Adam Giles as Chief Minister
Outcome: He is the first Aboriginal person to head an Australian government

2013: 7 September

Hon Tony Abbott becomes Prime Minister of Australia
Outcome: His Aboriginal policy declares that 'Australia will, in effect, have a prime minister for Indigenous affairs and a dedicated Indigenous affairs minister'
Hon Nova Peris becomes Senator for the Northern Territory
Outcome: She is the first Aboriginal woman to enter federal parliament

Continued

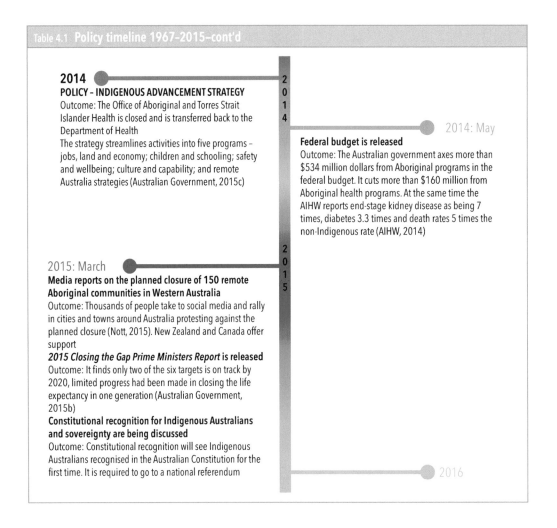

Table 4.1 Policy timeline 1967–2015–cont'd

2014
POLICY – INDIGENOUS ADVANCEMENT STRATEGY
Outcome: The Office of Aboriginal and Torres Strait Islander Health is closed and is transferred back to the Department of Health
The strategy streamlines activities into five programs – jobs, land and economy; children and schooling; safety and wellbeing; culture and capability; and remote Australia strategies (Australian Government, 2015c)

2014: May
Federal budget is released
Outcome: The Australian government axes more than $534 million dollars from Aboriginal programs in the federal budget. It cuts more than $160 million from Aboriginal health programs. At the same time the AIHW reports end-stage kidney disease as being 7 times, diabetes 3.3 times and death rates 5 times the non-Indigenous rate (AIHW, 2014)

2015: March
Media reports on the planned closure of 150 remote Aboriginal communities in Western Australia
Outcome: Thousands of people take to social media and rally in cities and towns around Australia protesting against the planned closure (Nott, 2015). New Zealand and Canada offer support
***2015 Closing the Gap Prime Ministers Report* is released**
Outcome: It finds only two of the six targets is on track by 2020, limited progress had been made in closing the life expectancy in one generation (Australian Government, 2015b)
Constitutional recognition for Indigenous Australians and sovereignty are being discussed
Outcome: Constitutional recognition will see Indigenous Australians recognised in the Australian Constitution for the first time. It is required to go to a national referendum

2016

Many students ask, '*Why do we have to learn this? It has nothing to do with health or our work in the future.*' This timeline demonstrates, however, that it has everything to do with health. One cannot look at the health status of Indigenous Australians without looking at the historical and political basis upon which the health outcomes have been constructed. There is a strong link between the colonisation process and the social and environmental factors that determine whether we will be healthy or not – the social determinants of health (Wilkinson & Marmot, 2003). Let us hope that with our new strategies we are not just moving the deck chairs around on a new state-of-the-art ship with the hope that it will be seen as something being done, when essentially it is still a ship, steered by a captain from the same type of political and cultural organisation – one who knows best – with the same imminent problems ahead of us, based on the same theories but using a new vessel within the same administration system.

This somewhat gruelling policy timeline demonstrates clearly the enormous number of reports, policies and reviews undertaken, the poor data collection processes that still today do not include all Australian states and the resulting poor health outcomes.

Indigenous stereotyping

Long after the theory of Social Darwinism was discredited, its underlying set of beliefs persisted in the Australian community. These beliefs created a number of stereotypes of Aboriginal people, which still exist today and are perpetuated by the media, who remain deficit-focused. School textbooks in the early 1970s portrayed Aboriginal Australians as 'simple child-like people', perpetuating the myth of low intelligence (Reynolds, 2001). Langton (2001) attributes the decline in Aboriginal employment numbers at mine sites since the 1970s as racist stereotypes perpetuating the myth that Aboriginal labourers are lazy. Yet the declining numbers only occurred once these workers were required by law to receive payment for their work. Numbers continue to remain low today.

This is not ancient history – what began over 200 years ago is still happening today. A fine example was the Northern Territory Intervention in May 2006, which resulted in weeks of political mud-slinging and front-page media reports that depicted all Aboriginal people as drunks and child molesters, therefore reinforcing the stereotype. Yet the government's solution to 'solve the Aboriginal problem', the details of which have been known to it for decades, was not to provide the necessary resources to overcome centuries of oppression and neglect, but to break down and destroy the town camps and remote communities, many of which are dry or alcohol-free communities. Children were removed, men were jailed, the police presence was increased and the rest were dispersed by bringing in the army.

Perhaps the underlying reason is that it would have meant exposing the indefensible record of neglect by both federal and Northern Territory governments over decades, compounded by our racist society (Allen, 2006). It seems easier for the

PAUSE AND THINK

Why, in 2006, were there communities in the Northern Territory with populations of over 2500 with no high school or policeman when they have over 1000 school-aged children?

Why has a community had no doctor for five years when the male life expectancy is 49 years?

Why didn't the media flesh out any of these issues?

Why in 2015 is the Western Australian government planning to close down over 100 remote Aboriginal communities?

media to maintain the negative stereotype of Aboriginal people as drunks, petrol sniffers and perpetrators of violence than it is to examine the ingredients to murder and sexual assault that are born out of poverty, boredom, alienation, discrimination, violence and a great sense of emptiness fuelled by alcohol, cannabis and inhalants (Lateline, 2006).

CONCLUSION

The timeline clearly demonstrates the huge amounts of data, reports and government inquiries that have been conducted, and the resulting health outcomes that show small improvements in health status during the 48-year period. Yet the data still, in 2015, only included four or sometimes five Australian states. The task of providing a national picture appears impossible due to the inconsistencies in data collection processes between the states and territories. This is a good example of institutional racism, whereby the collection of these data would provide an accurate national picture of the disadvantaged health status of Australia's Indigenous peoples. Or is this a good example of a lack of political will to make it happen? Maybe it is not in the best interest of the government to know, because then they would be compelled to do something significant about it, rather than move the deck chairs and the officers.

What is required is a human rights approach to address the health inequality of Indigenous Australians, the purpose of which is to enable Australia's Indigenous citizens to enjoy the highest attainable standard of health conducive to living a life with dignity (Human Rights and Equal Opportunity Commission, 2015). The human rights approach would:

- recognise the link between health status and systemic discrimination
- address the issue of how governments can make meaningful commitments
- address Indigenous health in a holistic manner that reflects the social determinants of health inequality
- build on the opportunities and challenges of applying the whole-of-government approach to Indigenous health in this country (Human Rights and Equal Opportunity Commission, 2005).

This requires a paradigm shift in the way in which we look at Indigenous health issues. It is also time to change the mantra.

Our current and continually recited mantra about Indigenous health statistics is not having an impact. It is washing over governments, funders, health service providers, students and the general public. It is not that we are unaware of these factors, issues and statistics – we have known about them for at least 40 years. The problem lies in the lack of political will to make it happen.

Twenty years ago in 1994 the first Social Justice Commissioner said:

We have all heard them – the figures of death and disability … Every few years the figures are repeated and excite attention. But I suspect that most

Australians accept them as being almost inevitable. A certain kind of industrial deafness has developed. The human element in this is not recognised. The meaning of these figures is not heard – or felt … The statistics of infant and perinatal mortality are our babies and children who die in our arms … the statistics of shortened life expectancy are our mothers and fathers, uncles, aunties and elders who lived diminished lives and die before their gifts of knowledge and experience are passed on. We die silently under these statistics.

(HUMAN RIGHTS AND EQUAL OPPORTUNITY COMMISSION, 2005, p. 11)

Let us hope that the Social Justice Commissioner will not be echoing these same sentiments in another two decades.

Discussion Points

1   Discuss the beliefs underlying the colonisation processes. Do these values still exist in Australia today? Discuss.

2   Why were Indigenous Australians moved onto missions and reserves?

3   What was the thinking of the day that supported the policies of Social Darwinism? Discuss.

4   Tutorial activity: refer to the policy timeline in Table 4.1. Ask each student to:

   - choose one report from the timeline
   - find the report in the library or on the internet
   - present a five-minute overview of the report and its findings to their tutorial group. Discuss with the group and make links between the report and the historical beliefs and values at the time.

References

Allen, S. (2006). Official response to Aboriginal child sexual abuse in Australia: more law and order. World Socialist Web Site. <http://www.wsws.org/en/articles/2006/05/abor-m22.htm> Accessed 30.10.15.

Attwood, B., Markus, A., Edwards, D., & Schilling, K. (1997). *The 1967 referendum, or when Aborigines didn't get the vote.* Canberra: Aboriginal Studies Press, Australian Institute of Aboriginal and Torres Strait Islander Studies.

Australian Bureau of Statistics (ABS). (2002). *Population – Aboriginal and Torres Strait Islander Population.* Canberra: ABS. <http://www.abs.gov.au/ausstats/abs@.nsf/0/BFC28642D31C215CCA256B350010B3F4?Open> Accessed 04.08.15.

Australian Bureau of Statistics & Australian Institute of Health and Welfare (AIHW). (1997). *The health and welfare of Australia's Aboriginal and Torres Strait Islander peoples.* Canberra: ABS and AIHW.

Australian Bureau of Statistics & Australian Institute of Health and Welfare. (2003). 4704.0 – *The health and welfare of Australia's Aboriginal and Torres Strait Islander peoples.* Canberra: ABS and AIHW.

Australian Bureau of Statistics & Australian Institute of Health and Welfare. (2005). 4704.0 – *The health and welfare of Australia's Aboriginal and Torres Strait Islander peoples.* Canberra: ABS & AIHW.

Australian Concise Oxford Dictionary. (2000). Melbourne: Oxford University Press.

Australian Government. (2015a). *Australian Indigenous cultural heritage.* Canberra: Australian Government. <http://www.australia.gov.au/about-australia/australian-story/austn-indigenous-cultural-heritage> Accessed 04.06.15.

Australian Government. (2015b). *Closing the Gap Prime Minister's Report 2015.* Canberra: Department of the Prime Minister and Cabinet, Australian Government. <http://www.dpmc.gov.au/sites/default/files/publications/Closing_the_Gap_2015_Report_0.pd> Accessed 04.08.15.

Australian Government. (2015c). *Indigenous advancement strategy.* Canberra: Australian Government. Department of the Prime Minister and Cabinet. <http://www.dpmc.gov.au/sites/default/files/files/ia/IAS%20Overarching.pdf> Accessed 05.06.15.

Australian Institute of Health and Welfare (AIHW). (1996). *Australia's health 1996.* Canberra: AIHW.

Australian Institute of Health and Welfare. (1997). *Annual Report AIHW: Aboriginal and Torres Strait Islander health and welfare information, 1996–97.* Canberra: AIHW. <http://www.aihw.gov.au/publications/corporate/ar96-7/ar96-7-c11.html#national_plan> Accessed 02.08.15.

Australian Institute of Health and Welfare. (2001). *Expenditures on health services for Aboriginal and Torres Strait Islander people 1998–99.* Canberra: AIHW.

Australian Institute of Health and Welfare. (2006). *National summary of the 2003 and 2004 jurisdictional reports against the Aboriginal and Torres Strait Islander health performance indicators.* Canberra: Standing Committee on Aboriginal and Torres Strait Islander Health, Statistical Information Management Committee, AIHW.

Australian Institute of Health and Welfare. (2014). *Australia's health 2014.* Canberra: AIHW.

Australian Institute of Health and Welfare & National Centre for Epidemiology and Population Health (NCEPH). (1998). *Expenditures on health services for Aboriginal and Torres Strait Islander people 1995–96.* Canberra: AIHW & NCEPH, Australian National University.

Australian Medical Association (AMA). (2006). *Australian Medical Association Report Card series 2006: Aboriginal and Torres Strait Islander Health.* Canberra: AMA.

Australian National Audit Office (ANAO). (2002). *Aboriginal and Torres Strait Islander health program follow-up audit report.* Canberra: ANAO.

Broome, R. (1982). *Aboriginal Australians.* Sydney: George Allen and Unwin.

Council for Aboriginal Reconciliation. (1994). *Sharing history: A sense for all Australians of shared ownership of their history.* Canberra: Australian Government Publishing Service.

Council for Aboriginal Reconciliation. (2001). *The final report of the Council for Aboriginal Reconciliation*, Appendix 5, Some reflections of Council members. Canberra: Council of Aboriginal Reconciliation.

Couzos, S., & Murray, R. (2003). *Aboriginal primary health care: An evidence based approach* (2nd ed.). Melbourne: Oxford University Press.

Department of Health and Aged Care (DHAC). (1996). *National Aboriginal and Torres Strait Islander hearing strategy.* <http://www.austlii.edu.au/au/other/IndigLRes/car/2000/16/appendices05.htm> Accessed 21.06.15.

Dudgeon, P., Oxenham, D., & Grogan, G. (1996). Learning identities and differences. In C. Luke (Ed.), *Feminisms and pedagogies of everyday life* (pp. 32–33). New York: State University of New York Press.

Eckermann, A. K., Dowd, T., Chong, E., Nixon, L., Gray, R., & Johnson, S. (2012). *Binan Goonj: Bridging cultures in Aboriginal health.* Chatswood NSW: Elsevier International.

Freemantle, J., Officer, K., McAullay, D., & Anderson, I. (2007). *Australian Indigenous health – within an international context.* Darwin: Cooperative Research Centre for Aboriginal Health.

Hollinsworth, D. (1998). *Race and racism in Australia* (3rd ed.). Katoomba NSW: Social Science Press.

Hollinsworth, D. (2010). Racism and Indigenous people in Australia. *Global Dialogue (Online)*, *12*(2), 1.

House of Representatives. (2000). *Health is life report: Report on the Inquiry into Indigenous health.* Canberra: Standing Committee on Families and Community Affairs, Commonwealth of Australia.

Human Rights and Equal Opportunity Commission (HREOC). (1997a). *Bringing them home report: Report of the national inquiry into the separation of Aboriginal and Torres Strait Islander children from their families.* Canberra: HREOC.

Human Rights and Equal Opportunity Commission. (1997b). *Bringing them home: A guide to the findings and recommendations of the national inquiry into the separation of Aboriginal and Torres Strait Islander children from their families.* Canberra: HREOC.

Human Rights and Equal Opportunity Commission. (2001). *Social justice report 2001.* Canberra: HREOC.

Human Rights and Equal Opportunity Commission. (2004). *Social justice report 2004: Chronology of events relating to the introduction of new arrangements for the administration of Indigenous affairs (2002–2004).* Canberra: HREOC.

Human Rights and Equal Opportunity Commission. (2005). *Social justice report 2005.* Sydney: HREOC.

Human Rights and Equal Opportunity Commission. (2006). *A statistical overview of Aboriginal and Torres Strait Islander peoples in Australia.* Sydney: HREOC. <http://www.humanrights.gov.au/publications/statistical-overview-aboriginal-and-torres-strait-islander-peoples-australia-social#fn158> Accessed 12.06.15.

Human Rights and Equal Opportunity Commission. (2015). *Human rights explained.* Sydney: HREOC. <https://www.humanrights.gov.au/education/human-rights-explained-index> Accessed 18.05.15.

House of Representatives Standing Committee on Aboriginal and Torres Strait Islander Affairs (HRSCoATSIA). (1994). *Justice under scrutiny: Report of the inquiry into the implementation by governments of the recommendations of the Royal Commission into Aboriginal Deaths in Custody.* Canberra: HRSCoATSIA, Australian Government Printing Service.

Kidd, R. (1997). *The way we civilise.* St Lucia Qld: University of Queensland Press.

Kidd, R. (2002). *Queensland stolen wages* (Fact sheet). Brisbane: Australians for Native Title and Reconciliation Queensland. <www.antarqld.org.au/05_involved/facts.html> Accessed 04.08.15.

Langton, M. (2001). *The nations of Australia.* Paper presented at An Alfred Deakin Memorial Lecture, 20th May 2001, Melbourne.

Lateline. (2006). Program reveals sexual abuse, violence in NT Indigenous communities. Lateline, Australian Broadcasting Commission.

National Aboriginal and Torres Strait Islander Health Council (NATSIHC). (2003). *National Strategic Framework for Aboriginal and Torres Strait Islander Health: Framework for action by governments.* Canberra: NATSIHC.

National Aboriginal Community Controlled Health Organisation (NACCHO). (2008). COAG a significant step forward. *Take Note NACCHOs News.* Canberra: NACCHO. <http://www.naccho.org.au/download/newsletters/TakeNote%20Newsletter_December_08%2019-12%20FINAL%20.pdf> Accessed 04.05.15.

National Aboriginal Health Strategy (NAHS) Evaluation Committee. (1994). *The National Aboriginal Health Strategy: An evaluation* (pp. 1–78). Canberra: Aboriginal and Torres Strait Islander Commission.

National Aboriginal Health Strategy (NAHS) Working Party. (1989). *National Aboriginal health strategy.* Canberra: Commonwealth of Australia, Australian Government Printing Service.

National Audit Office. (1999). *National Aboriginal Health Strategy: Delivery of housing and infrastructure to Aboriginal and Torres Strait Islander communities: Aboriginal and Torres Strait Islander Commission.* Canberra: Australian National Audit Office.

National Health and Medical Research Council (NHMRC). (1991). *Guidelines on ethical matters in Aboriginal and Torres Strait Islander health research.* Canberra: NHMRC. <http://www.nhmrc.gov.au/guidelines-publications/e11> Accessed 12.06.15.

National Health and Medical Research Council. (2002). *The NHMRC road map: A strategic framework for improving Aboriginal and Torres Strait Islander health through research and final report of community consultations on the NHMRC road map.* Canberra: NHMRC.

National Rural Health Alliance (NRHA). (2006). *Budget commitment to remote Indigenous stores.* Media release, NRHA, 14.5.06.

Nott, J. (2015). Convergence to help Aboriginal communities fight against communities' closure. *green left weekly.* <https://www.greenleft.org.au/node/58843> Accessed 04.08.15.

O'Donoghue, L. (2001). *Opening address.* Paper presented at the 5th Commonwealth Congress on Diahorrea and Malnutrition, 26th April 2001, Darwin, NT.

Office of Aboriginal and Torres Strait Islander Health (OATSIH). (2001). *Evaluation of the emotional and social wellbeing mental health action plan.* Canberra: Urbis, Keys and Young, for the Office of Aboriginal and Torres Strait Islander Health.

Ober, C., Peeters, L., Archer, R., & Kelly, K. (2000). Debriefing in different cultural frameworks: responding to acute trauma in Australian Aboriginal contexts. In J. Wilson

(Ed.), *Psychological debriefing: Theory, practice and evidence* (pp. 241–253). London: Cambridge University Press.

Office of Indigenous Policy Coordination (OIPC). (2006). *About OIPC*. Canberra: OIPC.

Royal Australian College of Ophthalmologists (RACO). (1980). *National trachoma and eye health program*. Sydney: RACO.

Reconciliation Australia. (2006). *Who is Reconciliation Australia?* Canberra: Reconciliation Australia. <https://www.reconciliation.org.au/> Accessed 04.08.15.

Reynolds, H. (1982). *The other side of the frontier*. Ringwood Vic: Penguin Books.

Reynolds, H. (1987). *Frontier: Reports for the edge of white settlement*. St Leonards NSW: Allen & Unwin Pty Ltd.

Reynolds, H. (1989). *Dispossession*. Sydney: Allen and Unwin.

Reynolds, H. (2001). *An indelible stain?: The question of genocide in Australia's history*. Melbourne Vic: Viking, Penguin Books.

Steering Committee for the Review of Government Service Provision (SCRGSP). (2005). *Overcoming indigenous disadvantage: Key indicators 2005*. Canberra: SCRGSP, Productivity Commission.

The Greens. (2010). *UN Report damns Australia's failure to end discrimination* [Press release]. Canberra: The Greens. <http://greensmps.org.au/content/media-releases/un-report-damns-australia%E2%80%99s-failure-end-discrimination> Accessed 04.08.15.

Thomson, N. (1991). A review of Aboriginal health status. In P. Trompf (Ed.), *The health of Aboriginal Australia* (pp. 37–79). Marrickville NSW: Harcourt Brace Jovanovich Group (Australia) Pty Ltd.

Wild, R., & Anderson, P. (2007). *Ampe Akelyernemane Meke Mekarle 'Little Children are Sacred'*. In our Law children are very sacred because they carry the two spring wells of water from our country within them. Report of the Northern Territory Board of Inquiry into the Protection of Aboriginal Children from Sexual Abuse. Darwin: Northern Territory Government.

Wilkinson, R., & Marmot, M. (Eds.), (2003). *Social determinants of health: the solid facts* (2nd ed.). Geneva: World Health Organization.. <http://www.euro.who.int/document/e81384.pdf> Accessed 09.05.15.

CHAPTER 5

PUTTING INDIGENOUS POLICY INTO PRACTICE – THE DOUBLE WHAMMY

Janie Dade Smith

My mother knows that I am home, at the water I am always home. Aunty and my brother, we are from the same people, we are of the Wiradjuri nation, *hard water*. We are of the river country, and we have flowed down the rivers to estuaries to oceans. To live by another stretch of water. Salt.

Even though this country is not my mother's country, even though we are freshwater, not saltwater people, this place still owns us, still owns our history, my brother's and my own, Aunty's too. Mum's. They are part of this place; I know now I need to find them.

When Billy and me lost our mother, we lost ourselves. We stopped swimming in the ocean, scared that we'd forget to breathe. Forget to come up for mouthfuls of air. We lost trust because we didn't want to touch something that was going to fall away. Like bubbles, too delicate, too fragile, too brief.

(TARA JUNE WINCH [WINNER OF THE DAVID UNAIPON AWARD FOR INDIGENOUS WRITERS], SWALLOW THE AIR, 2006, pp. 194–195)

Have you ever wondered why some people from meagre beginnings succeed in life and why other people from the same circumstances do not? What are the critical factors that make a difference between one person being able to realise their full potential as a human being and another, from the same beginnings, who never gets there? Life can be a series of activities of daily living punctuated by a series of critical moments that can define or change a life path.

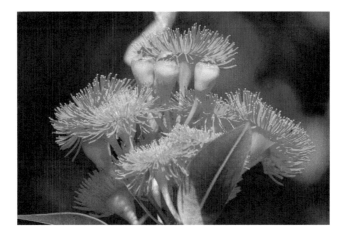

Source: Janie Dade Smith.

In 1954 a psychologist called Abraham Maslow studied positive human qualities and the lives of exemplary people. From this work he developed what is known as Maslow's Hierarchy of Needs, which is a way of measuring where people are at in their lives in terms of being able to be fully functioning and to realise their full potential as human beings – he calls this self-actualisation. However, one cannot achieve self-actualisation unless their basic needs are met first. This is important for health professionals to appreciate as it enables them to understand where a person or patient is at in their life and how to relate to them on their level.

This means if a person is unemployed it affects all aspects of their life. It affects their ability to eat good food, live in safe quality housing, buy good clothing and contribute to society. This affects their relationships and their self-respect and self-esteem and their health. Hence, they will never get past the first two basic levels of Maslow's Hierarchy of Needs – the basic needs of human survival. This means it will be difficult for them get out of the cycle of poverty into which they were probably born. Many Aboriginal and Torres Strait Islander peoples, especially those in remote areas, never get beyond the basic needs of the bottom two categories of Maslow's Hierarchy of Needs (Figure 5.1).

FIGURE 5.1 Maslow's Hierarchy of Needs.

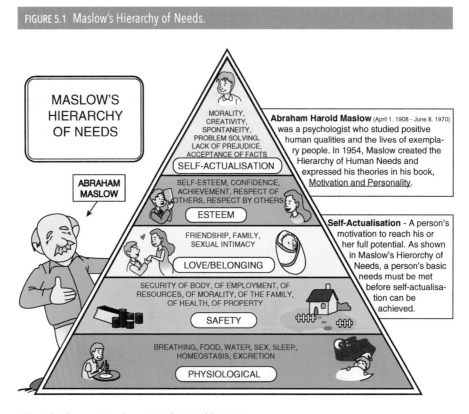

Adapted with permission from: © Tim's Printables 2015.

It would be easy in this chapter to do those things that other non-Indigenous people have done before me – to talk about the appalling health status, the oppressive history and the incredible statistics that affect Aboriginal and Torres Strait Islander Australians. But, while it would be remiss not to include these issues here, it is important, above all, to remind ourselves of what Indigenous Australians live with each day of their lives. This is their history today. In this chapter, therefore, I will attempt to put these issues into context using two real stories: both are about theft. The first is about theft of wages and the second is about theft of children. Both question the genocidal nature of these policies. This will enable you to understand the enormous burden that Indigenous Australians carry with them every day, and the significant challenges they face to break the cycle of poverty into which many were born.

In Chapter 4 we discussed some of the history of Aboriginal and Torres Strait Islander Australians. This chapter draws from this work and examines the effect that this history has had on Indigenous Australians' health today.

PUTTING POLICY INTO PRACTICE

There have been hundreds of policies and initiatives that have been put in place over the years to manage the lives of Aboriginal and Torres Strait Islander Australians. In 2015 there were two main campaigns running. The first is the Close the Gap Campaign, which commenced in 2007 and consists of a coalition of Aboriginal and Torres Strait Islander health bodies, leaders and mainstream health and human rights organisations campaigning together for health equality (Australians for Native Title and Reconciliation, 2015). They aim to close the gap in life expectancy of Aboriginal and Torres Strait Islander Australians by working in partnership; providing adequate infrastructure; securing adequate funding for education, nutrition and maternal and child health; and prevention and management of disease (Oxfam Australia, 2015). These are some pretty basic needs that fit into the bottom two levels of Maslow's hierarchy.

National Close the Gap Day. Video access through Student Consult.

The second campaign is for constitutional recognition, which aims to see recognition for the First Peoples of this land. Constitutional recognition is also seen as having a positive effect on Aboriginal and Torres Strait Islander peoples' social and emotional wellbeing by addressing disadvantage and protecting heritage and culture (Australians for Native Title and Reconciliation, 2015).

The following sections describe the strong links between policy and health outcomes and the current actions that are being undertaken to improve health outcomes. It is about the difference between giving people a 'hand-up' as opposed to a 'hand-out'.

PAUSE AND THINK

Why in 2016 are we still dealing with the provision of basic infrastructure, basic levels of education and nutrition and recognition of our First Nations peoples in our Constitution?

Wages policy

Storytelling is how we communicate as a group. Therefore, a small historical story will be used in this section to demonstrate the effect that policies, discussed in Chapter 4, had on Indigenous lives and the impact they are still having (Australian Government, 2015). There are many other, bigger stories that could be told – the theft of land, the theft of children and the theft of human rights. The story below – 'The sorriest of states' – is about the theft of wages, health and dignity that occurred in all Australian states. It has been chosen because it is a story that has only recently been told to the world by the historian Ros Kidd (Kidd, 1997, 2007), who so meticulously put the details together, and because many Indigenous Australians are still fighting this battle today. It is important that these stories are told and retold to give all Australians, and particularly health professionals, some insight into how rural, remote and Indigenous Australia was really put together, not on a sheep's back but on the backs of thousands of underpaid Indigenous Australians, and the effects that are still being lived today.

Story 1: The sorriest of states – stolen wages

As with much of the history of Australia, Queensland holds a special place as the state where the most elaborate practices of racism were executed (Kidd, 1997). This is therefore a Queensland story, which is largely told by two academics, historian Ros Kidd (Kidd, 1997) and Indigenous anthropologist Marcia Langton (Langton, 2002). It is told through their factual accounts of what Langton names the 'administration of racism' in which, she argues, lie the roots of present-day Aboriginal poverty, which is socially constructed.

Story 1: The sorriest of states – stolen wages—*cont'd*

For most of the 20th century there were two categories of Aboriginal Queenslanders, according to the now outdated theory of Social Darwinism:

1   those who theoretically shared the civil freedoms of other Australians
2   those who were 'under the Act'.

The *Protection Act* of Queensland was initially passed in 1897 and updated in 1939 and 1965. It specifically targeted Aboriginal people and introduced the most intensive regime of surveillance and intervention ever imposed by government. At the stroke of a pen, individuals and families could he forcibly extradited from their homes and confined to Aboriginal reserves. This was the fate of tens of thousands of Aboriginal people (Kidd, cited in Langton, 2002, p. 6).

The Labor Party governed Queensland for most of the first half of the 20th century (1915–29 and 1932–57). It was succeeded by the ultraconservative Country–Liberal Party (later the National Party), which was headed between 1968 and 1987 by Premier Joh Bjelke-Petersen.

Within the government was the Queensland Department of Aboriginal Affairs (DAA) which, between 1914 and 1986, appointed only three chief administrators (Kidd, 1997). The chief administrators exercised almost total control over the lives of thousands of Aboriginal Queenslanders, who had been brought from various clan groups onto government-run missions and reserves. 'They regulated freedom of movement, place of residence, employment, private savings and spending, marriage, adoptions and family cohesion' (Kidd, 1997). Their activities were based on their white ethnocentric views and a purposeful, knowing attempt to dispossess, domesticate, exterminate and dominate (Eckermann et al., 2012), which was supported by the state policy of the time. This resulted in a cycle of absolute poverty,* particularly for those in the more remote locations of Australia. Although this is not the only reason why most Indigenous Australians live in poverty, it formed a pattern for living based on inequity, oppression and discrimination, which resulted in a culture of poverty that still exists today.

Administering racism: 1913–2016
Let us look at a small part of what Langton terms 'the government theft of Aboriginal wages' over a 100-year period.

Early 1900s 'From 1904 the Queensland Government controlled all employment, wages and savings of Aboriginal Queenslanders, under compulsory labour contracts … workers' wages went direct to the police protector, apart from "pocket money"' (Kidd, 2002). 'Aboriginal workers could not use their own savings without departmental permission, which was frequently refused' (Langton, 2002).

Continued

Story 1: The sorriest of states – stolen wages—*cont'd*

1910 From 1910 the government took levies from the wages of people living on reserves and, from 1919, from those not living on reserves (Kidd, 2002). That year the government 'set pastoral wages at 66 per cent of the white wage' and every Aboriginal on a reserve was required to work a minimum of 32 hours per week for rations and shelter (Kidd, 1997; Kidd, 2002, p. 2).

Those 'under the Act' who did not work on reserves were contracted out to employment where, when and at whatever discounted rate of pay officials dictated. Their earnings went directly into government hands where they were subjected to a range of levies and taxes, in addition to the standard income tax paid by all Australian workers (Kidd, cited in Langton, 2002, p. 7).

1930s Malpractice with Aboriginal earnings was so entrenched that the minister centralised the savings accounts in Brisbane in 1933 in order to minimise fraud by police protectors (Kidd, cited in Langton, 2002). The government prevented these Queenslanders from seeing their bank passbooks. This remained policy until the 1970s, when many found, to their horror, that their balances showed little return after decades of compulsory work (Kidd, 1997; Langton, 2002). In 1934 the Act was revised to include all those with Aboriginal ancestry, who were then processed under the medico/hygiene policy (Kidd, 1997). In order to intensify surveillance, wage earners were allotted identification numbers, or 'dog tags' as they were known (Council for Aboriginal Reconciliation, 1994). In 1938 the missions reported that poverty was so entrenched that the grossly under-funded government grants for community development were being spent on rations (Kidd, 1997).

1940s During 1942 the department introduced a system of 'social history' cards that operated until 1972. The cards enabled more efficient surveillance of every Aboriginal person in the state (Kidd, 1997; Langton, 2002). 'In 1943 the government set up the Aboriginal Welfare Fund to receive wages, levies and profits from reserve enterprises to be used to develop enterprises on reserves' (Kidd, 2002, p. 2).

Lest we forget During the Second World War the department applied to the Army for the control of the service pay of more than 200 Aboriginal and Torres Strait Islander Queenslanders. They received only one-third of the white pay, which rose to two-thirds in 1944 (Kidd, cited in Langton, 2002). Aboriginal soldiers had to request permission to access their own savings – a request that was frequently withheld 'for their own good'. After the war, if servicemen returned to their home communities (under the Act), they were reduced to the indignity of a total loss of rights, primitive living conditions and chronic unemployment. For those hundreds of Aboriginal men working around Queensland during the war, the Australian Workers' Union successfully argued that they must be accorded full employment equality. However, the department retained control of all bank accounts and imposed multiple levies on their full wages (Kidd, 1997; Langton, 2002). After the war a comprehensive system of social security existed in Australia, except for Aboriginal people (North Australian Development Unit, cited in Langton, 2002).

1960s In 1968, the year following the referendum, the Queensland Government began the wage economy on reserves. 'Workers were paid 50 per cent of the state minimum wage' (Kidd 2002, p. 2), and were quarantined from industrial law by the writing of a regulation (Langton, 2002). When equal wages in the pastoral

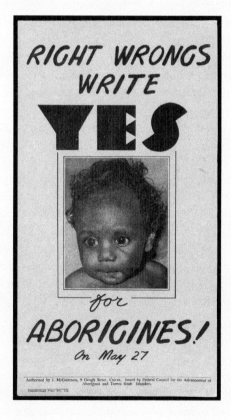

Reproduced with permission from: the National Library of Australia /Papers of Gordon Bryant 1917–1991. <http://museum.wa.gov.au/exhibitions/online/referendum/images/Right-wrongs -final.jpg>.

Continued

Story 1: The sorriest of states – stolen wages—cont'd

industry became law, forced contracting of Aboriginal employees ceased and many Aboriginal workers lost their jobs (Kidd, 1997; Langton, 2002). In 1966 the federal government signed the International Convention on Civil and Political Rights. This meant that all racially discriminatory legislation in Australia had to be eliminated. Queensland aggressively rejected federal pressure to lift restrictions, especially controls on the Aboriginal savings that were invested in high-interest Commonwealth bonds and hospital building programs (Kidd, cited in Langton, 2002). 'None of these benefits were returned to the account holders, most of whom were trapped in poverty' (Langton, 2002, p. 7).

1970s 'From 1971, forced confinement of Aborigines on reserves ceased' (Kidd, 2002, p. 2). From 1972, forced control over wages and savings account bank books ceased, although people had to request to be freed from financial management (Kidd, 2002). The state government remained intransigent with respect to Aboriginal citizenship rights, other than the right to vote. When Aboriginal people became eligible for equal wages, employers rejected Aboriginal labour and the state apparatus that had indentured Aboriginal people as rural labourers began to reduce the numbers of people on 'training wages', which were later called 'sit down money' (Kidd, cited in Langton, 2002). This caused a sharp increase in poverty and distress throughout rural Aboriginal populations (Langton, 2002). These events, in turn, forced Aboriginal people to attempt to obtain access to social security payments, such as the unemployment benefit. The federal government responded to the massive demand from Aboriginal people in the mid-1970s by devising a work-for-the-dole scheme for rural and remote Aboriginal communities – known as the Community Development Employment Program (CDEP) (Langton, 2002). 'From 1979 the Queensland Government knew that underpaying reserve workers was illegal' (Kidd, 2002, p. 2). When invalid, aged and widow pensions were introduced, authorities pocketed 66 per cent of the pensions of mission and settlement residents. The residue was distributed at the discretion of superintendents (Kidd, 1997; Langton, 2002).

1980s At the beginning of the 1980s the Aboriginal wage was 72 per cent of the state minimum (Kidd, 2002). In 1986 the government paid reserve workers only 75 per cent of the award (Kidd, 2002). In 1985, seven Palm Island workers started an action against the state government in the Human Rights and Equal Opportunity Commission for non-payment of legal wages (Kidd, 1997). In 1987 the government handed control of communities to Aboriginal Councils, whose budgets were insufficient to cover award rates. These communities are known as Deed of Grant in Trust Communities (DOGIT) (Kidd, 2002; Langton, 2002).

1990s In 1993 the Aboriginal Welfare Fund, which was commenced in 1942, totalled $8.6 million in unspent funds (Queensland Department of Aboriginal and

Torres Strait Islander Partnerships, 2003). In 1996 the Queensland government lost the Human Rights Commission case on under-award wages; it still refused to pay the suggested compensation of $7000 to each of the six Palm Island workers, who had proved 'deliberate, knowing and intentional' discrimination by the government (Kidd, 1997, p. 348; Kidd, 2002). The workers commenced Federal Court action. The government capitulated in 1997 (Kidd, 2002).

2000s In 2000 the Queensland (Beattie) Government 'made $25 million available to pay all workers, after losing several more cases on under-award wages, but it refused to include mission workers in the proposed payout' (Kidd, 2002; Langton, 2002, p. 2). 'The Queensland Aboriginal and Islander Legal Service Secretariat (QAILSS) collected testimony from over 2000 people who wanted to take action against the government for missing, unpaid and underpaid wages, misused trust funds, unpaid child endowment, workers' compensation and deceased estates' (Kidd, 2002, p. 2). 'In 2002, the Queensland Government offered $55.6 million to pay $4000 per person to some people, and $2000 per person to others, as a settlement for all claims on any of these matters' (Kidd, 2002, p. 2). Recipients were required to sign an agreement that they would not take legal action against the Queensland Government relating to controls over their wages and savings (Queensland Department of Aboriginal and Torres Strait Islander Partnerships, 2003).

2004 In 2004 a New South Wales cabinet report was leaked to the *National Indigenous Times*, which estimated that $69 million was still owing to 11 500 Aboriginal people whose wages, pensions, inheritances, lump sum entitlements and child endowment payments were placed in government trust accounts between 1900 and 1969 (Australian Catholic Social Justice Council, 2006). Victoria also started investigating these issues during the same year.

2006 Claims closed for Queensland's Indigenous wages and savings reparation. Less than half of the number of claims expected by government were lodged, with $35.87 million of the $55.6 million unclaimed. The Unfinished Business Report on stolen wages found that such practices were still in place in the 1980s (Creative Spirits, 2015).

2007 The West Australian Government announces an investigation into the extent of the stolen wages. The Victorian Government appoints an officer to sift through almost 100 years of records (Creative Spirits, 2015).

2008 Queensland establishes the Queensland Aboriginal and Torres Strait Islander Foundation with $10.8 million from the Aborigines Welfare Fund and $15 million of unspent funds from the Indigenous Wages and Savings Reparations Scheme to supply 100 scholarships worth $20 000 to young Aboriginal people (Nelson-Carr, 2008).

Continued

Story 1: The sorriest of states – stolen wages—cont'd

2012 The West Australian Government announces a repatriation scheme for people born before 1958 to apply for payments up to $2000 if they had experienced government control over their income (Creative Spirits, 2015).

2015 Australians for Native Title and Reconciliation (ANTaR) estimates that more than $1 billion in today's value was lost or stolen (Australians for Native Title and Reconciliation, 2015; Creative Spirits, 2015).

Today 'Aboriginal people have paid, with their own wages, for the oppression and incarceration they have suffered, both on and off the Aboriginal reserves and in their workplaces, in conditions not much better than slavery. They have only poverty to show for years of indentured labour under government management, which continued until only ten years ago. Aboriginal men and women working on missions and settlements never received legal rates of pay' (Langton, 2002, p. 7), and were not included in the payouts.

Added to this, Kidd found that the legal record clearly shows that the 'Queensland Government was constantly warned of systemic failures and of active and passive breaches of its duty as a legal trustee, but failed constantly to implement the necessary checks to prevent massive financial loss to its wards (of the state) over many decades. Aboriginal poverty is largely a construct of this system' (Kidd 2002, p. 1).

One Aboriginal stolen wages claimant, Marjorie Woodrow, said: *'We could have had our own homes from the wages we are owed, and had the ability to set things up for our children. It breaks your heart to see our children still struggling'* (Kidd, 2007, p. 6).

*A level of poverty in which only the minimal levels of food, clothing and shelter can be met.

The above story describes the policies in one Australian state, and includes only one aspect of the stories that could be told of Indigenous life at the time, and upon which many remote Indigenous communities were founded.

PAUSE AND THINK

There are a number of key points in this section that have contributed to the formation of stereotypes about Aboriginal people today. Discuss these stereotypes that you noted throughout.

What impact is being felt today by the next generation as a result of the reduction in Aboriginal labour and the CDEP program only paying training wages for a generation?

Why were governments so slow to act on repatriation of stolen wages, e.g. Western Australia in 2012?

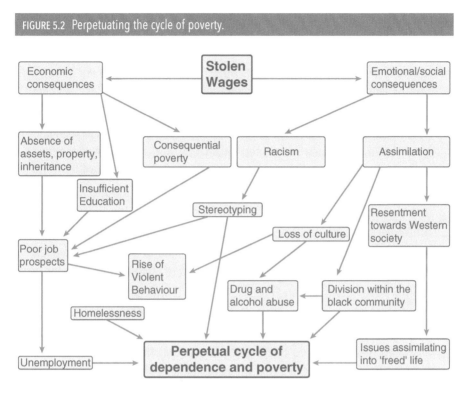

FIGURE 5.2 Perpetuating the cycle of poverty.

Adapted from: Smith, K. (2006). Queensland reparations offer for wages and savings: Community effects, reactions and responses.

Figure 5.2 clearly maps the effects on Aboriginal people of the stolen wages case, which is based on outdated policies, discrimination and institutional racism. Many Aboriginal people are still experiencing the impact and consequences of this government action (Australian Government, 2015). It also demonstrates how people cannot shift between the two basic levels of Maslow's Hierarchy of the basic needs of shelter, food, water and safety while they are still living in poverty. These issues have forced a passiveness in many remote Aboriginal peoples and a system of passive welfare dependency whereby many live in a house where no one has had to get up in the morning to go to work for two generations, and the cycle continues. It has become a permanent destination for many remotely located Aboriginal Australians who experience the resulting health outcomes. The consequences of this are felt in every sphere of life and nowhere more graphically than in the area of health.

The outcome

Indigenous lawyer and activist Noel Pearson has been lobbying for a change in the way the Australian Government handles welfare provided to unemployed, remotely located Indigenous peoples because of the level of passive welfare dependency that has resulted. He states:

> The irony of our newly won citizenship in 1967 was that, after we became citizens with equal rights and the theoretical right to equal pay, we lost the meagre foothold that we had in the real economy and we became almost comprehensively dependent upon passive welfare for our livelihood. So in one sense we gained citizenship and in another sense we lost it at the same time. Because we find thirty years later that life in the safety net for three decades and two generations has produced a social disaster. … And we should not be surprised that this catastrophe was the consequence of our enrolment at the dependent bottom end of the Australian welfare state. You put any group of people in a condition of overwhelming reliance upon passive welfare support – that is support without reciprocation – and within three decades you will get the same social results that my people in Cape York Peninsula currently endure. … So when I say that the Indigenous experience of the Australian welfare state has been disastrous I do not thereby mean that the Australian welfare state is a bad thing. It is just that my people have experienced a marginal aspect of that welfare state: income provisioning for people dispossessed from the real economy.
>
> (PEARSON, 2003)

This 'Sorriest of states' story about the administration of racism raises some key issues. First, it gives some insight into the ethnocentric views of absolute superiority that existed at the time. Second, it shows how government policy and our public institutions were built on disproven pseudoscientific theories and ethnocentric beliefs. Third, it demonstrates how the cycle of poverty began, which has resulted in passive welfare dependency and a culture that is based on a loss of identity and a sense of hopelessness and powerlessness to do anything about it – never getting past our basic human needs on Maslow's Hierarchy of Needs. Fourth, it shows how one dominant cultural group, through a lack of respect and tolerance, can judge and oppress another cultural group and try to make it fit into their own national pattern of thinking, on the basis of what they thought they knew about that group. The Queensland government, through this process of judgement, assumption, disrespect and intolerance, backed by pseudoscience, saw Aboriginal people as lesser human beings. This fostered the development of a cultural belief and value system, based on racism and stereotyping, which contributed to the greatest cultural conflict in Australian history. The health outcomes of this process are discussed in detail in Chapters 6 and 7.

WAS IT GENOCIDE?

There has been considerable debate in Australia as to whether the policies and legislation used to regulate the lives of Indigenous Australians were a form of attempted genocide. Genocide is a difficult and confronting subject – especially in Australia, the land of the 'fair go' – because it raises thoughts of the Holocaust and mass murder. Let us examine what it actually means, and look at one well-known Australian example: the assimilation policy and the Stolen Generations.

In 1944 Raphael Lemkin, the creator of the term 'genocide', defined it as 'a coordinated plan of different actions, aimed at the destruction of the essential foundations of the life of national groups, with the aim of annihilating the groups themselves' (cited in Human Rights and Equal Opportunity Commission, 1997b, p. 271). Genocide is directed against a national group as a whole although, while some of the actions may be directed against individuals, it is not in their individual capacity that they are attacked, but because they are members of a national group (Reynolds, 2001).

The actions of genocide include:

> a coordinated plan to disintegrate the political and social institutions of culture, of language, national feelings, religion, and of the existence of national groups and the destruction of personal liberty, health, dignity and the lives of the individuals.
>
> (LEMKIN, CITED IN HUMAN RIGHTS AND EQUAL OPPORTUNITY COMMISSION 1997b, p. 271)

Reynolds (2001) tells us that genocide has two phases. The first is the destruction of the national pattern of the oppressed group, for example by destroying their culture and traditions. The second is the imposition of the national pattern of the oppressing group, for example by imposing their own language and value systems.

Assimilation policy

Now let us look at the assimilation policy of the 1950s and 1960s. The assimilation policy was based on the assumption that Aboriginal Australians as a national group would attain the same lifestyle, customs, language and traditions as other Australians and that, since they refused to die out, they should lose their distinctive culture and language and develop value systems and beliefs that were 'more white'. The policy aimed to destroy 'the essential foundations' of Indigenous life (Human Rights and Equal Opportunity Commission, 1997b) and impose the dominant group's white national pattern of cultural norms. This policy persisted until the early 1970s – or the 1980s in some states – and continues to influence public attitudes and some official practices today (Human Rights and Equal Opportunity Commission, 1997b).

Story 2: The Stolen Generations

Let us examine the inquiry undertaken in 1997 by the Human Rights and Equal Opportunity Commission into the forcible removal of tens of thousands of Indigenous children – 'The Stolen Generations' – and compare it with the actions of genocide described by Lemkin above. The Human Rights Commission described the assimilation policy as genocidal in nature (Human Rights and Equal Opportunity Commission, 1997b).

The forcible removal of children was a 'nationally coordinated plan' that was endorsed by the government of the day. All 'rites and customs' that were seen as injurious to the welfare of Aboriginal children living on the reserves were prohibited; this included use of their own 'language' (Eckermann et al., 2012). The aim was to disintegrate Aboriginal culture and any 'political and social institutions' that existed in Indigenous society such as marriage customs, laws and social hierarchies. It destroyed the 'personal liberty' of Indigenous people through restrictive and paternalistic legislation that effectively denied them their citizenship rights and imposed 'foreign religious practices'. As a result, Indigenous Australians suffered sickness and Third World 'health problems' and lost their dignity; many 'lost their lives' through violence.

The United Nations Charter of 1945, the Universal Declaration of Human Rights of 1948 and the International Convention on the Elimination of all Forms of Racial Discrimination of 1965 all imposed obligations on Australia relating to the elimination of racial discrimination in all of its policies. Genocide was declared to be a crime against humanity by the United Nations Resolution of 1946. The Australian practice of Indigenous child removal involved both systemic racial discrimination and genocide as defined by international law. Yet it continued to be practised as official policy long after being clearly prohibited by treaties to which Australia had voluntarily subscribed (Human Rights and Equal Opportunity Commission, 1997b, p. 266).

Therefore, despite interventions from the United Nations, it took until the 1970s for the practice of child theft to stop. This and the many other policies of the day have had a long-term impact upon the ability of Indigenous Australians to trust the government, and police in particular, not to mention the long-term effects on their parenting, social skills and self-esteem.

PAUSE AND THINK

The issue of trust is an important one for all health professionals as it forms the basis of a therapeutic relationship. You can see from the above story and discussion why older Aboriginal people have trouble trusting people in positions of authority and how many have passed this on to younger generations.

Figure 5.3 provides an overview of the Stolen Generations and the impact this has had on these children. It does not, however, consider the mothers, fathers, sisters and brothers who also suffered as a result of these policies.

FIGURE 5.3 Australia's Stolen Generations.

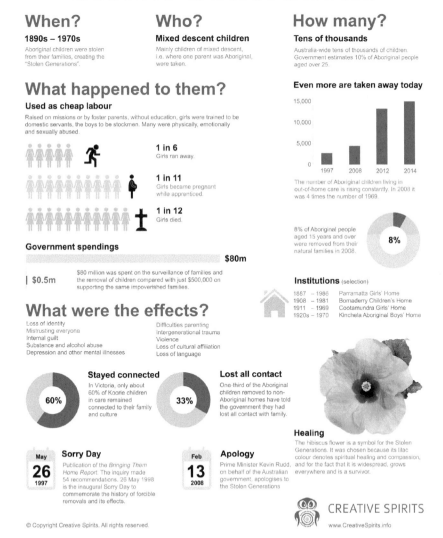

Adapted with permission from: Creative Spirits. <http://www.creativespirits.info/aboriginalculture/politics/a-guide-to-australias-stolen-generations>.

'SORRY' SEEMS TO HAVE BEEN THE HARDEST WORD

Much of the history of Indigenous Australia would make anyone weep. Common terminology in many reports and papers begins with words like 'appalling', 'bleak', 'worst', 'Fourth World', 'dominated' and 'oppressed' (Couzos & Murray, 2003; Henry, Houston, & Mooney, 2004; Human Rights and Equal Opportunity Commission, 1997a; Reynolds, 2001). This history, based on the principles of colonisation, dispossession and ongoing victimhood, continues to have an enormous impact upon the health of Indigenous Australians today, many of whom live in rural and remote Australia.

This is complicated by the fact that many Indigenous and non-indigenous Australians have had little opportunity to learn the history of Indigenous Australia during their years of schooling, when there was a focus on Burke and Wills, Captain Cook and other 'white' explorers. Many frequently say that 'all that' should be forgotten – that it is ancient history. However, it is not. Previous Australian Prime Ministers have used this as an excuse for 'not dwelling on the past', and have refused to apologise, despite the fact that the National Inquiry into the Separation of Aboriginal and Torres Strait Islander Children from their Families in 1997 recommended that an apology was imperative.

Although all state premiers did apologise in their state parliaments to the Stolen Generations between 1997 and 2001, it was not until 13th February 2008 that the then Prime Minister, the Honourable Kevin Rudd, made the historic 'Apology'. He apologised for past laws, policies and practices that devastated Australia's First Nations Peoples; and he said 'sorry' to the people, their forbearers and their families (National Sorry Day Committee, 2015). 'The Apology' was given from Parliament House, where thousands of Aboriginal and Torres Strait Islander people wept on the grounds, wrapped in each other's arms. It was broadcast across Australia, bringing the country to a standstill, with people in their homes, workplaces, schools and community gatherings stopping to watch the live broadcast. The Apology had enormous significance as it represented a public admission of the government's responsibility for the loss and separation from family, community, culture and land and the trauma experienced by the Stolen Generations (National Sorry Day Committee, 2015). This one spoken act was seen by Aboriginal and Torres Strait Islander peoples as an important stage in the journey of healing as it was an acknowledgement and mark of respect for their past.

The Apology Speech. Video access through Student Consult.

CONCLUSION – RECONCILIATION

Gandhi tells us that 'the road to the future lies over the bones of the past, on which we dare to tread and each must do what can be done' (Gandhi, cited in Brennan,

1992, p. 7). Therefore, this recognition of past injustices and the adverse effects it has had on the Indigenous population of Australia today is the basis of any meaningful reconciliation.

Indigenous leader Lowitja O'Donoghue (2010) argues that reconciliation also means Indigenous community control of services and systems; that is, bottom-up – not top-down – decision making. She states that individuals and organisations must be fully involved – not just consulted – in the initiation, design and implementation of programs; and that to do this in Australia requires a real head shift and real power shifts, not just a knee-jerk reaction to particular problems. This takes time, funding and a true commitment to act, advocate and work for significant change.

Reconciliation is about, at the very least, supporting a reconciling process jointly with Indigenous Australians, warts and all. It is about being open to working in a respectful and tolerant way that accepts and celebrates different cultural norms including different laws, institutional policies and traditions. This includes suspending judgement about those things that we do not understand, and constantly questioning our predisposition to seek security in those things that we feel we 'know' about other groups (Eckermann, 1991; Eckermann et al., 2012).

Accordingly, all activities should enhance Indigenous people's capacity to achieve what is important to them and contribute to their empowerment and the achievement of *their* objectives and priorities (O'Donoghue, 2010).

Discussion Points

1   Using Maslow's Hierarchy of Needs establish where you are at on the triangle. Discuss the factors that exist in your life that have assisted you to be in this position.

2   Why were Indigenous Australians moved onto missions and reserves?

3   Why do you think our governments have found it so difficult to apologise for the mistakes of the past? Discuss.

4   What has been the impact of the 'Apology' by the Honourable Kevin Rudd in 2008 on Aboriginal people? Discuss.

5   Discuss the stolen wages case. What do you think may have driven the thinking behind these policies at that time? Discuss.

6   What stereotypes of Indigenous Australians have resulted from the stolen wages case? Discuss.

7   Why do you think the Queensland Government did not include remote Indigenous Australians living on missions in the stolen wages payout?

8   Was the assimilation policy that resulted in the Stolen Generations a form of genocide? Use the criteria of genocide and establish whether it meets it.

As Australians we pride ourselves on giving 'a fair go'. We equate justice with a fair go for all, wherever they live and whatever their culture. With the best will in the world many Australians then equate justice with assimilation (Brennan, 1989) – a policy that was largely about being the same. We continue to want to treat everyone the same, but our world is more complex and justice is a complex phenomenon. The only way forward is to confront our past, appreciate difference, treat same cases equally and treat different cases differently (Brennan, 1989). But mostly we need to educate ourselves about the real history of Indigenous Australia, as told by Indigenous peoples, to understand the impact this has on current generations and their levels of trust and health. This is what will make our society richer in spirit, more diverse in nature and more just in the long run. It really is about a 'fair go' for all.

References

Australian Catholic Social Justice Council (ACSJC). (2006). *Stolen wages: An opportunity for justice?* Alexandria NSW: Australian Catholic Social Justice Council. <http://www.socialjustice.catholic.org.au/Content/pdf/2006_1_23stolen_wages_-_an_opportunity_for_justice.pdf> Accessed 25.05.15.

Australians for Native Title and Reconciliation. (2015). *Constitutional recognition and Close the Gap*. Brisbane: Australians for Native Title and Reconciliation. <http://antar.org.au/> Accessed 17.03.15.

Australian Government. (2015). *Closing the Gap Prime Minister's Report 2015*. Department of the Prime Minister and Cabinet. Canberra: Australian Government. <http://www.dpmc.gov.au/sites/default/files/publications/Closing_the_Gap_2015_Report_0.pdf> Accessed 15.07.15.

Brennan, F. Social justice, human and civil rights: How do they affect the delivery of health care in remote areas? 2nd Council of Remote Area Nurses of Australia National Conference, Canberra. Alice Springs: CRANA Inc. (1989).

Brennan, F. (1992). *Reconciling our differences*. Melbourne: Aurora Books.

Council for Aboriginal Reconciliation. (1994). *Sharing history: A sense for all Australians of shared ownership of their history*. Canberra: Australian Government Publishing Service.

Couzos, S., & Murray, R. (2003). *Aboriginal primary health care: An evidence based approach* (2nd ed.). Melbourne: Oxford University Press.

Creative Spirits. *Stolen wages timeline*. (2015). <http://www.creativespirits.info/aboriginalculture/economy/stolen-wages-timeline> Accessed 17.03.15.

Eckermann, A. K. (1991). *Aboriginal health: unit outline*. Armidale NSW: Department of Aboriginal and Multicultural Studies, University of New England.

Eckermann, A. K., Dowd, T., Chong, E., Nixon, L., Gray, R., & Johnson, S. (2012). *Binan Goonj: Bridging cultures in Aboriginal health*. Sydney: Churchill Livingstone, Elsevier.

Henry, B., Houston, S., & Mooney, G. H. (2004). Institutional racism in Australian health care: a plea for decency. *Medical Journal of Australia*, 180, 517–520.

Human Rights and Equal Opportunity Commission (HREOC). (1997a). *Bringing them home report: Report of the national inquiry into the separation of Aboriginal and Torres Strait Islander children from their families*. Canberra: HREOC.

Human Rights and Equal Opportunity Commission. (1997b). *Bringing them home: A guide to the findings and recommendations of the national inquiry into the separation of Aboriginal and Torres Strait Islander children from their families*. Canberra: HREOC.

Kidd, R. (1997). *The way we civilise*. St Lucia Qld: University of Queensland Press.

Kidd, R. (2002). *Stolen wages facts*. Brisbane: Australians for Native Title and Reconciliation. <https://www.antar.org.au> Accessed 08.04.03.

Kidd, R. (2007). *Hard labour, stolen wages: National report on stolen wages*. Brisbane: Australians for Native Title and Reconciliation.

Langton, M. A new deal? Indigenous development and the politics of recovery. Speech given at the Dr Charles Perkins oration ceremony. Australian Broadcasting Commission. (2002). <abc.net.au>.

National Sorry Day Committee. *The Apology to Australia's Indigenous peoples*. National Sorry Day Committee. (2015). <https://www.youtube.com/watch?v=aKWfiFp24rA> Accessed 19.03.15.

Nelson-Carr, L. *Fund to help young Indigenous Queenslanders close the educational gap*. Media statement, 25 November 2008. (2008). <http://statements.qld.gov.au/Statement/Id/61578> Accessed 26.09.2015.

O'Donoghue, L. (2010). *Launching of The Lowitja Institute* (edited speech). Adelaide: The Lowitja Institute. <http://www.lowitja.org.au/sites/default/files/docs/Lowitja_ODonoghue_brochure_2010.pdf> Accessed 17.07.15.

Oxfam Australia. (2015). *Why does the health gap exist?* Melbourne: Oxfam Australia. <https://www.oxfam.org.au/act/events/national-close-the-gap-day/> Accessed 18.03.15.

Pearson, N. (2003). *The enabling state*. Cairns: Cape York Institute. <http://sauer-thompson.com/archives/philosophy/cat_the_third_way.html> Accesed 18.03.15.

Queensland Department of Aboriginal and Torres Strait Islander Partnerships (QDATSIP). (2003). *Queensland Government reparations offer: wages and savings*. Brisbane: QDATSIP.

Reynolds, H. (2001). *An indelible stain?: The question of genocide in Australia's history*. Melbourne: Viking, Penguin Books.

Smith, K. *Queensland reparations offer for wages and savings: Community effects, reactions and responses*. (2006). <http://www.creativespirits.info/aboriginalculture/economy/stolen-wages> Accessed 17.03.15.

CHAPTER 6

WORKING WITH INDIGENOUS PEOPLE

Shannon Springer | Janie Dade Smith

I could run away again, I could run away from the pain my family hold. I could take the yarndi, the paint, the poppies, and all the grog in the world but I couldn't run from the pain and I couldn't run from my family either.

(TARA JUNE WINCH (WINNER OF THE DAVID UNAIPON AWARD FOR INDIGENOUS WRITERS), *SWALLOW THE AIR*, 2006, p. 195)

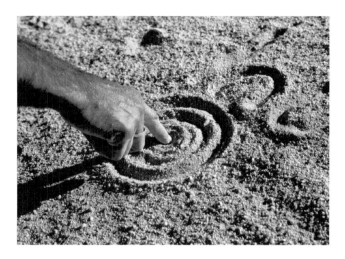

Reproduced with permission from: iStockphoto/Kerrie Kerr.

This chapter is different from the other chapters in this book. It is a first effort to look at health through a different lens, an Aboriginal lens. In it we define good health from an individual, Indigenous and health care provider perspective. We specifically look at the health of Indigenous people and their major chronic disease risk factors, without reciting the mantra of statistics and stereotypical views. We acknowledge the impact of colonisation and explore the health of people today. We then examine what it means for health professionals to work effectively with Aboriginal and Torres Strait Islander peoples and offer some consultation signposts and 12 practical principles for doing so.

The aim of this chapter is for you to develop awareness about the whole spectrum of enabling factors that contribute to good health and the positive contribution you can make as a health practitioner. Understanding the influences that our social circumstances have on feeling healthy, and living long disease-free lives, is essential to being an effective health practitioner.

WHAT IS GOOD HEALTH?

Looking at good health from a Western view point, we think about the absence of disease, having strong family connections, our work, managing daily stresses, eating well, exercising and playing with our kids. If we are among the dominant culture in a developed country then we probably will never be challenged to think much about it except, of course, if we get sick.

For some Indigenous Australians the concept of good health is different. Indigenous Australians – Aboriginal and Torres Strait Islander peoples – can struggle day-to-day with such concepts as losing their country, their spirituality, their language, not being employable, feeling like they have neither a strong culture nor identity. Many can be challenged about peace among their communities, premature disease, death and the health statistics we recite daily. Non-Indigenous Australians do not usually have to worry about a lack of good role models, racism or discrimination and the emotional impacts these may have on their children as they grow up. These aspects are taken for granted by the dominant culture and it is a privileged position to be in. We will explore a definition of health from an Indigenous perspective in the next section; however, there is no universal reality of health experienced by Indigenous Australians.

PAUSE AND THINK

It is difficult to talk about being healthy with your future Indigenous patients or clients without establishing an understanding of where health comes from.

- So what is health to you?
- What provides you with good health?
- What do your Indigenous patients see as good health for themselves, their families and community?
- If we are born into an unhealthy place, can we change that reality?

LOOKING BACK AND GOING FORWARD

Susan Graseck (2008) tells us that we need to explore the past if we want to understand the present and shape the future. Therefore, to not discuss the historical context that led to the current status of Indigenous health is a little like not talking about the elephant in the room, as many Aboriginal and Torres Strait Islander families continue to struggle in one way or another with the effects of this history today. It is also respectful and insightful to reflect on how we arrived at this point in time.

The effect of colonisation and the resulting negative views held by some non-Indigenous Australians has had a rippling impact across generations of Indigenous families and all aspects of their lives. Colonisation and the social policies that followed were a well-thought-out systematic process that dismembered a connected culture. This included the breaking up of families and the fracturing of their inherent 'knowledge lines' from one generation to the next. The dispossession of land and the removal of one's 'Country', separated Aboriginal peoples' spiritual connectives and their sense of belonging. This disconnection resulted in a deep sense of grief and loss and the foreign emotions of 'hopelessness and helplessness' in an otherwise connected community. This caused a loss of cultural values, language and social roles (Human Rights and Equal Opportunity Commission, 1997).

Let us unpack this concept of 'knowledge lines' and 'disconnection'. How we perceive and understand our reality from one moment to the next is influenced by layers of inherent social and cultural understandings. As we have seen in Chapter 3, every culture around the world passes on to the next generation their cultural beliefs, traditions and experiences. This passing on process gives rise to a wealth of inherent family and cultural knowledge. This information is more than just stories; it carries with it concepts that help us define and negotiate the changing social and environmental dimensions of life – our cultural template for living as a group. This inherent knowledge line also provides insight into the spiritual or scientific understandings that shape our belief systems, our values and our traditions. It determines what is 'normal' for us as a group of people and eventually forms the ether in which our own identity is born. This culmination of layered understandings gives us purpose: it orientates our moral compass, as well as our behaviours, values and subsequent emotional reactions to experiences.

To remove someone's sense of self, purpose and social connection in life generates a collapse of the protective mechanisms that hold families and their cultural values together. It was this collapse of culture and social order caused by colonisation that challenged the social and cultural ways of living and knowing. It resulted in successive generations of Indigenous children no longer being able to inherit an ordered and definable world that they were part of. No longer would they come to access thousands of years of ancestral knowledge. No longer would they have the skills passed down to them to know what it means to be self-sufficient. Instead, these tools of life rapidly decayed and gave way to a cycle of disempowerment and poverty and with it the formation of disease.

Despite the colonisation experience many Aboriginal and Torres Strait Islander people today remain very connected to their Country and maintain strong belief systems that are rooted in their land and culture. Hence, Aboriginal and Torres Strait Islander peoples remain one of the oldest living cultures in the world.

Aboriginal Community Controlled Health Organisations (ACCHOs) recognise these influences of the past and their potential impact on health today. As a result they have developed Social and Emotional Wellbeing Units to work with peoples to empower them to reconnect with their cultural practices and community and to develop skills in negotiating a way forward. Elders often play an active role in this process – sharing stories with generations about the land, their culture and their language. It may be helpful at this point to look at the 'Policy timeline' in Table 4.1 in Chapter 4, which outlines the many social policies that still affect people today.

One of the leading examples in identifying health issues that provided a pathway for change for Indigenous Australia was the development of the *National Aboriginal Health Strategy* in 1989. This document was developed by Aboriginal elders and leaders from across the country to negotiate what was needed to improve Indigenous health in Australia for the first time and provided a platform and impetus for change. A part of this process was defining 'health' from an Aboriginal perspective. In this report they defined health as a:

… holistic perspective, where it is not just the physical wellbeing of the individual but includes the social, emotional, cultural, and spiritual wellbeing of the whole community. This is a whole-of-life view and it also includes the cyclical concept of life–death–life.

(NATIONAL ABORIGINAL HEALTH STRATEGY
WORKING PARTY, 1989)

Although this report is now somewhat dated, the definition remains timeless as it emphasises how Indigenous Australians understand health as a holistic concept with the interconnected nature of health that has emerged from generations of lived experiences.

PAUSE AND THINK

Indigenous communities have suffered significantly from colonisation. How is an 'unwritten culture' affected by premature death and disease? Consider this quote:

I always say that when we lose an old person, we lose a library… language and culture. Lola Forester.

(FORESTER, UNKNOWN)

WHY SO MANY FUNERALS FOR OUR MOB?

All health professionals will at some time work with Indigenous Australians; therefore it is important that they feel prepared for this role. This not only includes understanding the history and the health statistics, but also how to work with others and organisations to 'close the life expectancy gap' between Indigenous and non-Indigenous people.

In 2013 there were an estimated 698 583 Aboriginal and Torres Strait Islander people living in Australia, who make up 3 per cent of the total population (Australian Bureau of Statistics, 2014). Most Indigenous people live in the suburbs, cities and large regional towns; 21 per cent live in remote or very remote areas compared with 1.7 per cent of the non-Indigenous population (Australian Institute of Health and Welfare, 2014a). Regardless of where Indigenous people reside, they continue to die at a younger age and suffer more illness and disability than their non-Indigenous counterparts, and these trends increase greatly with remoteness.

In this chapter we did not want to recite the mantra of appalling health statistics; this is done in Chapters 7 and 8. However, the sickening reality is, you can pick just about any disease or illness and expect that its incidence will be many times higher among Indigenous Australians. Therefore, in this chapter we will demonstrate this health gap by presenting three main graphical depictions. Figure 6.1 demonstrates clearly the 'health gap' in a snapshot of age-adjusted incidences on several measures of health against non-Indigenous rates: end-stage kidney disease, which occurs 7

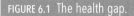

FIGURE 6.1 The health gap.

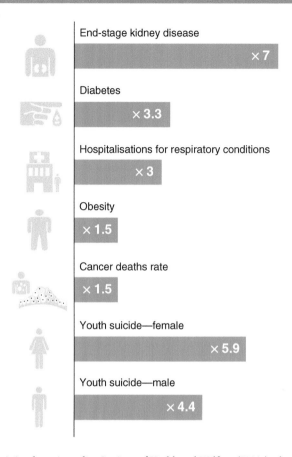

Adapted with permission from: Australian Institute of Health and Welfare. (2014a). <http://www.aihw.gov.au/australias-health/2014/not-faring-so-well/>.

times more frequently in Indigenous Australians; diabetes, 3.3 times; hospitalisations, 3 times; obesity, 1.5 times; cancer death rates, 1.5 times; and youth suicide rates, which are 5.9 times and 4.4 times for females and males, respectively (Australian Institute of Health and Welfare, 2014b). Figure 6.1 provides a powerful vision of how many times 'sicker' Indigenous Australians are in a range of measures when compared with the rest of the Australian community.

Now let us look at another important factor when considering Indigenous health – death rates. In Figure 6.2 it is not just the death rates to consider, but the ages when Indigenous people die compared with non-Indigenous Australians.

Figure 6.2 reports the age distribution of the proportion of deaths, by age and Indigenous status in five states – still in 2015 we do not have national Indigenous statistics (Australian Institute of Health and Welfare, 2014b).

FIGURE 6.2 Age distribution of the proportion of deaths, by age and Indigenous status in NSW, Qld, SA, WA and NT, 2007–2011.

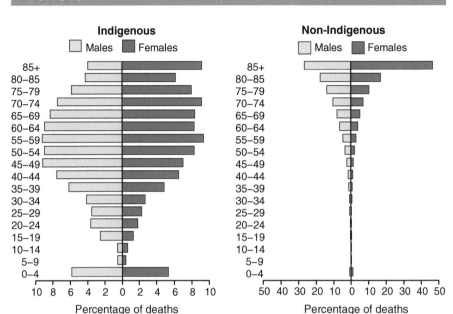

Note: Indigenous data for Vic, Tas and ACT were of insufficient quality for the reporting period.

Adapted with permission from: Australian Institute of Health and Welfare. (2014). *Australia's health 2014.* Australia's health series no. 14. Cat. no. AUS 178. Canberra: AIHW. <http://www.aihw.gov.au/WorkArea/ DownloadAsset.aspx?id=60129547777>.

You can see in Figure 6.2 that not only is there a much higher infant mortality rate – 5 times higher for Indigenous infants – but that this continues throughout life, where babies are also more likely to be underweight and children die at twice the rate of non-Indigenous children (Kildea et al., 2006). It also demonstrates clearly that Indigenous adults die at much higher rates at younger ages with the greatest difference being for the 35–44-year age group, which has a death rate that is 5 times the non-Indigenous rate (Australian Institute of Health and Welfare, 2014b; Kildea, Kruske, Barklay, & Tracy, 2010). This leaves a significant health gap and provides us with clear direction about where to place investment in order to make further health gains.

Figure 6.2 also provides a backdrop for the health profession regarding the physical and psychological health conditions that they can expect to see in the Indigenous setting, including the wide range of early onset chronic diseases often not seen in the same severity in everyday non-Indigenous practice. The amounts of chronic diseases that health care workers see in Indigenous health, along with the complex social circumstances that can accompany them, provide management challenges. This is why different models of health care are provided by Aboriginal Medical Services and why many health professionals are attracted to work in the field.

Figure 6.2 also provides a backdrop for Indigenous communities. Although we hear a lot about Indigenous health statistics, they represent real people with real families who have strong family and cultural connections with Indigenous families throughout Australia. This, coupled with the high mortality experienced in communities, can leave Indigenous people feeling like they are forever going to funerals. As one patient aged 54 years stated: *'Too many (funerals) hey....I'm sick of going to funerals for our mob! I'll only go to three a year; otherwise it gets me down too much...young ones too ... my age'.*

Dealing with 'sorry business' – family death – can be important to understand when working with Indigenous communities and families who have responsibilities to pay their respects to those who have passed. This is particularly so in regional, rural and remote settings where some Indigenous organisations may close the clinic out of respect.

PAUSE AND THINK

Consider the following quote from Aboriginal artist and teacher Yalmay Yunupingu (2014), winner of the National Indigenous Human Rights and Social Justice Award: *'We are still living in pain and trauma. We are in pain already and more and more pain is falling on top of us. It makes us feel weaker and weaker. People are getting sick, tired and stressed.'*

What is the Yalmay Yunupingu speaking about?

What impact does the continual burden of disease have on the Indigenous community?

What are the causes of the health gap?

The Australian Institute of Health and Welfare list the significant contributors to the health gap as being 'the complex interaction between the social determinants of health, such as unemployment and lack of education; and subsequent increases in behavioural risk factors, such as smoking and physical inactivity' (Australian Institute of Health and Welfare, 2014b; 2014c, p. 3).

Those working at the coal face with Indigenous people would also add that the health gap is caused by the accumulative stress of being poor, with few coping skills and resources in non-supportive environments, which compounds poverty. Other compounding factors that keep Indigenous people in poverty relate directly to the economic barriers that prevent people from tapping into the wider Australian society, such as owning your own home. Previous social policies have also influenced Indigenous people's educational attainment and employment opportunities, resulting in a cycle of welfare dependency for some.

For many, living in the grips of poverty can create a pressure cooker effect that can result in their feeling unable to escape the ongoing social burdens of life. This continual social influence can draw people into unhealthy behaviours such as abusing alcohol and drugs in their attempts to gain some temporary reprieve. Where communities experience widespread social disadvantage, unhealthy behaviours can easily become woven into community life, with regular drinking and gambling circles to pass the time. This is the result of not having the 'buffering cushions of life' that are typically found in privileged society, such as higher rates of employment, greater access to wealth and resources, inclusive social environments and greater access to education.

It is widely understood that people further down the social ladder run at least twice the risk of serious illness, incarceration and premature death, as those near the top (Wilkinson & Marmot, 2003). This is certainly so for Indigenous Australians, who die 10 years earlier than their non-Indigenous counterparts and make up 7 times the number of prisoners in our jails (Australian Bureau of Statistics, 2011).

It is important to note that, in 2014, 9264 Indigenous Australians were in prison, making up more than 27 per cent of all prisoners in Australia, though Indigenous Australians only make up 3 per cent of the total Australian population (Australian Bureau of Statistics, 2015). Between 2000 and 2010 in Western Australia and South Australia, Indigenous Australians were more than 20 times as likely to be imprisoned as non-Indigenous Australians (Australian Institute of Health and Welfare, 2011). Over that decade the Indigenous imprisonment rate increased by 54 per cent in Australia (see Figure 6.3). This is despite a Royal Commission into Aboriginal Deaths in Custody, which made 339 recommendations in 1994 to curb this disturbing trend (House of Representatives Standing Committee on Aboriginal and Torres Strait Islander Affairs, 1994).

Indigenous incarceration has been a sensitive area. As a result Indigenous leaders have responded and developed a range of community driven programs to deal with these issues. Queensland has developed 'Murri Watch', where Aboriginal and/or Torres Strait Islander people attend the needs of those in the police watch house, and 'Murri Court', which uses Aboriginal and Torres Strait Islander elders with judges to undertake hearings and apply appropriate punishments and rehabilitation programs for crimes of mainly young Aboriginal males. These programs are similar to those in other states where Indigenous people provide leadership in combating their community's problems. Engaging Indigenous people in this meaningful way, and funding such programs, are crucial in empowering Indigenous people to take control of their own lives.

Reading these health statistics can paint a very grim picture of Indigenous Australia, and some health professionals are turned off by the overwhelming statistics, negative stereotypes and long lists of 'dos and don'ts'. It would be easy to assume that most Indigenous people are walking around feeling sorry for themselves. This is not the case. Many Aboriginal and Torres Strait Islander peoples are proud and resilient. Most, despite the obvious burden of disease, approach their life and work with a sense

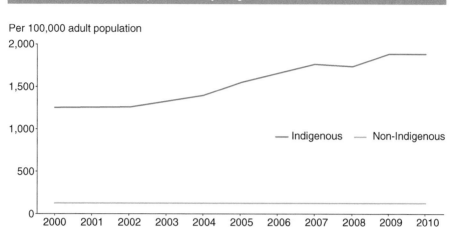

FIGURE 6.3 Trends in adult imprisonment, by Indigenous status, 2000–2010.

Note: Age-standardised to the 2001 Australian population.

Adapted with permission from: Australian Institute of Health and Welfare. (2011). *The health and welfare of Australia's Aboriginal and Torres Strait Islander people, an overview 2011* (p. 30). (Cat. no. IHW 42). Canberra: AIHW.

of humour and a willingness to improve the lives of their communities. This is important to remember for those who are thinking about working in the area.

IMPROVING INDIGENOUS HEALTH AND WELLBEING

Working in Indigenous health can be the best of worlds and the worst of worlds. It can be both rewarding and challenging to work with people through their complex social, emotional, physical and community health issues. It is an area where health professionals can assist in changing the lives of families and communities, not just individuals. It is therefore important to be able to interpret the impact of social issues on the high levels of chronic disease and how to influence and manage both.

People who are wedged in the cycle of poverty can often resort to more risky behaviours. The stress associated with this cycle, coupled with limited coping mechanisms, can funnel people towards drugs, excessive alcohol use and suicide. Those who have lived in a house where no one has ever had to get up in the morning to go to work for a whole generation have few good role models around employment and income management. Therefore, their ability to change, determine their own health or to remain in control of their own destiny, is greatly diminished – yet this is intrinsically a part of 'what it is to be healthy'. For example, it can be hard to change your smoking or binge drinking behaviours when you are using such behaviours to cope with stress about family violence or incarceration, or how you are going to pay next week's rent. Therefore, it is important to address a person's social and emotional reality as this can be the root cause of their behaviour. Working through people's social circumstances in this meaningful way will increase their susceptibility to change and enable them to live healthier lives.

Risky behaviours for chronic disease

Indigenous Australians suffer unacceptably high levels of chronic diseases, many of which are preventable. The top three risk-taking behaviours that significantly contribute to the burden of chronic disease among the Indigenous population include: 1) tobacco smoking, 2) obesity – associated with physical inactivity and poor diet, followed by 3) high blood cholesterol and alcohol consumption (Voss, Barker, Begg, Stanley, & Lopez, 2009). Voss et al. (2009) found that these risk factors account for 37 per cent of the total cause of premature death among Indigenous people. The implications of these findings are profound. They should speak to all health care providers about how simple health interventions can make a significant difference. This also has implications for policy makers about where to target prevention programs.

In Figure 6.4 it is important to note that alcohol is the fifth highest risk factor as fewer Indigenous Australians drink alcohol compared with non-Indigenous Australians (Australian Institute of Health and Welfare, 2011). However, those who do drink, often do so to harmful levels, causing significant illness to themselves, their families and communities.

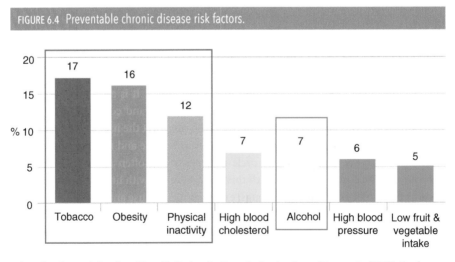

FIGURE 6.4 Preventable chronic disease risk factors.

Adapted with permission from: Voss, T., Barker, B., Begg, S., Stanley, L., and Lopez, A. (2009). Burden of disease and injury in Aboriginal and Torres Strait Islander peoples: the Indigenous health gap. *International Journal of Epidemiology, 38* (2), 470–477. <http://ije.oxfordjournals.org/content/38/2/470.full>.

Tobacco smoking

Smoking tobacco is the highest risk factor for chronic disease. In 2013 two out of every five Indigenous Australians over 15 years smoked, some 41 per cent, which is 2.6 times the smoking rate for non-Indigenous Australians (Australian Institute of Health and Welfare, 2014b). There are various smoking patterns that are important to note as they relate directly to poverty and the social determinants of health. Researchers found that those who are *less* likely to smoke include: those with higher incomes, those who have completed year 12 and those who are employed (Australian Bureau of Statistics, 2006). Therefore, what this means is, if you are poor, unemployed, have not completed year 12 and are Indigenous, you are more likely to smoke. This is important to know as it will assist health care planners to develop programs that impact these particular groups.

There have been a number of initiatives targeting these trends in tobacco smoking among Indigenous young people in particular (HealthInfonet, 2015). The decrease in smoking rates for Indigenous peoples from 49 per cent in 2002 to 41 per cent a decade later in 2012–13 may be partially attributed to such programs as well as the increased government tax on cigarettes. However, the Closing the Gap target of halving the smoking rates among Indigenous people by 2018 seems well off-track (Australian Government, 2015). This is not surprising considering the established links between smoking and education, employment and income standards. Therefore, health providers need to be mindful that reducing smoking rates cannot be easily separated from other important determinants of health such as keeping Indigenous children engaged in school, improving employment opportunities and addressing poverty (Australian Government, 2015).

Obesity

The second major chronic disease risk factor is obesity, which is strongly linked to physical activity and food consumption. The consumption of food is one of the fundamental needs of existence. However, the behaviours around what we eat, the availability of certain foods and our consuming patterns have brought us face-to-face with an obesity epidemic. According to the World Health Organization, humans are developing diseases such as type 2 diabetes, hypercholesterolaemia, dyslipidaemias, hypertension, cancer and subsequent vascular disease, and arthropathies as a direct result of obesity (Rippe & Library, 2012). Our social circumstances regarding where we live, how we live and our incomes influence our behaviours and our subsequent food consumption decisions (Cheadle, Rauzon, & Schwartz, 2014; Ferreira et al., 2010; Perianova, 2012).

The relationship between obesity and income, education, employment and food security is complex (Jones & Hernandez, 2012). Evidence suggests that obesity has increased across the spectrum of the community, from the wealthiest to the poor populations, except for those in extreme poverty (World Health Organization, 2008). However, it is those who have the lowest income and least education that have the highest prevalence of obesity. Inequity and poverty are seen as solid indicators for obesity (Ferreira et al., 2010; Jones & Hernandez, 2012; Usfar, Lebenthal, Atmarita, Soekirman, & Hadi, 2010).

Responding to the obesity issues facing Indigenous communities in Australia is not as easy as simply providing health education. Getting affordable access to healthy fresh produce can be logistically difficult and expensive, especially in remote areas where the cost of food can make up more than half of the weekly income for many Indigenous Australians (Burns & Friel, 2007; Burns & Thomson, 2006; Erasmus, Kuhnlein, & Spigelski, 2013; HealthInfonet, 2014). Wider public health measures are needed to help food stores be seen as an essential service rather than just a small business (Lee, Leonard, Moloney, & Minniecon, 2009; Northern Territory Department of Health and Community Services, 2007). Good modelling of improving access to healthy food has been demonstrated in the Northern Territory where remote food stores have come together to increase their purchasing power. This has resulted in stores reducing their overhead costs and transferring lower priced healthier foods on to remote consumers (Northern Territory Department of Health and Community Services, 2007).

In many areas Aboriginal and Torres Strait Islander people continue to practise traditional hunting and gathering of foods. Access to traditional hunting grounds, from the sea to the land, is an important element in this context. There are many benefits to maintaining hunting and gathering practices including better diets and strengthening of traditional practices that maintain culture.

Individual health care providers may find it difficult to feel that they can make an impact on people's diets, particularly in some Indigenous communities where there are many health issues to deal with. However, by understanding what affordable foods are available to most people, and educating people about portion sizes and food preparation practices, health professionals can play a significant role in sustainable improvement in dietary consumption.

Physical inactivity

Physical inactivity is the third highest risk factor for chronic disease. Almost one-third, 30 percent, of Indigenous children and 66 per cent of Indigenous people over 15 years were overweight or obese in 2012–13 (Australian Institute of Health and Welfare, 2014b).

In the rural, remote and Indigenous context there are several potential barriers to physical activity. Some of these barriers are associated with living in a rural or remote community where there are few available walking paths, or where there are personal safety concerns. There is also a perception of feeling 'shame' (embarrassment) to exercise in public in small communities where everyone knows who you are. Discrimination, access to travel to and from sporting events, insurance and equipment costs are also disincentives to participate in sport. Some Indigenous people also see good health as of community and family importance rather than for the individual. Therefore, activities that foster cultural practices and community wellbeing can prove to be more inclusive, motivating and supportive. Many

Aboriginal Community Controlled Health Organisations have recognised this and have developed programs that include group yoga classes, cultural walks and hunting and gathering activities.

At this point it is sufficient to say that the reasons behind these health disparities are complex. Many of these overlapping issues are confounded further by the lack of access to culturally appropriate health care, culturally appropriate preventative programs and fragmented governmental approaches. However, given the picture painted above, incremental improvements are emerging and primary health care workers are ideally positioned to contribute to making significant improvements to health outcomes.

GOVERNMENT AND ORGANISATIONAL LEADERSHIP

There have been many attempts by various governments to respond to the inequalities suffered by Australia's Indigenous peoples (Council of Australian Governments, 2009; National Aboriginal Health Strategy Working Party, 1989; National Health Priority Action Council, 2006). Government attempts have been hampered by the natural four-year political cycle, lack of long-term planning, piecemeal ad-hoc funding arrangements and programs based on biomedical systems and 'body parts' funding rather than holistic approaches (Houston, 2009). This has been compounded by a lack of genuine partnerships with Indigenous communities, who have struggled to communicate the complex interconnected nature of the issues facing them. For example, it is impossible to talk about improving long-term health outcomes without talking about increased access to educational opportunities, sovereignty, targeted housing arrangements, overcrowding, improving culturally appropriate health services and meaningful employment opportunities.

The Australian Government's response to health had previously been a siloed or compartmentalised approach, until 2007 when the 'Closing the Gap' Campaign was developed and launched by Catherine Freeman, Ian Thorpe and the then Prime Minister, the Honourable Kevin Rudd. The 'Closing the Gap' Campaign, which is now led by the Council of Australian Governments (CoAG) (Australian Government, 2015), fostered a bipartisan approach with planned health targets and dedicated funding for a decade from 2013 to 2023. There are five priorities: 1) producing healthy babies, 2) getting kids to school, 3) getting adults into employment, 4) improving access to health care and 5) making Indigenous communities safer for people to live, work and raise their families in (Australian Government, 2015). The overall targets of the campaign are to:

- close the life expectancy gap within a generation (by 2031)
- halve the gap in mortality rates for Indigenous children under five years within a decade (by 2018)
- ensure access to early childhood education for all Indigenous four-year-olds in remote communities within five years (by 2013)

- halve the gap in reading, writing and numeracy achievements for children within a decade (by 2018)
- halve the gap for Indigenous students in year 12 attainment rates (by 2020)
- halve the gap in employment outcomes between Indigenous and non-Indigenous Australians within a decade (by 2018) (Australian Government, 2015).

While some targets were on track in 2015 many others are not, such as literacy and numeracy rates, closing the gap in life expectancy and halving the gap in employment rates (Australian Government, 2015). Indigenous Australians have seen many of these policies, strategies, agreements and targets over the decades. However this 'blue print for action' could be different as it has bipartisan government support, with set funding and targets spanning over more than a decade, rather than the four-year governmental cycle. It will be important that Indigenous communities are consulted through every stage of this process.

PAUSE AND THINK

What can health practitioners do to work towards change and make a contribution to improving health outcomes?

Why had no targets been set prior to 2007?

PROVIDING ACCESS TO APPROPRIATE HEALTH SERVICES

What do we mean when we talk about appropriate health service models for Indigenous health? When we get sick we usually see our local doctor, nurse or emergency department for a diagnosis of our medical issue or concern. We usually receive effective health care to fix the problem, and often life goes on until the next time we get sick again.

Imagine this situation

Imagine yourself as a health professional working in a medical practice where your patients are booked every 10 minutes. Now imagine that every patient you see has three complex uncontrolled chronic diseases, with multiple medications, and a psychological issue. Plus, each patient needs a faecal occult blood screening test or Pap smear, as well as health promotion advice about their smoking behaviour. You can see that it would be nearly impossible to provide culturally safe, efficient and effective health care in this practice.

Indigenous health for the most part is like this: a complex combination of many competing issues with an added layer of social disadvantage.

In order to make the health professional's role and the patient's health care culturally safe, efficient and effective, it becomes important to look at the model of care and how it is delivered – meaning that the person sees the right health professional, at the right time, in the right place and in a manner that is affordable, safe and culturally appropriate.

Aboriginal community controlled services

The most effective type of health service for Indigenous peoples has been found to be the comprehensive primary health care approach (Department of Health and Aged Care, 2001). This approach is about *how* we do it – how we approach health – within the whole health care system, as opposed to *what* we do. The way we approach health has been found to have a greater impact upon a person's health than what we actually do. The primary health care approach is a social approach to health that is about ensuring that everyone in the Australian community, irrespective of their culture, environment, ethnic background or place of residence, has a right to *affordable, accessible* and *appropriate* health care. Primary health care is a holistic approach to health development. It is based on social justice, equity, community participation, social acceptability, cultural safety and trust, and links with the social determinants of health (Johnson cited in Eckermann et al., 2012). It has been found to empower people to be self-reliant and improve health outcomes.

In the 1970s Indigenous Australians responded to their continual lack of culturally appropriate health care and their inability to find services that understood their circumstances and would work in a holistic and culturally sensitive way. A handful of Indigenous and non-Indigenous community leaders led the formation of the first Aboriginal Community Controlled Health Service in Redfern, Sydney, in 1971. This display of self-determination and leadership set in motion the development of Aboriginal Community Controlled Health Services throughout the country. Today there are over 130 Aboriginal Community Controlled Health Services across Australia, which are represented by the National Aboriginal Community Controlled Health Organisation (NACCHO). There are many benefits to working in this sector as a health professional as the work is in multidisciplinary teams that are well supported by the organisation. These organisations provide services to any person, Indigenous or non-Indigenous, and they are greatly valued by the community. Aboriginal Medical Services provide a wide range of services and programs including:

- acute medical care – general practitioners
- chronic disease management programs
- allied health services – dietitians, podiatrists, occupational therapists, physiotherapists, diabetic educators, exercise physiologists, optometrists, psychologists, Aboriginal health practitioners, social workers
- nurses and midwives
- pharmacists
- specialist services – paediatricians, cardiologists, endocrinologists, nephrologists
- smoking cessation programs

- exercise programs
- cooking programs
- women's and men's groups and gender-specific clinics
- Centrelink direct access programs
- housing programs
- social and emotional wellbeing units – including Stolen Generation Workers
- *Ngangkari* – traditional healers
- antenatal programs
- child health, mums and bubs and vaccination programs
- sexual health programs and health workers.

While this list is by no means exhaustive, nor universal to all Aboriginal Medical Services, you can appreciate the comprehensive and holistic nature of these services. Although these Aboriginal Medical Services provide culturally appropriate comprehensive primary care, for arguably the most marginalised sector of the population, mainstream health services continue to act as the largest point of care for Indigenous people (Australian Government, 2009). Therefore, the care of Indigenous people does not just belong to Aboriginal health organisations. It is a whole of health sector responsibility – and you can play a part regardless of where you may choose to work within the Australian health care system.

Here are two relatively recent examples of Indigenous models of care in Queensland. Apunipima – Cape York Health Council was established in Cairns in 1994. Apunipima is the largest community controlled health organisation in Queensland with over 150 staff who deliver comprehensive primary health care services to 11 Cape York communities through their Healthy Lifestyles and Family Health programs. Apunipima adheres to a family-centred model of comprehensive primary health care, which sees clients as people embedded in families and communities (Apunipima, 2015). Their teams include: Aboriginal and Torres Strait Islander health practitioners, outreach midwives, podiatrists, audiologists, physiotherapists, dietitians and nutritionists, diabetes nurse educators, paediatricians and GPs, who travel throughout the Cape.

The second is the Institute for Urban Indigenous Health (IUIH), which was established in 2009. The Institute integrates four Community Controlled Health Services in south-east Queensland, by working in partnership with health care providers, research bodies, academia, government departments and other community-based agencies. They aim to improve the health of the urban Indigenous population and ultimately close the gap in life expectancy between Indigenous people and non-Indigenous people. Their model of service delivery, known as the 'IUIH Model of Care', represents a customised, system-based approach. It is designed and led by Aboriginal and Torres Strait Islander people to ensure the delivery of accessible, efficient, effective and appropriate comprehensive primary health care (Institute for Urban Indigenous Health, 2015).

Accessing appropriate safe care

Let us now consider 'points of care' throughout the health care system for Indigenous peoples. We can think about 'access barriers' to health care under the three objectives below, where we have listed a few examples of how organisations and government have attempted to overcome these barriers.

1   **Getting patients to see the right health professional at the right time.**
   - At times it is not possible or feasible to get patients to travel from their homes, towns or camps to health care services. The use of tele-health, transport and outreach services has helped bridge this gap.
   - Home visiting is valuable, particularly with home medication reviews where a pharmacist visits the client to review their medications and provide education to improve compliance.
   - There are a number of care plan arrangements, and the development of the 'Aboriginal and Torres Strait Islander Health Check', (known as the 715 Health Check in the community), which allows patients to be referred to allied health professionals, is an attempt to overcome the financial barriers to access.

2   **Getting patients to feel comfortable and safe.**
   - There are many examples of patients travelling past their local general practice to get to their closest community controlled health service to seek care, as they feel more comfortable and safe there.

3   **Linking patients with Indigenous specific programs.**
   - Some general practices have also employed Aboriginal Health Practitioners to improve their capacity to provide culturally appropriate health care; and many have implemented better processes to help identify Aboriginal and/or Torres Strait Islander patients and link them to Indigenous specific programs.
   - There are a number of government programs that link people with health promotion and clinical programs such as: the mums and bubs programs – improving antenatal care; tackling smoking programs; and vaccination programs.
   - The Close the Gap program for medications allows Indigenous patients to access more pharmaceutical prescriptions by allowing Indigenous people to pay concession card prices for medications, or receive free medication if they are on a health care or concession card.

The current trends in health care access are positive and show an increase in the number of Aboriginal and Torres Strait Islander Health Assessments, general practice management plans, team care arrangements and allied health items being claimed through the Medicare system (Council of Australian Governments, 2014). However, elective surgery rates for Indigenous Australians are close to half those for other Australians; and Indigenous women had higher rates of service than Indigenous men, confirming that men are a hard-to-reach population (Council of Australian Governments, 2014). As fewer Indigenous people are covered by private health insurance, they were found to be twice as likely to visit casualty, and are half as likely to visit a dentist (Council of Australian Governments, 2014). Of concern is that those who have identified as Indigenous on their hospital admission form were found to be significantly less likely to receive a diagnostic investigation or a principal procedure recorded for the same conditions as their non-Indigenous counterparts, despite their burden of disease (Cunningham, 2002).

Evidence suggests Indigenous patients are presenting to services at the same rate as the non-Indigenous population (at a rate of 1.1). At face value, one could see that as good and equitable. However, given the avoidable death rates shown in Figure 6.5, it is obvious that Indigenous Australians need to be accessing health care services at a much higher rate than their non-Indigenous counterparts to prevent premature death (Australian Health Ministers Advisory Council, 2012b). We can see in Figure 6.5 that the top line represents the avoidable mortality rates (2008–12) and the lower line represents the access to health care rate (in 2013–14). Access to health care did not increase despite the likelihood of preventable death. This key finding is important for all health professionals to understand as it indicates the need for more frequent and regular health checks, more regular screening, health promotion and more aggressive treatment.

FIGURE 6.5 Comparing avoidable mortality rate ratios (2008–12) with accessing health care rate ratios (2013–14) by age group.

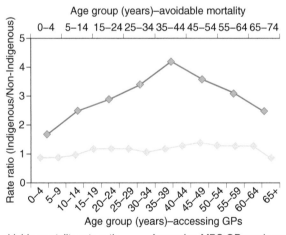

Note: Avoidable mortality rate ratio includes people aged 0–74 years, NSW, Qld, WA, SA, and NT.

Source: AIHW analysis of National Mortality Database and Medical Benefits Division, Department of Health Medicare Data. Aboriginal and Torres Strait Islander Health Performance Framework 2014 Report © Commonwealth of Australia 2015. Licensed from the Commonwealth of Australia under a Creative Commons Attribution 3.0 Australia Licence. The Commonwealth of Australia does not necessarily endorse the content of this publication.

These data also speak of the workforce capacity and the additional resources required in responding to this disease burden.

EFFECTIVE COMMUNICATION IN INDIGENOUS HEALTH CARE

In the past, mainstream primary health care professionals have been found to be poorly equipped to work effectively in a cross-cultural context or to deal with the complex multiple morbidities and specific illnesses that are prevalent in Indigenous communities (Department of Health and Aged Care, 2001). This situation still exists today. Therefore, to be able to respond to this situation and to work towards improving Indigenous health outcomes, it is essential that health professionals develop the skills to work more effectively, respectfully and safely in the cross-cultural context. In this section we provide you with some advice about how this could be done to assist you in the future. It should also be read in conjunction with Chapter 3, which discusses cultural safety.

Effective cross-cultural interactions depend on seeing the patient or client as the 'expert in the room'. Unlike an acute emergency situation, where immediate action is required to save a life, health care in the community context should unfold with the full participation of the patient. Only they, the patients, possess a real understanding of their social reality, which has brought them to this point in their illness or disease process. Therefore, in order to understand their reality and be an effective 'agent for change', health professionals may have to change their usual communication approach. Communication takes conscious effort and continual reflection and, while it can be difficult and time consuming at the outset, getting it right is a powerful tool.

The consultation

Most people, not only those who are Indigenous, value the effort that goes into establishing mutual respect and rapport prior to sharing their personal information. As health practitioners we often think that our position of trust is a given, and that we achieve it automatically upon graduation. This is not true. Trust needs to earned, fostered and maintained throughout the therapeutic relationship in the primary health care setting. Given the history of Indigenous Australia, trust is more vital than ever in this situation. Making a conscious effort to establish trust and rapport on the first encounter, and at the beginning of every consultation, will go a long way to fostering both therapeutic relationships and the influence you can have on the patient's decisions.

Communication is more than understanding the patient and their illnesses. It is more than being able to explain management plans, investigations and medications to patients. Effective communication can allow patients to link their social and cultural circumstances to their illness or disease and can result in greater behaviour change. Helping patients understand this complex interaction can provide them with an empowering sense of control over their illness or disease experience.

The usual way in which we encounter people and their illness or disease begins by questioning 'why they have come to see us at this point in time'. This is often followed by a detailed history of the presentation, gaining further insights into their past medical history, medications, family history and their social context, before performing an examination. It is a systematic way of working through issues in order to not miss key aspects of that person's history and their clinical presentation. It is an effective way to quickly assess an acute situation.

However, in the community context, acute illness may not be the presenting factor. Patients are often seen in the community context for a variety of reasons, such as having a check-up; getting medical advice about what they have heard from media, the internet or their family or friends; stress; or a simple medication review. While our systematic approach works well to address 'our' medical agenda, how does it look to the patient when we dive into the disease process in the first minute of each encounter? Often this may portray a disease-focused approach with little regard for the individual and their social circumstances at this point in time. For example, it would be easy to immediately focus on a blood glucose level of 15 mmol/L, a blood pressure of 182/98 mmHg and the large diabetic ulcer on the leg of a 50-year-old Aboriginal lady. Within the first minute of noting these findings, our medical minds move effortlessly into second gear. Unconsciously, we begin to think about the appropriateness of her medications and compliance, her renal function, peripheral vascular disease, asymptomatic ischaemic heart disease et cetera. We are distracted enough that we have overlooked the critical need to **establish trust and rapport**. Although this can seem distant to the presenting problems, making a conscious effort to understand this person and their social reality will help in the long-term management of this patient. Think of the missed opportunity by not establishing that this lady is a traditional owner of the Country where you're working, a board director of the Aboriginal Medical Service you are employed by and a busy grandmother of eight children with little time for herself.

It might be helpful to see, as in Figure 6.6, the unfolding of a consultation in the community context as like spirals that start with big open understandings about each other. Then, when certain thresholds of trust are achieved, one can branch off into small spirals representing more sensitive information. Often these spirals of information sharing need to accumulate over a number of consultations before you really begin to understand what makes this person 'tick'. Communication can be difficult in some cross-cultural contexts, and many different techniques might need to be employed to **allow patients to open up to you**.

In this spiral process, it is easy to talk about where the person has come from historically and traditionally and to talk about their families, work and other hobbies such as cultural mentoring, football or cooking. This indirect conversation style forms the perception that you might be interested in them as a person, rather than just a disease. It will also give you an idea of the social and local politics of the community in which you are working. Remember that your patients or **clients are the experts** in this area.

FIGURE 6.6 Consultation spirals.

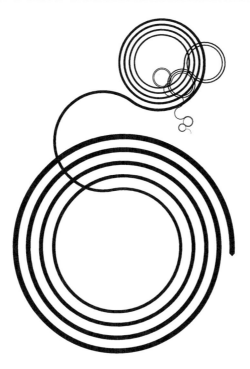

Adapted with permission from: Context Free/Curran Kelleher.

The key consideration in this patient's journey is that they feel comfortable, engaged and connected to the health service. Regardless of how trivial things may seem to you, patients need to feel comfortable to return to that service. In some instances, it is essential to recognise that a **therapeutic relationship with the service** is more important than forcing a medication change or other intervention at that point in time. At times you may need to acknowledge that a therapeutic relationship is not happening and actions to connect patients to other care providers may be required – this is difficult when practising in a rural or remote region when you may be the sole provider. Even though time will always be a constraint, **reflective thinking** can help you recognise how you can improve your communication and identify where it may have gone wrong.

Some patients may find it especially difficult to communicate about issues such as complex social and emotional wellbeing issues; this is particularly so for men suffering from mental health issues, distress and poly-substance use. So, a less direct approach may be required. In most cultures men are not a health-seeking population and often find it hard to talk about themselves. Also people may find it difficult to articulate and describe their emotions and subsequent behaviours as they often do not know the right words. It is not often that we connect the dots in our own lives and assign meanings to things we may feel or do. All we may know is how we feel. This is even more difficult for those people with English as a second or third language, which is common in some Indigenous communities less impacted by colonisation. In these contexts the Aboriginal Health Practitioner is key to understanding and communicating and negotiating aspects of health care.

Useful communication tips

So what is useful? Where people seem challenged or unable to describe issues, I find it is often easier to use general **open-ended questions** such as: '*... You know....I see a few blokes around here who seem a bit lost, down and not themselves, they pick up bad habits like glue sniffing – it's like they're depressed...there must be a lot of stress around here for people?*'

This approach removes an interrogation-like perception. Patients may recognise what is happening around them, more so than what may be happening within themselves. This approach can provide an indirect and unchallenged opportunity to relate to the notion or dismiss it. It can provide the patient with some permission to speak about their behaviours with some social context so that you may understand them. It can provide them with permission to speak about what they see are their problems in the third person and not feel personally challenged. This sort of communication style takes some knowledge of the problems in the local area. Therefore, getting a brief of both the clinical and sociocultural dynamics of the community is a helpful communication stimulator.

Putting such comments out there can be followed by an **uncomfortable pause** or silence before a patient opens up. It is important not to perceive silence as a sign of non-communication or a marker of disengagement. Often in Western culture we feel uncomfortable with silence and try to fill it with meaningless words. Allow people time to respond.

Providing context to questions through '**signposting**' is a good way to prevent people from developing a negative association with a question and you. Remember the historical aspects of Indigenous people – it is likely you may not be trusted at the outset, and people may be suspicious about why you are asking such questions and where you're heading. Patients may be more comfortable answering questions more accurately if they have some idea where the consultation may be heading, for example:

Signpost: '*At this clinic we offer specific programs to Aboriginal and Torres Strait Islander people*'.

Question: '*Do you identify as being Aboriginal and/or a Torres Strait Islander?*'

If we did not signpost this question, some people may feel very uneasy about why you are asking this question about their Indigeneity, or feel they may be discriminated against.

Signposting is also useful in taboo situations where male and female roles may need to be separated. Depending on your community, some people will allow you to talk about opposite sex health, but not perform any procedures and examine them, though some people may not even allow you to discuss it, for example:

Signpost: '*At this clinic we have female doctors and nurses who do the Pap smear tests for lady's business*'.

Question: '*Do you remember if you have had one before?*'

This sort of questioning allows female Indigenous patients to be 'more truthful', rather than assume that you as a male may imply that you might do this test today. Getting an honest answer allows you to make the appropriate steps to link patients to important screening and health care.

So that patients do not feel judged, rapport can be built further. Think about a non-judgemental disclaimer question that does not imply a paternalistic approach, for example:

…'*Some people I see forget to take their tablets for lots of different reasons – how have you been going?*'

versus

'*Your BP is high, and you have protein in your urine, and your HbA1C is 10 per cent – have you been taking your medication?*'

It is also helpful to use non-medical jargon when trying to gather information or explain your diagnosis, treatment and/or follow-up.

The patient's familiarity with health facilities and their previous experiences, including that of other family members, will influence their behaviour and their level of communication. If you are new to a practice, hospital or organisation, and find it difficult to engage with Indigenous patients, perhaps speak with other Indigenous workers or the patients themselves about what has happened before. Sometimes previous death, shame or local politics might be a barrier to engaging and communicating.

It is important that you get some idea of the **family dynamics and kinship roles** when working with any particular community. This influences communication and will also impact on certain management decisions and working out who speaks on behalf of whom. This is particularly important when working with children and their caregivers. Be mindful that the adult presenting with the child may not be the biological father or mother of that child. There are many diverse roles undertaken by extended family and children can have many brothers, sisters, mothers, fathers or grandparents.

Other taboo situations that may arise and influence the underlying patient management are past issues of stolen generations, black magic, deaths in the community and the use of people's names and strong religious beliefs.

Remember, many Aboriginal people have heard what others think they should do to be healthy and, frankly, they are sick of it. Indigenous people strongly believe the solutions to their current health issues lie within the hands of the people who understand their reality, and not the expert practitioner born out of successive trans-generational privilege. This paradoxical way of thinking challenges the biomedical model where the health provider is the expert on the disease and its treatment, especially when in a hospital context. Practising health care in this comprehensive cross-cultural primary health care paradigm takes a level of humility, maturity and interpersonal adjustment by the practitioner.

TWELVE PRINCIPLES FOR WORKING EFFECTIVELY WITH AUSTRALIAN INDIGENOUS PEOPLES

Many students ask for the recipe book on working in an effective and culturally safe way with Indigenous peoples and communities. There is no such book, and such lists of 'dos and don'ts' should be avoided because of the different customs, practices and histories of the approximately 500 different Indigenous groups in Australia. These customs, practices and histories also differ greatly among the various states and territories. There are, however, some general principles that we have developed to assist you to build strong working relationships when interacting with Aboriginal and Torres Strait Islander peoples, communities and organisations in a culturally safe way.

As you become more experienced in working with Indigenous peoples and communities you might like to add to the following 12 principles or even refine them.

Principle 1: Stand back, be quiet, listen, hear and wait You are not the expert in this relationship and you might be surprised by what you learn if you constantly adopt this principle. Things are not always as they seem. This principle requires acknowledgement that your views stem from your own lived experience and set of values, priorities and beliefs. Remember, listening and hearing are two different skills.

Principle 2: Get to know the local community Learn the names of the traditional owners, the elders and key Indigenous organisations in the community. Quietly introduce yourself when the moment arises. Have an interest in finding out about the history and language, and make sure you are open to learning. Appreciate the privileged position you are in and do not expect that you have a right to know about the culture and its people. Often, when the community sees that you are interested, they will become more open and accepting. Respect the sharing of knowledge and experience you gain about the culture, and remember it is not yours to own.

Principle 3: Be respectful at all times Be open to different understandings, beliefs, values, practices and norms. Acknowledge that there is a 'difference' and respect it. Instead of asking questions when people are telling their stories, listen and reflect on the teachings and clarify meaning at a later time. Always maintain confidentiality and be respectful, particularly of older people and community leaders.

Principle 4: Find a local cultural mentor for advice and guidance This might be an Aboriginal health practitioner or other community member, who will often find you before you are able to identify them. Having a mentor might also be vital for your survival while you live and work in an Indigenous community. Respect their advice and seek their guidance as required. The Royal Australian College of General Practitioners identifies and appoints cultural mentors for their doctors in training. These mentors assist the doctors to reflect upon what they have learnt, advise on local culture, advocate for the local community without making the learner feel guilty or criticised, support the learner and affirm good attitudes when things go wrong (Abbot, Dave, Gordon, & Reith, 2014). You may also need a non-Indigenous mentor to assist you in translating or discussing some of the issues you identify.

Principle 5: Have an open heart This is probably the most important principle. If people can see that you are trying, and are being open to understanding, then they will be open and accepting. This is how trust is established. Do not expect everything you want when you want it. Be patient, not imposing. People will open up to you when they feel comfortable to do so – when they are ready and can sense your openness.

Principle 6: Don't assume you know because you are experienced If you have worked in an Aboriginal or Torres Strait Islander community before, it does not mean that you understand this community or its people. In fact, the aware novice is often more culturally safe than the experienced worker who may think they understand – they may have actually stopped listening, hearing, learning and understanding. There is an old saying in remote practice: 'If you have seen one remote community, then you have seen one remote community.' They are all different. The same could be said when working with different groups of Indigenous Australians. This process of not seeing yourself as the authoritarian begins a transformative 'unlearning' of sorts about what you thought you know about treating patients and their illness in the community context. Such a process can often feel uncomfortable while you adjust to being still, listening and turning to your patients to find the answers to their own realities.

Principle 7: Communication in practice is King Effective cross-cultural interaction depends on seeing the patient as the 'expert in the room'. Only they, the patients, possess the real understanding of their social realities that have bought them to this point. To understand their reality and be an effective agent for change, develop and build the skill to communicate. This takes a conscious effort and continual reflection. While it can be difficult and time-consuming at the outset, getting it right will be the most powerful tool you will possess.

Principle 8: Don't participate in racist behaviour Sometimes we are paternalistic, patronising or covertly racist without even realising it, as we all function from our own set of cultural practices, values and beliefs. Telling racist jokes and name calling, even in jest, is offensive and perpetuates many of the myths and stereotypes we are trying to change in this society. Racism is illegal misconduct and is punishable by law (Australian Government, 1975).

Principle 9: Learn to laugh at yourself and with others at you See the funny side of things. We all make mistakes and in cross-cultural environments this is a given. Expect to do so – it will make you look human! Indigenous peoples are often extremely generous and forgiving and will probably laugh with you. Seek advice from your patients about how you could have done this better and reflect and learn.

Principle 10: The health status The Indigenous peoples you are working with, and the families that they go home to every night, are living with the statistics that we recite daily. Make sure you are aware of the statistics and health priorities and be cognisant of the impact these may have not only on their day, but on their lives.

Principle 11: Community control When working in a community-controlled organisation, you are a tool that is being used by the community to achieve a goal. You have one set of skills that they require. When you have used these skills there are many other things for the community to think about, and they probably will not involve you. Leave your ego at home. You are not the senior manager in this setting and it is unlikely that you ever will be. The power of decision making will always rest with the community and things will be done as they determine. This might be different from what you are used to, and the setting of priorities may not sit well with your own. See this as an opportunity to learn rather than to teach. Remember principle 1 – *stand back, be quiet, listen, hear and wait.* Do not dictate how things should be done. If you cannot do this, it is OK to not work in community control.

Principle 12: Be cognisant of the cycle of staffing Indigenous Australians are constantly educating and re-educating non-Indigenous Australians about their culture, values and beliefs. This can be exhausting to do again and again as the staff continually turn over, and many burn out. This is more often evident in remote communities where Indigenous staff might be performing the education process on a monthly basis. Be patient, stand back, wait, listen, hear, don't judge and have an open heart. You will never be the expert and you alone will not 'save these people' – so get over that now. As the saying goes, 'the more you get to know, the more you realise how much you have to learn'. If you can do these things you are halfway there. You never know, it might be the place where you may find your own humanity, embrace it and good luck!

CONCLUSION

We hope that you read this chapter to gain an awareness of Indigenous Australians' health and because you have a passion to help people. Although we have not covered all aspects about Indigenous people and their health in this chapter, we did make a conscious effort to view health through an historical lens, which is critical to understand when working in this area. We then drew out some insights about opportunities to improve Indigenous health and offered some guidance on how to develop therapeutic alliances and communicate with Indigenous patients and communities to achieve better health outcomes.

It is fitting to finish this chapter on a positive note. There are many moving stories occurring all over this great country where both Indigenous and non-Indigenous people are working together to drive social and economic development, and they are achieving the goals of equality, equity and better health outcomes. There have been many Aboriginal and Torres Strait Islander forerunners who created innovative ways to change the realities of their peoples and their country. One of the first was *David*

Unaipon (born 1872) – a famous Aboriginal inventor and writer who is pictured on the $50 note; others include *Edward Koiki Mabo* (born 1965) – a Mer (Murray) Island man who famously overturned the legal doctrine of terra nullius ('land belonging to nobody') in a Landmark Land Rights case for all Indigenous people and *Neville Bonner* (born 1922) – the first Aboriginal member of the Parliament of Australia. This legacy has continued to present day leaders such as *Professors Noel Pearson, Marcia Langton, Noel Hayman, Patrick Dodson* and *Pat Dudgeon* and Australian of the Year and footballer *Adam Goodes* and Olympian *Cathy Freeman* and many more. Whether in health, education, employment, housing, sport, child care, native title or justice, Indigenous people continue to lead change to achieve brighter futures for all Australians.

Indigenous health can be a rewarding area to work in. It provides many opportunities for health professionals to challenge themselves and make a contribution. While Indigenous people continue to drive this process there have been many non-Indigenous champions who have stood shoulder-to-shoulder with the First Australians to achieve their endeavours. The challenge for you is: will you be one of these champions? Will you advocate for better health for your future Indigenous patients in the face of inequality or inequity or racism? Our hope is that after reading this you will be inspired to do so!

Discussion Points

1   There are many significant days that are remembered and celebrated by Indigenous Australians. Identify these significant days and establish what they mean. Perhaps there is a possibility for you to be a part of these events and work towards reconciliation.

2   Using the 12 principles for working effectively and the tips for consulting above, establish what you would do differently next time you are consulting with an Indigenous Australian.

References

Abbot, P., Dave, D., Gordon, E., & Reith, J. (2014). What do GPs need to work more effectively with Aboriginal patients? Views of Aboriginal cultural mentors and health workers. *Australian Family Physician*, 43(1), 58–63.

Apunipima. Cairns: Apunipima Cape York Health Council. (2015). <http://www.apunipima.org.au/about> Accessed 01.08.15.

Australian Bureau of Statistics (ABS). (2006). *National Aboriginal and Torres Strait Islander health survey 2004–05*. Canberra: ABS. <http://www.abs.gov.au/ausstats/abs@.nsf/mf/4715.0> Accessed 27.07.15.

Australian Bureau of Statistics. (2011). 4517.0 – *Prisoners in Australia, 2008*. Canberra: ABS. <http://www.abs.gov.au/ausstats/abs@.nsf/Previousproducts/4517.0Main%20

Features22008?opendocument&tabname=Summary&prodno=4517.0&issue=2008&num =&view=> Accessed 27.07.15.

Australian Bureau of Statistics. (2014). *Aboriginal and Torres Strait Islander population may exceed 900,000 by 2026*. Canberra: ABS. <http://www.abs.gov.au/ausstats/abs@.nsf/ Latestproducts/3238.0Media%20Release02001%20to%202026?opendocument&tabname =Summary&prodno=3238.0&issue=2001%20to%202026&num=&view=> Accessed 03.03.15.

Australian Bureau of Statistics. (2015). 4517.0 –*Prisoners in Australia, 2014*. Canberra: ABS. <http://www.abs.gov.au/ausstats/abs@.nsf/Lookup/by%20Subject/4517.0~2014~Main%20 Features~Prisoner%20characteristics,%20Australia~4> Accessed 27.07.15.

Australian Government. (1975). *Racial Discrimination Act*. Canberra: Commonwealth of Australia.

Australian Government. (2009). *Primary health care reform in Australia report to support Australia's first National Primary Health Care Strategy*. Canberra: Australian Government.

Australian Government. (2015). *Closing the Gap Prime Minister's Report 2015*. Canberra: Department of the Prime Minister and Cabinet, Australian Government. <http://www .dpmc.gov.au/sites/default/files/publications/Closing_the_Gap_2015_Report_0.pdf> Accessed 27.07.15.

Australian Health Ministers Advisory Council (AHMAC). (2012a). *Aboriginal and Torres Strait Islander health performance framework 2012 report*. Canberra: AHMAC.

Australian Health Ministers Advisory Council. (2012b). *National strategic framework for rural and remote health*. Canberra: AHMAC.

Australian Institute of Health and Welfare (AIHW). (2011). *The health and welfare of Australia's Aboriginal and Torres Strait Islander people, an overview 2011*. (Cat. no. IHW 42) Canberra: AIHW. <http://www.aihw.gov.au/WorkArea/DownloadAsset.aspx?id =10737418955> Accessed 27.07.15.

Australian Institute of Health and Welfare. (2014a). Chapter 7 Indigenous health. In *Australia's health 2014*. Canberra: AIHW. <http://www.aihw.gov.au/australias-health/2014/ indigenous-health/#t7> Accessed 27.07.15.

Australian Institute of Health and Welfare. (2014b). *Australia's health*. Canberra: AIHW. <http://www.aihw.gov.au/WorkArea/DownloadAsset.aspx?id=60129547777> Accessed 16.09.15.

Australian Institute of Health and Welfare. (2014c). *Not faring so well: Australia's health 2014*. Canberra: AIHW. <http://www.aihw.gov.au/australias-health/2014/not-faring-so-well> Accessed 27.07.15.

Burns, C., & Friel, S. (2007). It's time to determine the cost of a healthy diet in Australia. *Australian and New Zealand Journal of Public Health*, 31(4), 363–365.

Burns, J., & Thomson, N. (2006). Summary of Indigenous health: overweight and obesity. *Aboriginal and Islander Health Worker Journal*, 30(5), 11.

Cheadle, A., Rauzon, S., & Schwartz, P. M. (2014). Community-level obesity prevention initiatives. *National Civic Review*, 103(1), 35–39.

Council of Australian Governments (CoAG). (2009). *National strategy for food security in remote Indigenous communities*. Canberra: CoAG. <www.coag.gov.au/sites/default/files/ nat_strat_food_security.pdf> Accessed 27.07.15.

Council of Australian Governments. (2014). *Healthcare in Australia 2012–13: Five years of performance*. Canberra: CoAG Reform Council.

Cunningham, J. (2002). Diagnostic and therapeutic procedures among Australian hospital patients identified as Indigenous. *Medical Journal of Australia*, 176(2), 58–62.

Department of Health and Aged Care (DHAC). (2001). *Better health care: Studies in the successful delivery of primary health care services for Aboriginal and Torres Strait Islander Australians.* Canberra: DHAC.

Eckermann, A. K., Dowd, T., Chong, E., Nixon, L., Gray, R., & Johnson, S. (2012). *Binan Goonj: Bridging cultures in Aboriginal health.* Chatswood NSW: Elsevier International.

Erasmus, B., Kuhnlein, H. V., & Spigelski, D. (2013). *Indigenous peoples' food systems and well-being: Interventions and policies for healthy communities: FAO/CINE.* Rome: Food and Agriculture Organization of the United Nations Centre for Indigenous Peoples' Nutrition and Environment.

Ferreira, V. A., Silva, A. E., Rodrigues, C. A. A., Nunes, N. L. A., Vigato, T. C., & Magalhães, R. (2010). Inequality, poverty and obesity. Ciência & saúde. *Ciênc. saúde Coletiva*, 15(1), 1423–1432.

Forester, L. (unknown). Bold and beautiful. *Koori Mail 470.*

Graseck, S. (2008). Explore the past to understand the present and shape the future. *Social Education*, 72, 367–370.

HealthInfonet. (2014). *Concern about the high cost of fresh produce in remote communities.* Perth: Edith Cowan University, Australian Indignous Health Infonet. <www.healthinfonet.ecu.edu.au/about/news/1931> Accessed 22.05.15.

HealthInfonet. (2015). *Tackling Indigenous smoking measure.* Perth: Edith Cowan University, Australian Indigenous Health Infonet. <http://www.healthinfonet.ecu.edu.au/key-resources/programs-projects?pid=1112> Accessed 22.05.15.

House of Representatives Standing Committee on Aboriginal and Torres Strait Islander Affairs. (1994). *Justice under scrutiny: Report of the inquiry into the implementation by governments of the recommendations of the royal commission into Aboriginal deaths in custody.* Canberra: House of Representatives Standing Committee on Aboriginal and Torres Strait Islander Affairs, Australian Government Printing Service.

Houston, S. (2009). Cultural security as a determinant of Aboriginal health. In H. Keleher & C. McDougall (Eds.), *Understanding Health*. Melbourne: Oxford University Press.

Human Rights and Equal Opportunity Commission (HREOC). (1997). *Bringing them home report: Report of the national inquiry into the separation of Aboriginal and Torres Strait Islander children from their families.* Canberra: HREOC.

Institute for Urban Indigenous Health (IUIH). (2015). *A new model.* Brisbane: IUIH. <http://www.iuih.org.au/About/A_New_Model> Accessed 02.08.l5.

Jones, M. A., & Hernandez, F. E. (2012). *Food security: Quality management, issues and economic implications.* New York: Nova Publishers.

Kildea, S., Humphrey, M., Sherwood, J., Paterson, B., Finn, M., Black, D., et al. (Ed.) (2006). Maternal mortality in Aboriginal and Torres Strait Islander women. In J. King & E. Sullivan (Eds.), *Maternal Deaths in Australia 2000–2002.* Canberra: Australian Institute of Health and Welfare..

Kildea, S., Kruske, S., Barklay, L., & Tracy, S. (2010). Closing the Gap: How maternity services can contribute to reducing poor maternal infant health outcomes for Aboriginal and Torres Strait Islander women. *Rural and Remote Health (Online)*, 10, 1383, <http://www.rrh.org.au>.

Lee, A. J., Leonard, D., Moloney, A. A., & Minniecon, D. L. (2009). Improving Aboriginal and Torres Strait Islander nutrition and health. *Medical Journal of Australia*, 190(10), 547.

National Aboriginal Health Strategy Working Party. (1989). *National Aboriginal health strategy*. Canberra: Commonwealth of Australia, Australian Government Printing Service.

National Health Priority Action Council (NHPAC). (2006). *National chronic disease strategy*. Canberra: National Health Priority Action Council, Australian Government Department of Health and Ageing.

Northern Territory Department of Health and Community Services (NTDHCS). (2007). *Northern Territory market basket survey, 2006*. Darwin, NT: Department of Health and Community Services. <digitallibrary.health.nt.gov.au/.../10137/338/1/Market_basket_2006 .pdf> Accessed 27.07.15.

Perianova, I. (2012). *The polyphony of food: Food through the prism of Maslow's pyramid*. Cambridge: Cambridge Scholars Publishing.

Rippe, J. M., & Library, E. B. (2012). *Obesity: Prevention and treatment*. Hoboken NJ: CRC Press.

Usfar, A. A., Lebenthal, E., Atmarita, A., Soekirman, E., & Hadi, H. (2010). Obesity as a poverty-related emerging nutrition problems: the case of Indonesia. *Obesity Reviews*, 11(12), 924–928.

Voss, T., Barker, B., Begg, S., Stanley, L., & Lopez, A. (2009). Burden of disease and injury in Aboriginal and Torres Strait Islander Peoples: the Indigenous health gap. *International Journal of Epidemiology*, 38(2), 470–477.

Wilkinson, R., & Marmot, M. (Eds.), (2003). *Social determinants of health: The solid facts* (2nd ed.). Geneva: WHO. <http://www.euro.who.int/document/e81384.pdf> Accessed 27.07.15.

World Health Organization. (2008). *The world health report 2008: Primary health care now more than ever*. xiv. Geneva: WHO. <http://www.who.int/whr/2008/whr08_en.pdf> Accessed 27.07.15.

Yunupingu, Y. *Keynote speaker: Human rights and social justice award*. (2014). Paper presented at the National Indigenous Human Rights Awards. <http://www.concern edaustralians.com.au/media/NIHRA_2014_Yalmay_Yunupingu_speech.pdf> Accessed 27.07.15.

CHAPTER 7

REMOTE INDIGENOUS HEALTH

Janie Dade Smith

Like slavery and apartheid, poverty is not natural. It is
man-made and it can be overcome and eradicated by the
actions of human beings.

(NELSON MANDELA)

When Australians think of remote Indigenous Australia many automatically think of the Northern Territory, its ochre deserts, Uluru, Kakadu…and the stories they heard during 2007 about the 'Northern Territory Intervention'. There is something about 'The Intervention' that is implanted in our brains. It resulted from a report on sexual abuse of Indigenous children in remote areas (Wild & Anderson, 2007). It resulted in a highly political package of changes to welfare provision, law enforcement, land tenure and other measures that were forcibly introduced by the Australian

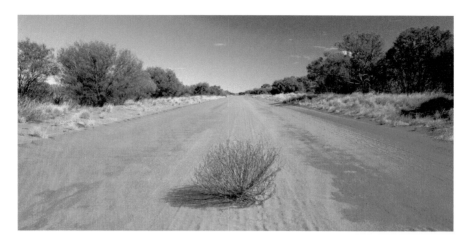

Reproduced with permission from: iStockphoto/Wellyboots.

Government. The then Prime Minister, the Honourable John Howard, sent in the army and police under the title of The Northern Territory Emergency Response. There are many stories the Australian community could tell about remote Indigenous people, but they would be based on the stereotypical views they formed or reinforced during this time … as that is all they know. It also reinforces what they 'think they know' about remote Indigenous people, though few have ever experienced remote Australia.

Remote Australia makes up over three-quarters of the landmass of this great nation. It is a place of enormous diversity and, just like the temperature, everything is magnified in the remote context. Remote communities are characterised by geographical isolation, cultural diversity, socioeconomic inequality, health inequality, resource inequity and a full range of climatic conditions. Floods, cyclones, lack of transport, resources and a lack of political will for change further heighten the isolation experienced by these communities.

The largest remote and very remote population is made up of Aboriginal and Torres Strait Islander Australians. Indigenous Australians represent 16 per cent and 45 per cent of all people living in remote and very remote areas, respectively, many of whom live in what are called 'discrete remote Indigenous communities' (Australian Institute of Health and Welfare, 2014b).

There are 1212 discrete remote Indigenous communities in Australia. These communities are defined by their 'geographic location bounded by physical and legal boundaries and made up of predominantly Indigenous people, with housing and infrastructure that is either owned or managed on a community basis' (Australian Institute of Health and Welfare, 2014a). This means that those living there cannot own their property. The locations are either part of these people's original homelands, outstations or they are the locations where the policies of the day forcibly removed them to missions and reserves. It is these very outstations that the Western Australian Government was trying to move Indigenous people from in 2015 (Gordon, 2015). This history differs greatly between the states. One thing that does not differ greatly is the much poorer health status of the people, which worsens with geographical remoteness.

INDIGENOUS HEALTH

The health of Indigenous Australians, no matter how one tries to view the statistics, is a national and international embarrassment. When compared with that of other international indigenes such as Canada's First Nations people and New Zealand's Māoris, who were colonised under the same ethnocentric principles, the health status of Australian Indigenous peoples remains the worst in the First World on many indicators (Australian Institute of Health and Welfare, 2009). Aboriginal leader Lowitja O'Donoghue (1999) states that: 'It is almost as if Australia has two nations: the haves and the have-nots'.

PAUSE AND REFLECT

Why today, in a First World country, are Indigenous Australians so impoverished, especially those living in remote areas?

How has this situation been allowed to become so serious?

Why do Indigenous Australians continue to have the worst health in the world on some indicators?

In Chapters 4 and 5, we delved into some of Australia's Indigenous history. The legacy of this history lives on today in the health of many remotely located Indigenous Australians. Rather than reciting a continual mantra of statistics to try to explain the health of Indigenous Australians, in this chapter we will use a story to demonstrate how these statistics impact upon the daily lives of remote people, to illustrate the burden of disease they carry. We will then examine why these health inequities exist by comparing Australian Indigenous conditions with those affecting indigenous peoples in other First World countries. Finally, we will explore the reasons why investigations into the issues have been ineffective in changing the health status of remote Indigenous Australians.

The story 'Stella and Rob live in Nabvana' is based on the latest statistics available, largely from the Australian Institute of Health and Welfare and the Australian Bureau of Statistics, as well as on scenarios that are common in many discrete remote Indigenous communities in northern Australia today. The characters and the community, however, are fictitious. The story is based on a primary health care approach to health, which emphasises equity, equality, affordability, appropriateness, accessibility and social and economic justice, issues discussed in detail in other chapters.

Note: This story has been made into a teaching tool in the e-book. It provides an innovative approach to applying the statistics to real life today for many remote

Story 3: The remote scenario – Stella and Rob live in Nabvana

Part 1: Welcome to Nabvana

Nabvana is a small community in the tropical coastal country of Northern Australia. The community was established as an Aboriginal reserve in 1949 under state government rule. It was reclassified in 1985 as a Deed of Grant in Trust (DOGIT*) community. Nabvana has a population of about 1200 people. Ninety-five per cent are Indigenous and come from five different clan groups who were historically grouped together 'under the Act', when the government formed the reserve. The remaining 5 per cent of the population are non-Indigenous; they provide some of the educational, health and other services in the town.

Nabvana looks picturesque as it is on the ocean with lots of palm trees blowing in the breeze. The community has a local council building, a community store that sells food and a few kids' clothes, a takeaway shop, a flash new hospital building surrounded by a big fence and a police station. Opposite is a school that takes students up to year 10, a big football field, a post office that also provides banking services between 10 a.m. and 3 p.m. Monday to Friday, a club that is open from 6 pm to 8 pm, a wharf for fishing and about 150 houses and around 30 other dwellings. Electricity and water are available in most of the houses, but they are constantly unreliable, and Nabvana did not pass the water safety testing in 2015. There are four big new houses in town: one for the chairperson of the community council, one for the visiting doctor who works there three days a week, one for the two nurses who work at the hospital and one for transient church people, teachers, linguists and other visitors who come in and out of the community. There is also an airstrip, which was sealed in 2010 and has recently had lights installed for night-time landings and medical evacuations. There is a big building out near the airport for the new electricity supply though, as it keeps breaking down, most people have not changed over and still rely on the community generator, or their own diesel generators, for electricity.

*In 1984 the running of the Aboriginal reserves was handed back to local Indigenous people instead of being administered by state governments. That year, Queensland established a system of community-level land trusts to own and administer former reserves under a special title called a Deed of Grant in Trust (DOGIT). Each trust area became a local government area with incorporated Aboriginal councils, with representatives who were elected every three years to manage the community's affairs.

Indigenous peoples and could serve as a discussion starter about the social determinants of remote Indigenous health.

Remote infrastructure: The facts

FACT: *Housing* In 2006, 17 177 permanent dwellings existed in 1187 discrete remote Indigenous communities housing some 92 960 Indigenous people. Seventy-six per cent (13 105) of these permanent dwellings were in very remote areas with another 1828 (11 per cent) in remote areas. Four percent lived in temporary dwellings – caravans, tin sheds and humpies, and were in need of permanent housing. In 2008, 85 per cent of remote Indigenous people were renting (Australian Bureau of Statistics, 2010a). The average weekly rent in remote areas increased by 38 per cent between 2001 and 2006 (Australian Bureau of Statistics, 2007). Only 8 per cent of houses are privately owned (Australian Bureau of Statistics, 2010a).

FACT: *Water* Bore water is the most common form of drinking water in 58 per cent of remote communities. Only 18 per cent of discrete remote Indigenous communities are connected to the town water supply (Australian Bureau of Statistics, 2007). Water restrictions are frequently reported in remote communities due to equipment breakdown.

FACT: *Electricity* Community generators are the most common source of electricity supply in remote communities, and are used by 32 per cent of the population. Only 23 per cent have state-supplied electricity and 15 per cent use domestic generators (Australian Bureau of Statistics, 2007). In 2006, 32 discrete Indigenous communities had no organised electricity supply (Australian Bureau of Statistics, 2007). Power interruptions are common.

FACT: *Sewerage* A total of 1969 people were affected by a lack of sewerage facilities and 25 discrete Indigenous communities had no organised sewerage system in 2006. Half the communities had septic tanks with leach drains, which were the most common type of sewerage system (Australian Bureau of Statistics, 2007). Fifty-nine per cent of communities reported sewerage overflows or leakages due almost entirely to maintenance and support problems (Australian Bureau of Statistics, 2007). Any overflow or leakage of sewage can impact on the health of a community by providing conditions where diseases spread rapidly.

FACT: *Basic maintenance* One-third of community-owned or managed dwellings needed either repairs or replacement in 2010. Of those repaired 21 per cent were due to faulty construction, 71 per cent were routine maintenance and only 9 per cent were due to damage by tenants (Pholeros, 2013). Equipment breakdown of community electricity supply affected 52 per cent of remote Indigenous communities and was the second leading cause of electricity interruptions next to storms (Australian Indigenous HealthInfoNet, 2008). Electrical breakdown affects refrigeration of food, lighting, washing of clothes and contact with the outside world.

There is no particular industry in Nabvana, though there is good fishing and a small and growing craft centre. Two artists in the community have made it big in the city and act as mentors for some of the gifted young people. There is a mine about 150 kilometres away, but it has not employed many local people for the past 20 years. Apart from those who are employed to provide the services in the community, most people are unemployed, work for the Remote Jobs and Communities Program (RJCP) or are on a pension. On the RJCP program they do a variety of work, such as community development work and council work, two or three days per week.

The local shop tries hard and flies in fresh fruit and vegetables every Thursday. Usually by Monday or Tuesday there are only a few very ripe bananas left, along with the tinned or frozen food. The diabetes workers from the health centre have been working with the shop manager to improve the food selection, though many of the old people still buy what they have always bought over the years. There is another shop called Nick's Place, run by an ex-miner. He sells smokes, bread, milk, lollies, cold soft drinks, hot chips and fried chicken legs. Recently, the diabetes workers told him that they would get the whole community to boycott his shop if he did not start selling some healthier takeaway foods. Nick now sells hamburgers and sandwiches and does a roaring trade at night around suppertime, especially on pay week.

On pay week about half of the men and a third of the women have a drink at the local club, which is open for two hours, five days a week. The grog is twice the price that it is in Fairville, the closest regional town. Sometimes some of the men drive down and pick it up in their truck and sell it at greatly inflated prices to the people in the town. The community council members get very angry and come down heavily on sly groggers.

Some of the men drink too much, and many become violent. There is a safe house for women to go to when their husbands have been drinking and become violent. It is run by a small group of older, respected women known as the Night Patrol.

Employment, food and grog: The facts

FACT: Unemployment The unemployment rate of Indigenous Australians is about 17.2 per cent – three times the national average of 5.5 per cent (Australian Bureau of Statistics, 2014a). The unemployment rate in remote Indigenous communities is much higher.

FACT: CDEP or RJCP In 2008 remote Indigenous Australians were 8 times more likely than other Indigenous Australians to be employed by the Community Development Employment Project (CDEP) and half as likely to be employed in non-CDEP work (Australian Institute of Health and Welfare, 2008b). In July 2013, the CDEP program was replaced by the Remote Jobs and Communities Program (RJCP) (Australian Bureau of Statistics, 2013a, 2014b).

FACT: Access to food Indigenous Australians have undergone rapid dietary change from a fibre-rich, high-protein, low saturated fat 'traditional' diet to one that is high in refined carbohydrates and saturated fats. Remote communities often do not have access to an affordable healthy diet that includes basic fruit and vegetables. This has led to a predisposition to high levels of preventable diet-related chronic conditions including renal disease, heart disease, diabetes and obesity, which are reaching epidemic levels (Australian Health Ministers' Advisory Council, 2011).

FACT: Cost of food Basic food costs in remote communities are often more than double those in capital cities, due primarily to high transport and storage costs (Council of Australian Governments, 2009). Expensive foods and low incomes mean that the food budget can represent 50 per cent of the total Indigenous household income in remote areas, compared with a national average of 15 per cent (Australian Indigenous HealthInfoNet, 2014c).

FACT: Alcohol consumption Indigenous people are less likely to drink alcohol than non-Indigenous people and 23 per cent have never consumed alcohol (Australian Indigenous HealthInfoNet, 2014b). Half of Indigenous men and one-third of Indigenous women drink alcohol compared with two-thirds of non-Indigenous men and half of non-indigenous women. Those Indigenous people who do drink are more inclined to drink to dangerous levels (Australian Indigenous HealthInfoNet, 2014b).

FACT: Violence against women Hospitalisation rates of Indigenous women due to assault and family violence are 35 times those of other Australian women (Al-Yaman, Van Doeland, & Wallis, 2006). Indigenous women in remote areas were subjected to family violence at rates up to 45 times higher than non-Indigenous women and 1.5 times higher than Indigenous women in urban areas. The rates of sexual assault experienced by remote and rural Aboriginal women were 16 to 25 times higher than for other women (Lievore, 2003).

Part 2: Rob and Stella's house

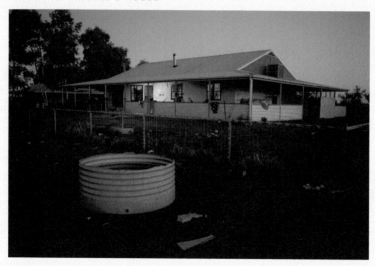

Source: © Amy Toensing/National Geographic Creative/Corbi

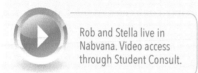
Rob and Stella live in Nabvana. Video access through Student Consult.

At No. 12 Third Street, on the outskirts of Nabvana, live a couple called Stella (aged 26) and Rob (aged 30). They have two children, George (four) and Henrietta (seven). Stella is 35 weeks pregnant with their third child, who she secretly hopes will be another lovely little girl just like Henrietta. Also living with them are Stella's mother, Doris, and her brother, Julian, who is 18 years old and always in trouble. Sometimes on pay week her sister Rowena comes and stays over with her two kids. Stella's Dad died from a heart attack last year. He was 52 years old.

Rob's family all live in Nabvana, too, and sometimes his relatives and their kids come over and stay, but not so often since Doris has been living there. You see, Stella fell in love with Rob but he was from a different clan group, and at times there is a lot of fighting between the families, as they think Stella should have married the man her parents chose for her to marry, an old man from her own clan group. It caused a lot of trouble at the time.

Stella works part-time at the local school as a teacher's aide and she loves her job. She attended school up to year 10 and always wanted to be a teacher. She enrolled in the remote area teacher education program to gain a teaching qualification but a lot of it was done over the internet, which was very slow and unreliable and could only be accessed at the local school. It was just too hard with the kids to look after as well. Stella would love Henrietta to be a qualified teacher one day, and come back and work in Nabvana. But that would mean she would have to leave her family and community to do years 11 and 12 and then go to university for an additional three years, plus she's heard it's really expensive, so it probably won't happen. Rob works for the RJCP three days a week. This week he's working with the Community Council painting the new hoist they have installed on the wharf.

Lifestyle and education: The facts

FACT: Overcrowding An average of 8.1 people lived in each multi-family remote Indigenous household in 2008 compared with an average 2.6 people per household in non-Indigenous households (Australian Bureau of Statistics, 2012). Overcrowding increased with remoteness, affecting half of remote people, compared to 13 per cent in major cities (Australian Bureau of Statistics, 2012). In 2008, 48 per cent of Indigenous people in remote areas were in need of additional bedrooms, compared to 20 per cent in regional areas and 13 per cent in major cities (Australian Bureau of Statistics, 2010a). Overcrowding can put stress on bathroom, kitchen and laundry facilities, as well as on sewerage systems. It is linked to the spread of infection and disease and also causes high levels of psychological distress (Australian Bureau of Statistics, 2010).

FACT: Life expectancy The average life expectancy for Indigenous Australian men is 69.1 years and it is 73.7 years for women, which were 10.6 years and 9.5 years less than the life expectancies of non-Indigenous males and females, respectively. This varies greatly between the states and with geographical location, with life expectancy reducing with remoteness (Australian Institute of Health and Welfare, 2014e). The average life expectancy for men in some communities in the Northern Territory and South Australia is as low as 52 and 48 years, respectively (Australian Bureau of Statistics, 2013b; Australian Indigenous HealthInfoNet, 2013).

FACT: Cardiovascular disease Indigenous Australians in remote areas were significantly more likely to suffer from heart and/or circulatory diseases compared to those in non-remote areas (18 per cent compared with 11 per cent) (Australian Bureau of Statistics, 2014f). They will also die at twice the rate from ischaemic heart disease as other Australians (Australian Bureau of Statistics, 2015b). Heart disease is the primary cause of death for Indigenous Australians (Australian Bureau of Statistics, 2015b).

FACT: Family violence Twenty-three per cent of remote Indigenous people over 15 years of age reported being subjected to physical or threatened violence in the previous 12 months, which is ten times the urban rate (Australian Bureau of Statistics, 2012). Remote Indigenous people have double the family violence, assault and sexual assault rates compared to those living in urban areas (Australian Bureau of Statistics, 2012).

FACT: Access to education To access late secondary and tertiary education, remote children have to leave their families and live in larger regional towns or cities. In 2010, the retention rate for Indigenous students in Year 11 was 21 per cent less than that of non-Indigenous students. Indigenous Australians were less than half as likely as non-Indigenous Australians to have completed Year 12 in 2008 (Australian Institute of Health and Welfare, 2011a). Urban Indigenous people were more likely to have a qualification; those living in major cities were 3 times as likely to hold a Bachelor degree or above as those living in remote areas (Australian Bureau of Statistics, 2011a).

FACT: Maternal education Maternal education is a key determinant of the health status and survival of a child. Three-quarters of Indigenous carers of children aged 0–14 years had not completed Year 12, and only one-third of carers had completed Year 9 or below (Australian Institute of Health and Welfare, 2011a). These factors impact on health literacy and the health status of the children.

FACT: Internet access in remote communities Only 13 per cent of Indigenous Australians living in very remote areas had access to the internet compared with 53 per cent of Indigenous people living in major cities (Australian Bureau of Statistics, 2010b).

Stella is becoming anxious because next week she has to go into town and wait until her baby is born. All women in remote communities have to go into town at 36 weeks and wait in a hostel until they go into labour. But today Stella has had a few pains and fears it will be like the time she had George and that the baby will come early. Maybe that will be good, she thinks, as she is nervous about having to stay in a hostel with all those other people for such a long time. She also worries about who will look after Henrietta and George properly because, even though Rob has stopped drinking, last time when she wasn't there he started again.

Her Mum, Doris, is too sick and cranky to look after the kids properly. She is a diabetic with kidney problems and poor eyesight and she has trouble getting around. She also has to go into Fairville for a few days herself during that time for an appointment with the renal specialist. The specialist thinks Doris will probably have to start on dialysis soon, like several of her relatives from Nabvana South where they have their own dialysis unit.

Also, without Stella's income it will be difficult to cope financially. However, she doesn't want to go in yet, not before Rob's Auntie's funeral on Friday.

Diseases of poverty: The facts

FACT: Income In 2006, the mean equivalised gross household income for Indigenous people was $460 per week, which was 62 per cent of the equivalised gross income ($740) for non-Indigenous people (Australian Bureau of Statistics, 2010c). Indigenous people in very remote areas earned $329 per week compared with $539 per week for Indigenous people living in major cities (Australian Bureau of Statistics, 2010c). There were also state variations: Indigenous Australians living in the Northern Territory received only 41 per cent of the average equivalised gross household income of non-Indigenous Territorians ($288 and $694 per week, respectively), yet Indigenous Tasmanians received 77 per cent of the average income of other Tasmanians ($379 and $491 per week, respectively) (Australian Bureau of Statistics, 2006).

FACT: Diabetes Diabetes has doubled worldwide since the 1980s and Indigenous people are three times more likely to suffer diabetes (Australian Bureau of Statistics, 2014f; McDermott, McCulloch, Campbell, & Young, 2007). In very remote areas diabetes is twice as prevalent among Indigenous people (14 per cent) as it is in urban Indigenous people (7 per cent), and it is extremely high in Torres Strait Islanders (Australian Bureau of Statistics, 2014e; McDermott et al., 2007). Remote people were half as likely to be effectively managing their diabetes as urban people (Australian Bureau of Statistics, 2014f). In 2012 diabetes was the second leading cause of death of Indigenous Australians, while their age standardised death rate was 7 times higher compared to non-Indigenous Australians (Australian Bureau of Statistics, 2015a). Three-quarters of Indigenous diabetics have type 2 diabetes and the incidence is higher for younger Indigenous people (Australian Indigenous HealthInfoNet, 2014b). Diabetes is the second most common cause of chronic kidney failure, and causes a range of complications including cardiovascular disease, eye damage, ulceration and gangrene (Australian Institute of Health and Welfare, 2010).

FACT: Renal disease Indigenous Australians suffer epidemic proportions of renal disease, which is strongly associated with socioeconomic disadvantage. In remote and very remote areas, the rates of end-stage renal disease were almost 18 times and 20 times higher for Indigenous Australians when compared with the non-Indigenous population (Australian Health Ministers' Advisory Council, 2011). In 2008, 88 per cent of all Indigenous patients registered with the Australia and New Zealand Dialysis and Transplant Registry relied on dialysis compared to 55 per cent of non-Indigenous Australians. However, only 12 per cent of Indigenous patients received a kidney transplant, compared with 45 per cent of non-Indigenous patients (Australian Health Ministers' Advisory Council, 2011).

Stella sees the visiting aero-medical doctor on Thursday afternoon. The doctor tells Stella that she needs to come back on the plane with her that night, as she may be in very early labour and it will be safer and more cost-effective to transport her then. Stella goes home to get her things and say goodbye to her family, who come to wave her off. Henrietta cries; she will miss her mother, but George is fascinated by the aeroplane and wants to go too.

Stella delivers her baby boy, Arnold Francis Luke, at 2 a.m. on Friday. He is a lovely little boy who weighs 1650 grams. Stella thinks he looks just like George when he was born. He has a bit of trouble breathing, so he has to go to the neonatal nursery where they put tubes all over his body. Stella is very worried about him. When they move her down to the ward, she goes out on the veranda for a smoke and bumps into a relative of Rob's who is a patient in one of the other wards. 'It's nice to see a familiar face,' she thinks. Stella tries to ring Rob and tell him about the baby. She has to ring Marcie at the Community Council office and leave a message for Rob, as they don't have the phone on at home. She knows the whole community will know by the end of the day, now that Marcie knows. She misses her family and is very worried about Rob now, especially with his Auntie's funeral that afternoon. Marcie tells Stella that her brother Julian has been arrested again, this time for taking the police paddy wagon for a drive when he was stoned. She knows that this means he will probably go to jail this time. She worries for him, as he has been very down lately.

The next 10 days are touch-and-go for Arnold. He is more premature than anticipated, and he is having some breathing problems. Because of this he is having trouble breastfeeding and is fed via a nasogastric tube. The midwife makes sure Stella expresses her breasts because it is important for Arnold's survival that he is breastfed when he goes home. As Stella is just a bit anaemic, the doctor says she can go home and come in to feed Arnold. 'Doctors never understand that it's not quite that easy if you don't come from Fairville,' she thinks as she averts her eyes. She reluctantly goes off to live at the hostel and comes in to feed Arnold during the day.

Birth, lifestyle and death: the facts

FACT: Maternal mortality Stella, as an Indigenous woman, was 3 times more likely to have died during childbirth than other expectant mothers. The most common causes of maternal death in Indigenous women are sepsis and cardiac conditions (Australian Institute of Health and Welfare, 2011c).

FACT: Premature birth incidence Arnold was twice as likely as other Australian babies to be of low birth weight (Australian Institute of Health and Welfare, 2014d). Low birth weight is associated with socioeconomic disadvantage, maternal nutrition, smoking and illness. These babies are more prone to ill health, inhibited growth and cognitive development during childhood and more vulnerable to chronic diseases in adulthood. The low birth weight rate was 3 times higher for Indigenous compared to non-Indigenous babies in very remote areas (Australian Institute of Health and Welfare, 2014d).

FACT: Smoking incidence Forty-one per cent of Indigenous Australians aged 15 years and over smoke on a daily basis, which is double the non-Indigenous rate. This rate is significantly higher in remote areas where 50 per cent of Indigenous people smoke compared with 38 per cent in non-remote areas (Australian Bureau of Statistics, 2014c). This was attributed to the significantly higher smoking rates among young Indigenous people in remote areas. Smoking is slightly more prevalent in men, with 43 per cent of Indigenous men and 39 per cent of Indigenous women currently daily smokers (Australian Bureau of Statistics, 2014c).

FACT: Substance abuse Indigenous Australians have twice the rate of death due to psychoactive substance use. The hospitalisation rate due to substance abuse was over twice that of other Australians, which is an indicator of psychological illness and distress in a community (Australian Institute of Health and Welfare, 2011b). Indigenous people living in urban areas were more likely to have used an illicit substance than those in remote areas (Australian Bureau of Statistics, 2014d).

FACT: Detention Indigenous Australians are 13 times more likely to be jailed than other Australians, accounting for 27 per cent (9264) of the total prisoner population in 2004 (Australian Bureau of Statistics, 2011b). Indigenous women account for 29 per cent and Indigenous men 24 percent of the total female and male prison populations, respectively (Australian Institute of Criminology, 2010). There has been a 53 per cent increase in incarceration numbers in the past decade (Australian Bureau of Statistics, 2015c).

FACT: Suicide Indigenous suicide rates were almost double the non-Indigenous Australians rates between 2008 and 2012 (Australian Bureau of Statistics, 2015b). Indigenous youth suicide rates were 5.9 times higher for females and 4.4 times higher for males (Australian Institute of Health and Welfare, 2014f). Cluster suicides often take place in remote communities, and their rates are much higher for the 25–34-year-old age group (Steering Committee for the Review of Government Service Provision, 2014). The rates of non-fatal hospitalisations for intentional self-harm in Indigenous people increased with remoteness.

Part 3: Arnold's remote health story – looking through the crystal ball
During the next 28 days, the neonatal period, Arnold is 1.8 times more likely to die than other Australian babies. If he was born in Western Australia or the Northern Territory, the likelihood of his dying would increase by 2 or 3.8 times, respectively (Australian Institute of Health and Welfare, 2013b). By the time he reaches his fourth birthday he will be 3.8 times more likely to have contracted meningococcal disease (Australian Indigenous HealthInfoNet, 2014a) and 3 times more likely to be hospitalised for pneumonia (Australian Institute of Health and Welfare, 2011a). If he was born in Western Australia his likelihood of pneumonia would be 14 times more likely (Carville et al., 2007); if he was born in Central Australia he would have contributed to the highest reported incidence of pneumonia in the world (O'Grady et al., 2010). Arnold would be 3.2 times more likely to have been hospitalised for respiratory conditions, 2.8 times more likely to be hospitalised for infectious and parasitic diseases and 4 times more likely to be hospitalised for skin diseases compared to non-Indigenous infants (Australian Bureau of Statistics, 2010d).

Between his birth and fourth birthday, Arnold will be 50 times more likely to be hospitalised for hepatitis A (MacIntyre et al., 2007), twice as likely to be admitted to hospital for asthma and 12 times more likely to be hospitalised for rheumatic fever or rheumatic heart disease, with the Northern Territory having one of the highest incidences in the world (Australian Institute of Health and Welfare, 2013b). He will have an over 90 per cent chance of contracting otitis media (Australian Institute of Health and Welfare, 2014c) and will be nearly 4 times more likely to be diagnosed with a hearing loss or deafness between birth and 14 years than non-Indigenous children (Australian Bureau of Statistics, 2010d).

Between his fifth and fourteenth birthdays Arnold will be growing more slowly and be shorter than his cousin who lives in the city, and have a one-in-five chance of being anaemic (Li, Guthridge, Tursan d'Espaignet, & Paterson, 2007). He will also be 43 times more likely to present to hospital with malnutrition compared to non-Indigenous children in this age group. Between his fifth and fourteenth birthdays, he will be 20 times more likely to suffer from scabies (Li et al., 2007), which may become infected and lead to glomerulonephritis or rheumatic heart disease. He will have a much greater likelihood of suffering learning difficulties at school due to his hearing problem.

Throughout his childhood he will be half as likely to attend school, and have a 35 per cent chance of reaching the national reading benchmark for year 7 students if he lives in the Northern Territory, compared to his cousin who lives in the city (Australian Government, 2015a). Arnold will be more than twice as likely to die by the age of 14 than other Australian males (Australian Institute of Health and Welfare, 2011a).

Between receiving a new football for his fourteenth birthday and adulthood, Arnold will be twice as likely to be a smoker, 45 times more likely to have been involved in family violence, five times more likely to be admitted to hospital due to assault (Australian Institute of Health and Welfare, 2014g), 13 times more likely to be jailed and 7 times more likely to commit suicide, probably by hanging, than other Australian males (Australian Institute of Health and Welfare, 2014g).

Should he survive, by the time Arnold marries his true love, Cynthia, at 25 years and they settle in Nabvana and have their four children, there is a 90 per cent chance that he will mostly work for the RJCP program. Throughout his adult life Arnold will be 3 times more likely to suffer from type 2 diabetes (Australian Bureau of Statistics, 2014f) and be hospitalised 3.4 times more often than other Australian males for this disease (Diabetes Australia, 2013), which could also lead to renal disease. Arnold will be 3–4 times more likely to die from chronic kidney disease, for which he will be treated with long-term haemodialysis, and he will be about one-quarter as likely to receive a renal transplant as other Australians (Australian Institute of Health and Welfare, 2011d). If he lives in the Northern Territory he will die at about 52 years; if he lives in remote South Australia he will die at about 48 years (Australian Bureau of Statistics, 2013b; Australian Indigenous HealthInfoNet, 2013).

During Arnold's lifetime he will be likely to have attended more than 40 funerals. He will have earned 65 per cent less than the average Australian and have paid twice the price for his food and goods during his life. Despite the fact that Arnold will have lived with 3–4 times the amount of health disadvantage than other Australians, and had far less access to health care professionals throughout his life, the amount that will have been spent on his health care will be similar to that for other Australians in low-income groups (Australian Institute of Health and Welfare, 2013a). Like his parents before him Arnold is less likely to ever get to play on a level playing field unless something is done to break the cycle of poverty and disadvantage – the poverty trap – that he was born into.

SPINNING OUT OF CONTROL

This story about Rob and Stella's family provides an overview of the life and future of an Indigenous family living in a very remote Indigenous community today. It raises issues that are directly related to living in poverty and not being able to break the cycle. It draws out those issues that impact upon our health – the social determinants of health – such as our health status at birth; our access to education, housing and food; whether we have a clean water supply, sewerage... and mostly if we have a job – because with a job comes an income, which gives us some choice and control over our life. Breaking the poverty cycle impacts on all aspects of our lives and makes us feel good about ourselves. It emphasises the distinction between the rich and the poor – if you are rich you are going to live longer and be healthier than if you are poor.

Arnold's remote health story provides an overview of his future life trajectory, which is largely generic for Indigenous people in very remote Australia. Figure 7.1 demonstrates:

- the initial predetermining factors that will impact upon the health of a child, which are compounded by remoteness, access to services and institutional racism
- the impacts that the social determinants have upon the health status of a child born today and throughout their life cycle into adulthood
- the downward and increasing spiral that spins out of control if something is not put into place to break the cycle of poverty and disadvantage
- the resulting health effects and early death.

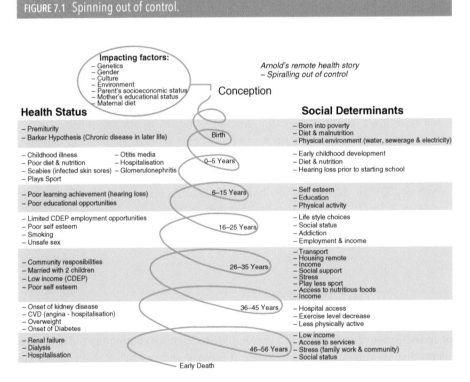

FIGURE 7.1 Spinning out of control.

Developed by: Jacinta Elston and Janie Dade Smith.

HEALTH EXPENDITURE

It would seem from the above story that the cost of providing health care to Rob, Stella, Arnold and their family would be considerably more than is spent on other Australians, due to the burden of disease they suffer and their remote geographical location. That would seem like a 'fair go'. However, this is not necessarily the case.

The health expenditure on Aboriginal and Torres Strait Islander people is measured by the amount spent in four areas, on: 1) admitted hospital services (there are very few hospitals in remote areas), 2) grants provided mainly to support Aboriginal Medical Services, 3) the Medical Benefits Scheme and 4) the Pharmaceutical Benefits Scheme, where the latter two are difficult to access in remote areas (Australian Institute of Health and Welfare, 2013a). For every dollar spent per non-Indigenous Australian in 2010–11, $1.52 was spent per Indigenous Australian. More was spent on hospital services for those in remote and very remote areas where $2.68 was spent per person. This varied with remoteness whereby in cities $3899 was spent per Indigenous person, and in remote and very remote areas $6616 was spent per Indigenous person (Australian Institute of Health and Welfare, 2013a). This was largely due to the costs of renal dialysis, which accounted for the largest proportion of expenditure – 11 per cent or $195 million. This was closely followed by $191 million spent on mental and behavioural disorders; maternal, neonatal and nutritional conditions, which made up 8 per cent; and unintentional injuries, which made up another 8 per cent (Australian Institute of Health and Welfare, 2013a). The total health expenditure for potentially preventable hospitalisations was double the non-Indigenous rate and was largely due to chronic conditions such as pulmonary disease and diabetes complications (Australian Institute of Health and Welfare, 2013a).

When we consider the burden of disease suffered by remote Indigenous Australians, these are very modest amounts of expenditure. This is especially so when we consider the cost of delivering services to and from remote communities, which are compounded by geographical issues such as the cost of resident and fly-in fly-out health professionals, climate issues and transport to hospital for the patient and a family member. Yet Indigenous Australians are between 2 and 12 times sicker on every health indicator, are twice as likely to be hospitalised and are much more likely to live further from a range of health services and facilities than other Australians.

Indigenous Australians also access health services in ways that are different from other Australians. Larger amounts are spent on patient transport, public hospital care, mental health and public health services (Australian Institute of Health and Welfare, 2008a). Smaller amounts are spent on Medicare, the Pharmaceutical Benefits Scheme, residential aged care and private health services than for other Australians (Australian Institute of Health and Welfare, 2008a). These three factors combined – inequitable levels of health, different health service access patterns and holistic understandings of health – indicate the critical need for different approaches to be used.

INTERNATIONAL COMPARISON

Looking at Indigenous health statistics it is difficult to really understand how they compare with those for other Australians, as they are so high on all indicators. Also not all states, let alone all countries, collect data in the same way, so we are not comparing apples with apples. What is common is that all Aboriginal populations in New World nations have been colonised and these health factors are a direct link between them as a result of colonisation. All countries also report concerns in the quality of data collected, much of which was collected prior to the 1980s, and they report an undercounting of Indigenous mortality data and an underestimation of the size of disparities that exist so that the data should be used with caution (Freemantle, Officer, McAullay, & Anderson, 2007). On this basis and to gain some perspective, let us examine an international comparison with other indigenous groups.

There are about 350 million indigenous people in more than 70 countries in the world, and they represent more than 5000 separate language and cultural groups (Australian Government, 2015b). Their life expectancy at birth is 10–20 years less than for the non-indigenes of their respective populations, and maternal mortality rates and infant mortality rates are between 1.5 and 3 times greater than their respective national averages (Freemantle et al., 2007). The state of health of indigenous people worldwide shows a consistent pattern of lower life expectancy. It also shows that those in rich countries have higher life expectancies than those in poor countries. In First World countries these life expectancies have all increased significantly over the past 20 years. The country that lags well behind is Australia (see Figure 7.2).

Native Americans in the United States and Canada, Māori people in New Zealand and Indigenous Australians all have similar histories. They were all colonised and dispossessed of their land; they all make up a minority of the total population and became displaced and marginalised within what is now a First World nation. They also all suffer excessive levels of cardiovascular disease, diabetes and renal disease. However, while other nations are improving in this regard, Australian rates remain the highest in the world on some indicators.

PAUSE AND THINK

Why does a First World country like Australia, one that prides itself on a 'fair go', still have significant sections of its population living with contaminated water, poor sanitation, unsafe housing, lack of basic food and poverty?

These are the very conditions that we know contribute to ill health, and can be prevented. Yet our governments continue to do what their forebears did: minimise and gloss over the past. In 2015 there was a move to close down 100 remote Indigenous communities in Western Australia, which sounds similar to actions in the past. What is the rationale behind this proposed action, which smells of money and iron ore?

FIGURE 7.2 The age standardised mortality rates by indigenous status of Australia, New Zealand and USA, 1996–2006. *Note*: Canadian data were not available for comparison.

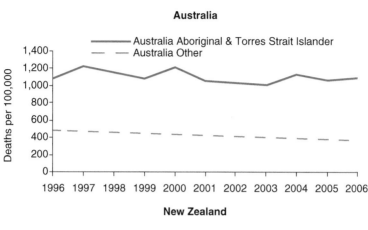

Australia

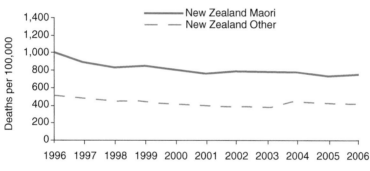

New Zealand

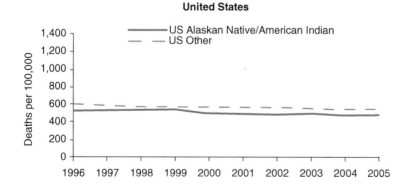

United States

Notes

1. Australia data are for Western Australia, South Australia and the Northern Territory combined.
2. Rates are diectly age-standardised to the World Standard Population 2001–2025.

Source: AIHW analysis of National Mortality Database; Statistics New Zealand; United Departmend of Heath and Human Services.

MORTALITY RATES

Mortality rates are only one indicator of the health of a population, but death rates are important indicators of health (Australian Institute of Health and Welfare, 2014e). When we compare the mortality rates of the three groups in Figure 7.2, we find that the Māori people and Native Americans have made rapid gains in health and life expectancy over the past two decades, though new evidence is emerging that this is plateauing. This is largely thought to be due to the increasing incidence of diabetes in Indigenous populations (Elston & Ring, 2005). When we compare the three groups we find that Australia's Indigenous population suffers a higher infant mortality rate and a lower life expectancy than the indigenous populations in New Zealand, Canada and the United States (Australian Institute of Health and Welfare, 2009).

The mortality rates for Indigenous Australians, however, are equivalent to those observed 30 years ago for Māoris and Native Americans. Death rates for Indigenous Australians are currently 2 times those of the Native Americans, and 1.3 times those of the New Zealand Māori. Australian Indigenous mortality rates for ischaemic heart disease and cerebrovascular disease are also 2 times and 3 times higher than for Native Americans, respectively; 3 times and 2 times higher compared to Native Canadians and Americans, respectively, for chronic obstructive pulmonary disease; and 2.8 times and 1.3 times the rate for injury and poisoning (Freemantle et al., 2007).

One concerning factor is the extremely high maternal mortality rate for Indigenous Australian mothers. Kildea, Kruske, Barkley & Tracy (2010) found that this maternal mortality rate was 5.3 times greater than for other Australian women and 2–3 times the rate of women in Malaysia and Sri Lanka. They also found that Indigenous women in remote areas had double the maternal mortality rates (Kildea et al., 2010). The authors warn that this could be an undercount as 27 per cent of cases did not record Indigenous status. This rate of maternal death was greater than both Sri Lanka (19:100 000) and Malaysia (18:100 000). These are the 'two countries that have strived to ensure locally based skilled attendant care at the primary care level and successfully and dramatically reduced their mortality rates in consecutive years', something Australia has not done nor plans to do (Kildea et al., 2010, p. 3). Yet maternal mortality rates were not included as a Close the Gap Report target by the Australian Government in 2015.

Figure 7.3 highlights the enormous disparity between Indigenous and non-Indigenous health outcomes, and builds a case for doing things differently in Australia (Kildea et al., 2010).

Infant mortality

Infant mortality is an internationally recognised measure of the general health and wellbeing of a population. It is a good indicator of the health of the mother, the quality of her antenatal care and obstetric services and the care of the infant in hospital and at home in the community (Australian Institute of Health and Welfare, 2006). High infant mortality is directly associated with poor socioeconomic conditions, meaning

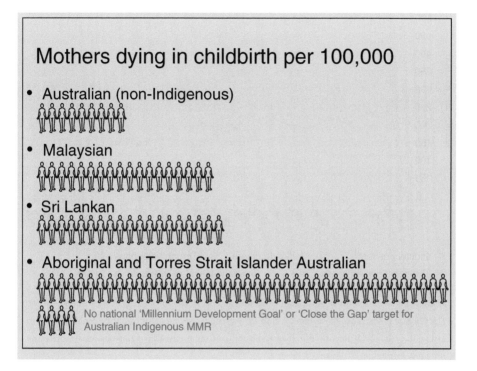

FIGURE 7.3 Maternal mortality rates of Aboriginal and Torres Strait Islander women compared with all Australian non-Indigenous women, Malaysian and Sri Lankan women 2000–2002.

Adapted with permission from: Kildea, S., Kruske, S., Barkley, L., & Tracy, S. (2010). 'Closing the Gap': how maternity services can contribute to reducing poor maternal infant health outcomes for Aboriginal and Torres Strait Islander women. *Rural Remote Health, 10*(3), 1383. <http://www.rrh.org.au/articles/subviewnew.asp?ArticleID=1383>.

that babies born into poor families are more likely to die in infancy than those from wealthier families.

The Indigenous infant mortality rates in Australia (see Figure 7.4) are 1.4 times those of the New Zealand Māori, 1.8 times those of the Canadian First Nations people and 1.3 times those of Native Americans (Australian Institute of Health and Welfare, 2009). Australian Aboriginal and Torres Strait Islander babies are also dying at 2 times the rate of non-Indigenous Australian babies (6.1 and 3.4 per 1000 live births, respectively) (Australian Bureau of Statistics, 2014g). Yet again, this only includes data from five states due to the dearth of data collection systems. This also varies with geographical location, with the Northern Territory maintaining extremely high infant mortality rates. Research undertaken by Kildea et al. (2010) found that, in Western Australia between 1980 and 2001, Indigenous infants living in remote areas died from

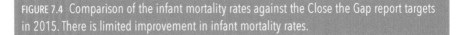

FIGURE 7.4 Comparison of the infant mortality rates against the Close the Gap report targets in 2015. There is limited improvement in infant mortality rates.

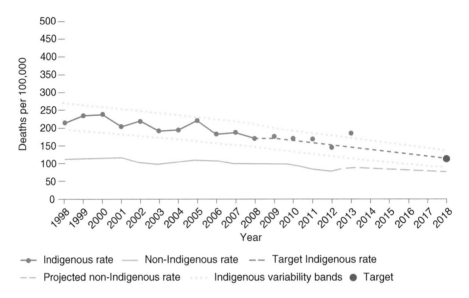

Adapted with permission from: Australian Government. (2015). *Closing the Gap Prime Minister's Report 2015.* Canberra: Australian Government. <https://www.dpmc.gov.au/sites/default/files/publications/Closing_the_Gap_2015_Report.pdf>. Licensed from the Commonwealth of Australia under a Creative Commons Attribution 3.0 Australia Licence.

infection at 7.5 times the rate of other remote infants and 5 times the rate of rural infants. They call for a model similar to the successful Inuit model in Canada – where they use a 'collaborative community development approach to care, local employment, on-site midwifery training, integration of knowledge with western knowledge, the involvement of men, a risk screening process that includes social and cultural risks in addition to biomedical risks' and an interdisciplinary perinatal committee that reviews each woman's case at 32–34 weeks gestation and creates a care plan for birth (Kildea et al., 2010). Interestingly, it has been found that, if the father is involved in the birth on the land, the incidence of domestic violence is greatly reduced (Downing, 2015).

BREAKING THE POVERTY CYCLE

When we examine the possible reasons for these enormous discrepancies, we find a few key issues that together can contribute to the cause. First is the issue of a treaty. The Treaty of Waitangi, signed in 1840, is central to the relationship between Māoris and other New Zealanders. The USA and Canada also established treaties for Native Americans. While these were often abused, they played a useful role in the development of health services and in social and economic issues for the indigenous peoples in those countries (Ring & Firman, 1998). Australia has no such treaty, since the land was regarded as terra nullius. The issue of a treaty has been on the agenda for more than a decade, 234 years after settlement.

Second, Kunitz (1992) identified several aspects of Australian postcolonial Indigenous experience that may have contributed to the lack of improvement in health status. These are largely related to government input. Kunitz (1992) describes how handing over the responsibility for native affairs to the state governments was rather like using a fox to guard the chickens, as state governments have even more direct conflicts of interest over land rights than do federal governments. In particular, he notes the long-term effects of the official assimilation policy, which gathered different tribal groups together, removed their children and actively discouraged the establishment of specialised Indigenous health programs. This has resulted in a lack of Indigenous control over health and health services (Kunitz 1992). These factors are compounded in more recent times by the poorly coordinated state-versus-federal competition for funds for Indigenous health and the merry-go-round of funding management.

Thus, we have an Indigenous Australia where there is no formal treaty, managed by policies that have been described as both racist and genocidal in nature (Hollinsworth, 1998). The results are poorly coordinated state and federal programs that provide insufficient funding to deal with the problems and show a lack of commitment to change. This leaves Indigenous Australians with a lack of control over their lives and the sense of hope that such control creates, which in turn determines their health status.

INDIGENOUS STATISTICS

To add insult to injury, the data that are used to allocate resources for Indigenous health in Australia include less than half of the Indigenous population. There are several causes for this. First, 'before 1971 people who were considered to be more than 50 per cent Aboriginal (in terms of their genetic profile) were excluded from the official population figures' (Australian Bureau of Statistics, 2000, p. 1). Second, unlike in other First World nations, the 'race' of the population was not recorded until 1986. Consequently, what is available only goes back 30 years and there are enormous state variations. This is in spite of the Taskforce on Aboriginal Health Statistics in 1984, which reached agreement with all states and territories, except Queensland, to identify Aboriginal Australians in a number of health statistics collections (Couzos & Murray, 2003). Additionally, Torres Strait Islanders were only added as a separate entity in 2003 (Australian Bureau of Statistics, 2003).

Yet in 2015, many reports from our two major sources of information – the Australian Bureau of Statistics and the Australian Institute of Health and Welfare – still only include Indigenous data from four or sometimes five Australian states. The three main challenges in data collection relate to Aboriginal and Torres Strait Islander identification between data collections, surveying just 3 per cent of the total

Australian population, especially when 24 per cent of the Indigenous population live in remote and very remote areas (Australian Institute of Health and Welfare, 2015). Therefore, most reports state that there are variations and probable underestimations and that it is difficult to point to trends with confidence. This remains an issue of natural justice. This lack of data raises the risk that attention and resources will be directed at the problems measured in those states with the lowest population size, instead of in those that constitute the greatest burden of disease (Couzos & Murray, 2003).

It remains concerning that the way in which we allocate resources is based on these statistics, when many of the sickest people in this country are not being recorded in the national health statistics.

GOOD REMOTE STORIES

There is, however, much good work being done in some of these remote communities. The most successful interventions that have been found to impact upon health outcomes have three common features – 'they are developed by the community in partnership with those who are best placed to support and advise; they respond to community priorities and are well resourced and involve community at all levels' (Freemantle et al., 2007). You will also note that these are all focused on where the impact will have the most effect for the future – our children.

At the Cherbourg community in Queensland, the (then) state school principal Chris Sarra used a new approach with the motto 'strong and smart', which introduced a number of new ways of approaching education. This was mostly done through the expectation that the students could and would achieve academic outcomes that were just as good as any other children in the state. This initiative saw a 94 per cent reduction in absenteeism and dramatic improvements in literacy levels within two years (Sarra, 2006).

The 'Strong Women, Strong Babies, Strong Culture' project in the Northern Territory targets young pregnant women through education and antenatal care. It promotes better health and nutrition in order to reduce the incidence of low birth weight babies. This project has proven to be very successful; it is operated by a whole network of Indigenous workers in bush communities and camps assisted by dietitians. It is now credited as having a significant impact on improving child mortality rates, increasing mean birth weight and reducing prematurity (Freemantle et al., 2007). A similar program is being conducted in Kalgoorlie in Western Australia through the Ngunytju Tjitji Pimi Corporation, which is staffed by Aboriginal Health Practitioners who provide culturally appropriate and accessible antenatal care.

In Western Australia a health promotion and health education program was developed to prevent sudden infant death syndrome (SIDS) in Aboriginal communities. The program is evidence-based and uses a collaborative management model (Freemantle et al., 2007).

In Derby in Western Australia the Jalaris Aboriginal Corporation conducts a community controlled and operated outreach service and kids club, which works with mainstream health services to respond to the health and education needs of the community (Freemantle et al., 2007). They do this by daily outreach at an education centre for children at most risk of truancy.

On Badu Island in the Torres Strait, interagency partnerships have strengthened primary school students' educational outcomes by creating real employment for their families. Through the work of the Council and others in training and employing local people in areas such as carpentry, 133 new houses have been built on the island in the past decade. This has reduced their CDEP payments by almost 20 per cent; also, local money is staying in the community rather than disappearing down south to southern crews (Osborne, 2003). This activity provides role models for the children, who then work harder, as it gives them a sense of purpose in life. This results in better educational outcomes, reduced poverty and restored community self-esteem.

Initiatives such as these are successful because they start from the local Indigenous people's needs as determined by them, and put the control for the everyday outcomes in their hands. The people can consequently measure their own success.

The 'no school no pool' initiative is also making an impact on the health, education and behaviours of kids in remote Burringurrah in Western Australia. The pool is not only a place to cool off, it is associated with health benefits to the skin and ears, affords an exercise routine, provides social support and sport, and it is changing behaviours with support from the local elders.

No School No Pool. Video access through Student Consult.

CONCLUSION

Remote Australia is the place that thousands of people visit each year because of its rich heritage, fascinating animals and diversity of nature. One would think, therefore, that Australian governments would invest in and nurture remote Australia for future generations to enjoy. Yet it is the place of the have-nots. 'Remote' means 'a far-away place', and remote health is easy for governments to ignore, since it happens in a far-away place. It is not something they have to drive past every day on their way home from work.

These 2012 discrete remote Indigenous communities originated largely as a result of restrictive and paternalistic government policies that placed different clan groups of Indigenous Australians together on the assumption that they were going to die out. There was little consideration that the clan groups (over 500 of them) were different, with different laws and cultural practices that prevented them from intermarrying and living harmoniously together. The policies of the day were based on the assumption that everyone should be the same; there was no place for difference. Yet it was on the basis of difference – cultural difference – that these clan groups were moved together in the first place.

Pearson (2000) tells us that these factors have taken a decisive toll on his people, their relationships and their values, and that these remote communities have become havens of social problems, violence and passive welfare dependency, which seem so overwhelming that no one knows where to begin. In the past decade these communities have largely been handed back to Indigenous control. However, along with their children, traditions and rich cultural practices, the communities have also had their laws, self-respect, dignity and health stolen. Yet in 2015 we witnessed the Western Australian Government trying to close down over 100 small remote communities. As Johnson (1992, p. 157) reminds us, without the basic ingredients for health – such as dignity and self-respect – 'then no matter what services are supplied their health status will not change'. Nor will health care if it is imposed and does not deal with the societies' priorities, as set by them and in partnership with them.

What is required are poverty cycle breakers if overall health outcomes are to be improved. This means health dollars need to be spent in those areas that can actually improve health and reduce poverty. Health systems need to be restructured in consultation with some of the best Indigenous thinkers in this land to ensure they meet the real needs of remote Indigenous peoples. This means a national approach that minimises the levels of bureaucracy, makes our systems appropriate and contributes towards those factors that actually affect health – the social determinants of health. This will mean a real commitment to being prepared to treat cultural, geographical and health difference with difference, and handing back control of health to the people whose health is being acted upon, supported by strong leadership. Funding should be invested based on 'real' population numbers as determined by Indigenous inhabitants; the different morbidity and mortality levels, which are three times greater than other Australians; geographical and cultural difference; different health access patterns; and processes that enable people to make their own mistakes, warts and all. This means real action based on the evidence.

Obvious starting points include:

- ensuring the national Indigenous health statistics are accurate and include all Australian states and territories
- getting children back into schools where there is an expectation by both students and teachers that they will strive and be successful
- prioritising and supporting initiatives that provide 'real' work opportunities that can create real long-term sustainable employment in remote communities, where people can also learn a trade
- developing positive discrimination policies whereby government tenders for remote communities can only be won by those who must employ 80 per cent local Indigenous people as they work towards a 'real' qualification
- investing in the provision of education and training that results in real qualifications in areas of need – plumbing, technicians, builders, electricians, teachers, small business entrepreneurs, health professionals and child care workers
- supporting these initiatives with career structures that recognise 'culture' as a qualification, and award wages and conditions that provide long-term work and treat difference with difference

- providing tax exemptions for those working in remote communities to help reduce the cycle of poverty
- supporting fully government-subsidised transportation costs for food, goods and services
- prioritising educational opportunities for girls and funding boarding school opportunities
- building infrastructure in remote communities – swimming pools and shared walkways – to encourage physical activity
- educating health professionals in using a population health model and in providing appropriate prevention, early detection and management of chronic disease
- providing significant government and industry investment.

As a minimum this must include: working towards safe living and housing environments such as a clean water supply, affordable nutritious food, adequate educational opportunities and the provision of basic services, which are managed by the Indigenous people at affordable prices.

This translates as community-controlled services that are run and managed by Indigenous people, for Indigenous people, based on the community's needs, as determined by them. A 'warts-and-all' approach that gives Indigenous people control over

Discussion Points

1 Discuss the story 'Rob and Stella Live in Nabvana'.
   - Discuss the facts that surprised you in this story.
   - Why do you think the people had not been employed at the local mine site for 20 years?
   - Discuss the role of the diabetes workers and the night patrol.
   - Why is it so important that Arnold is breastfed when he returns to the community?

2 What are the differences in the New Zealand and Canadian indigenous experiences that have resulted in improved health outcomes? What does Australia have to learn from these initiatives? Discuss.

3 Why don't Indigenous Australians have a treaty? How could a treaty contribute towards improved Indigenous health status in Australia? What are the major obstacles to success? Discuss.

4 How could primary health care and community-controlled approaches to health contribute to improvements in remote Indigenous health? Discuss.

5 What have been the impact and outcomes of the Northern Territory Intervention? Discuss.

their own affairs and allows them to make their own mistakes is what is needed. We could learn from the National Movement of Tanzania, which found that 'any action that reduces a person's say in determining their own affairs or running their own lives is not development and retards them, even if action brings them a little health and a little more bread' (1972, cited in Johnson 1992, p. 157).

These are some of the early steps that can be taken to improve the health of remote Aboriginal and Torres Strait Islander Australians, to bring them out of the spiral of disadvantage and poverty and back onto a level playing field. It is the decent, fair and 'just' thing to do.

References

Al-Yaman, F., Van Doeland, M., & Wallis, M. (2006). *Family violence among Aboriginal and Torres Strait Islander peoples*. Canberra: AIHW. <http://www.aihw.gov.au/WorkArea/DownloadAsset.aspx?id=6442458606> Accessed 14.07.15.

Australian Bureau of Statistics (ABS). (2000). *History of Indigenous statistics*. Canberra: ABS. <http://www.abs.gov.au> Accessed 14.07.15.

Australian Bureau of Statistics. (2003). *Population characteristics of Aboriginal and Torres Strait Islander Australians: 2001 Census*. Canberra: ABS. <http://www.abs.gov.au> Accessed 07.06.06.

Australian Bureau of Statistics. (2006). 4102.0 – *Australian social trends, 2004*. Canberra: ABS. <http://www.abs.gov.au/AUSSTATS/abs@.nsf/2f762f95845417aeca25706c00834efa/f62e5342be099752ca256e9e0028db17!OpenDocument> Accessed 14.07.15.

Australian Bureau of Statistics. (2007). 4710.0 – *Housing and infrastructure in Aboriginal and Torres Strait Islander communities, Australia, 2006*. Canberra: ABS. <http://www.abs.gov.au/ausstats/abs@.nsf/Latestproducts/4710.0Main%20Features42006?opendocument&tabname=Summary&prodno=4710.0&issue=2006&num=&view> Accessed 17.07.15.

Australian Bureau of Statistics. (2010a). 4714.0 – *National Aboriginal and Torres Strait Islander social survey, 2008*. Canberra: ABS. <http://www.abs.gov.au/AUSSTATS/abs@.nsf/Latestproducts/4714.0Main%20Features102008?opendocument&tabname=Summary&prodno=4714.0&issue=2008&num=&view#PARALINK1> Accessed 17.07.15.

Australian Bureau of Statistics. (2010b). *Indigenous statistics for students*. Canberra: ABS. <http://www.abs.gov.au/websitedbs/cashome.nsf/89a5f3d8684682b6ca256de4002c809b/3edb51e4239d3689ca25758b00127e66!OpenDocument> Accessed 17.07.15.

Australian Bureau of Statistics. (2010c). *Indigenous statistics for schools*. Canberra: ABS. <http://www.abs.gov.au/websitedbs/cashome.nsf/4a256353001af3ed4b2562bb00121564/65317b8f86968271ca25758b0011e956!OpenDocument> Accessed 17.07.15.

Australian Bureau of Statistics. (2010d). 4704.0 – *The health and welfare of Australia's Aboriginal and Torres Strait Islander peoples, 2008*. Canberra: ABS. <http://www.abs.gov.au/ausstats/abs@.nsf/0/866417CB91E3D978CA2574390014B2B2?opendocument> Accessed 17.07.15.

Australian Bureau of Statistics. (2011a). 4102.0 – *Australian social trends, March 2011*. Canberra: ABS. <http://www.abs.gov.au/AUSSTATS/abs@.nsf/Lookup/4102.0Main+Features50Mar+2011> Accessed 17.07.15.

Australian Bureau of Statistics. (2011b). 4517.0 – *Prisoners in Australia, 2008*. Canberra: ABS. <http://www.abs.gov.au/ausstats/abs@.nsf/Previousproducts/4517.0Main%20

Features22008?opendocument&tabname=Summary&prodno=4517.0&issue=2008&num =&view=> Accessed 17.07.15.

Australian Bureau of Statistics. (2012). 4704.0 – *The health and welfare of Australia's Aboriginal and Torres Strait Islander peoples, October 2010.* Canberra: ABS. <http://www.abs .gov.au/AUSSTATS/abs@.nsf/lookup/4704.0Chapter25Oct+2010> Accessed 17.07.15.

Australian Bureau of Statistics. (2013a). *Aboriginal and Torres strait Islanders peoples' labour force outcomes, Australian social trends, November 2013.* Canberra: ABS. <http://www.abs .gov.au/ausstats/abs@.nsf/Lookup/4102.0Main+Features20Nov+2013#CDEP> Accessed 17.07.15.

Australian Bureau of Statistics. (2013b). 3302.0.55.003 – *Life tables for Aboriginal and Torres Strait Islander Australians, 2010–2012.* Canberra: ABS. <http://www.abs.gov.au/ausstats/ abs@.nsf/Latestproducts/A80BD411719A0DEECA257C230011C6D8?opendocument> Accessed 17.07.15.

Australian Bureau of Statistics. (2014a). 4102.0 – *Australian social trends, November 2013.* Canberra: ABS. <http://www.abs.gov.au/ausstats/abs@.nsf/Lookup/4102.0Main +Features20Nov+2013#PARTICIPATIONANDUNEMPLOYMENT> Accessed 17.07.15.

Australian Bureau of Statistics. (2014b). 4102.0 – *Australian social trends, November 2013.* Canberra: ABS. <http://www.abs.gov.au/ausstats/abs@.nsf/Lookup/4102.0Main+Features 20Nov+2013#CDEP> Accessed 17.07.15.

Australian Bureau of Statistics. (2014c). 4727.0.55.001 – *Australian Aboriginal and Torres Strait Islander health survey: First results, Australia, 2012–13.* Canberra: ABS. <http:// www.abs.gov.au/ausstats/abs@.nsf/Lookup/39E15DC7E770A144CA257C2F00145A66 ?opendocument> Accessed 17.07.15.

Australian Bureau of Statistics. (2014d). 4727.0.55.001 – *Australian Aboriginal and Torres Strait Islander health survey: First results, Australia, 2012–13.* Canberra: ABS. <http:// www.abs.gov.au/ausstats/abs@.nsf/Lookup/DE7BD4BEC2293FD4CA257C2F00145B19 ?opendocument> Accessed 17.07.15.

Australian Bureau of Statistics. (2014e). 4727.0.55.006 – *Australian Aboriginal and Torres Strait Islander health survey: Updated results, 2012–13.* Canberra: ABS. <http://www.abs .gov.au/ausstats/abs@.nsf/Lookup/by%20Subject/4727.0.55.006~2012%E2%80%9313 ~Main%20Features~Heart%20and%20circulatory%20diseases~9> Accessed 17.07.15.

Australian Bureau of Statistics. (2014f). 4727.0.55.003 – *Australian Aboriginal and Torres Strait Islander health survey: Biomedical results, 2012–13.* Canberra: ABS. <http:// www.abs.gov.au/ausstats/abs@.nsf/mf/4727.0.55.003> Accessed 17.07.15.

Australian Bureau of Statistics. (2014g). 3302.0 – *Deaths of Aboriginal and Torres Strait Islander Australians, Australia, 2013.* Canberra: ABS. <http://www.abs.gov.au/ausstats/ abs@.nsf/Lookup/39E15DC7E770A144CA257C2F00145A66?opendocument> Accessed 22.09.15.

Australian Bureau of Statistics. (2015a). 3303.0 – *Causes of death, Australia, 2012.* Canberra: ABS. <http://www.abs.gov.au/ausstats/abs@.nsf/Lookup/by%20Subject/3303.0~2012 ~Main%20Features~Diabetes%20(E10-E14)~10018> Accessed 17.07.15.

Australian Bureau of Statistics. (2015b). 3303.0 – *Causes of death, Australia, 2012.* Canberra: ABS. <http://www.abs.gov.au/ausstats/abs@.nsf/Lookup/by%20Subject/3303.0~2012 ~Main%20Features~Leading%20Causes%20of%20Aboriginal%20and%20Torres%20 Strait%20Islander%20Deaths~10015> Accessed 17.07.15.

Australian Bureau of Statistics. (2015c). 4517.0 – *Prisoners in Australia, 2014.* Canberra: ABS. <http://www.abs.gov.au/ausstats/abs@.nsf/Lookup/by%20Subject/4517.0

~2014~Main%20Features~Prisoner%20characteristics,%20Australia~4> Accessed 17.07.15.

Australian Government. (2015a). *Closing the Gap Prime Minister's Report 2015*. Canberra: Australian Government. <https://www.dpmc.gov.au/sites/default/files/publications/Closing _the_Gap_2015_Report.pdf> Accessed 17.07.15.

Australian Government. (2015b). *Indigenous peoples of the world*. Canberra: Australian Government. <http://www.australia.gov.au/about-australia/australian-story/indigenous -peoples-of-the-world> Accessed 17.07.15.

Australian Health Ministers' Advisory Council. (2011). *Aboriginal and Torres Strait Islander Health Performance Framework report 2010*. Canberra: Australian Health Ministers' Advisory Council. <http://www.health.gov.au/internet/publications/publishing.nsf/Content/health -oatsih-pubs-framereport-toc/$FILE/HPF%20Report%202010august2011.pdf> Accessed 14.07.15.

Australian Indigenous HealthInfoNet. (2008). *Review of the impact of housing and health -related infrastructure on Indigenous health*. Perth: Australian Indigenous HealthInfoNet, Edith Cowan University. <http://www.healthinfonet.ecu.edu.au/determinants/physical -environment/reviews/our-review> Accessed 14.07.15.

Australian Indigenous HealthInfoNet. (2013). *Mortality*. Perth: Australian Indigenous HealthInfoNet, Edith Cowan University. <http://www.healthinfonet.ecu.edu.au/health-facts/ overviews/mortality> Accessed 14.07.15.

Australian Indigenous HealthInfoNet. (2014a). *Overview of Australian Indigenous health status, 2013*. Perth: Australian Indigenous HealthInfoNet, Edith Cowan University. <http:// www.healthinfonet.ecu.edu.au/uploads/docs/overview_of_indigenous_health_2013.pdf> Accessed 14.07.15.

Australian Indigenous HealthInfoNet. (2014b). *Summary of Australian Indigenous health, 2013*. Perth: Australian Indigenous HealthInfoNet, Edith Cowan University. <http:// www.healthinfonet.ecu.edu.au/uploads/docs/summary-2013.pdf> Accessed 14.07.15.

Australian Indigenous HealthInfoNet. (2014c). *Concern about the high cost of fresh produce in remote communities*. Perth: Australian Indigenous HealthInfoNet, Edith Cowan University. <http://www.healthinfonet.ecu.edu.au/about/news/1931> Accessed 14.07.15.

Australian Institute of Criminology. (2010). *Data on prisons*. Canberra: Australian Institute of Criminology. <http://www.aic.gov.au/publications/current%20series/rpp/100-120/ rpp107/06.html> Accessed 14.07.15.

Australian Institute of Health and Welfare (AIHW). (2006). *National summary of the 2003 and 2004 jurisdictional reports against the Aboriginal and Torres Strait Islander health performance indicators*. Canberra: Standing Committee on Aboriginal and Torres Strait Islander Health and Statistical Information Management Committee, AIHW. <http:// www.aihw.gov.au/WorkArea/DownloadAsset.aspx?id=6442458590> Accessed 17.07.15.

Australian Institute of Health and Welfare. (2008a). *Australia's health 2008*. Canberra: AIHW. <http://www.aihw.gov.au/WorkArea/DownloadAsset.aspx?id=6442453674> Accessed 17.07.15.

Australian Institute of Health and Welfare. (2008b). *Aboriginal and Torres Strait Islander Health Performance Framework, 2008 report: Detailed analyses*. Canberra: AIHW. <http:// www.aihw.gov.au/WorkArea/DownloadAsset.aspx?id=6442458630> Accessed 17.07.15.

Australian Institute of Health and Welfare. (2009). *International Group for Indigenous Health Measurement, 2006*. Canberra: AIHW. <http://www.aihw.gov.au/WorkArea/Download Asset.aspx?id=6442458735> Accessed 17.07.15.

Australian Institute of Health and Welfare. (2010). *Contribution of chronic disease to the gap in adult mortality between Aboriginal and Torres Strait Islander and other Australians.* Canberra: AIHW. <http://www.aihw.gov.au/WorkArea/DownloadAsset.aspx?id=10737418922> Accessed 17.07.15.

Australian Institute of Health and Welfare. (2011a). *The health and welfare of Australia's Aboriginal and Torres Strait Islander people, an overview 2011.* Canberra: AIHW. <http://www.aihw.gov.au/WorkArea/DownloadAsset.aspx?id=10737418955> Accessed 17.07.15.

Australian Institute of Health and Welfare. (2011b). *Substance use among Aboriginal and Torres Strait Islander people.* Canberra: AIHW. <http://www.aihw.gov.au/WorkArea/DownloadAsset.aspx?id=10737418265> Accessed 17.07.15.

Australian Institute of Health and Welfare. (2011c). *Maternal deaths in Australia 2006–2010.* Canberra: AIHW. <http://www.aihw.gov.au/WorkArea/DownloadAsset.aspx?id=60129548375> Accessed 17.07.15.

Australian Institute of Health and Welfare. (2011d). *Chronic kidney disease in Aboriginal and Torres Strait Islander people 2011.* Canberra: AIHW. <http://www.aihw.gov.au/WorkArea/DownloadAsset.aspx?id=10737420068> Accessed 17.07.15.

Australian Institute of Health and Welfare. (2013a). *Expenditure on health for Aboriginal and Torres Strait Islander people 2010–11: An analysis by remoteness and disease.* Health and welfare expenditure series No. 49, Cat. no. HWE 58. Canberra: AIHW. <http://www.aihw.gov.au/WorkArea/DownloadAsset.aspx?id=60129544363> Accessed 14.07.15.

Australian Institute of Health and Welfare. (2013b). *Aboriginal and Torres Strait Islander Health Performance Framework 2012: Detailed analyses.* Canberra: ABS. <http://www.aihw.gov.au/WorkArea/DownloadAsset.aspx?id=60129543818> Accessed 14.07.15.

Australian Institute of Health and Welfare. (2014a). *Discrete Indigenous community, identifying and definitional attributes.* Canberra: AIHW. <http://meteor.aihw.gov.au/content/index.phtml/itemId/268994> Accessed 14.07.15.

Australian Institute of Health and Welfare. (2014b). *Remoteness and the health of Indigenous Australians: Australia's health 2014.* Canberra: AIHW. <http://www.aihw.gov.au/workarea/downloadasset.aspx?id=60129548150> Accessed 14.07.15.

Australian Institute of Health and Welfare. (2014c). *Ear disease in Aboriginal and Torres Strait Islander children.* Canberra: AIHW. <http://www.aihw.gov.au/uploadedFiles/ClosingTheGap/Content/Our_publications/2014/ctgc-rs35.pdf> Accessed 14.07.15.

Australian Institute of Health and Welfare. (2014d). *Birthweight of babies born to Indigenous mothers.* Canberra: AIHW. <http://www.aihw.gov.au/WorkArea/DownloadAsset.aspx?id=60129548200> Accessed 14.07.15.

Australian Institute of Health and Welfare. (2014e). *Mortality and life expectancy of Indigenous Australians: 2008 to 2012.* Canberra: AIHW. <http://www.aihw.gov.au/WorkArea/DownloadAsset.aspx?id=60129548468> Accessed 14.07.15.

Australian Institute of Health and Welfare. (2014f). *Australia's health 2014.* Canberra: AIHW.

Australian Institute of Health and Welfare. (2014g). *Indigenous child safety.* Canberra: AIHW. <http://www.aihw.gov.au/WorkArea/DownloadAsset.aspx?id=60129548256> Accessed 14.07.15.

Australian Institute of Health and Welfare. (2015). *Indigenous statistics quality and availability.* Canberra: AIHW. <http://aihw.gov.au/indigenous-statistics-quality-availability/> Accessed 14.07.15.

Carville, K. S., Lehmann, D., Hall, G., Moore, H., Richmond, P., de Klerk, N., et al. (2007). Infection is the major cause of the disease burden in Aboriginal and non-Aboriginal

Australian children. *Pediatric Infectious Disease Journal*, 26, 210–216. <http://www.ncbi
.nlm.nih.gov/pubmed/17484216> Accessed 14.07.15.

Council of Australian Governments (CoAG). (2009). *National strategy for food security in
remote Indigenous communities.* Canberra: COAG. <https://www.coag.gov.au/sites/default/
files/nat_strat_food_security.pdf> Accessed 14.07.15.

Couzos, S., & Murray, R. (2003). *Aboriginal primary health care: An evidence based approach*
(2nd ed.). Melbourne: Oxford University Press.

Diabetes Australia. (2013). *Aboriginal and Torres Strait Islanders and Diabetes Action Plan.*
Canberra: Diabetes Australia. <http://www.healthinfonet.ecu.edu.au/key-resources/
bibliography/?lid=25838> Accessed 22.07.15.

Downing, R. Birthing in the bush overseas: models that work, 13th National Rural Health
Conference, Darwin, 24–27th May 2015. (2015).

Elston, J., & Ring, I. Indigenous mortality in the US, Canada, New Zealand and Australia:
little progress in 20 years? (2005). Paper presented at the International Network of
Indigenous Health knowledge and Development, 2nd biennial meeting, Vancouver, Canada.

Freemantle, J., Officer, K., McAullay, D., & Anderson, I. (2007). *Australian Indigenous health
– within an international context.* Darwin: Cooperative Research Centre for Aboriginal
Health. <https://www.lowitja.org.au/sites/default/files/docs/AustIndigneousHealthReport
.pdf> Accessed 14.07.15.

Gordon, M. (2015, March 16). Outstations message: closing remote communities will 'finish
Broome'. *Sydney Morning Herald*, <http://www.smh.com.au/federal-politics/political-news/
outstations-message-closing-remote-communities-will-finish-broome-20150315-144i8s
.html> Accessed 14.07.15.

Hollinsworth, D. (1998). *Race and racism in Australia.* Katoomba, NSW: Social Science
Press.

Johnson, S. (1992). Aboriginal health through primary health care. In R. Pratt (Ed.), *Issues in
Australian Nursing 3* (3rd ed., pp. 151–170). South Melbourne: Churchill Livingstone.

Kildea, S., Kruske, S., Barkley, L., & Tracy, S. (2010). 'Closing the Gap': how maternity
services can contribute to reducing poor maternal infant health outcomes for Aboriginal and
Torres Strait Islander women. *Rural and Remote Health*, 10(3), 1383. <http://www.rrh.org.au/
articles/subviewnew.asp?ArticleID=1383> Accessed 14.07.2015.

Kunitz, S. J. (1992). *Disease and social diversity: The European impact on the health of
non-Europeans.* New York: Oxford University Press.

Li, S., Guthridge, S. L., Tursan d'Espaignet, E., & Paterson, B. A. (2007). *From infancy to
young adulthood: Health status in the Northern Territory 2006.* Darwin: Department of
Health and Community Services, Northern Territory. <http://digitallibrary.health.nt.gov.au/
dspace/bitstream/10137/84/1/infancy_to_young_adulthood_2006.pdf> Accessed 14.07.15.

Lievore, D. (2003). *Non-reporting and hidden recording of sexual assault: An international
literature review.* Canberra: Australian Institute of Criminology, Commonwealth of
Australia. <http://www.aic.gov.au/media_library/archive/publications-2000s/non-reporting
-and-hidden-recording-of-sexual-assault-an-international-literature-review.pdf> Accessed
14.07.15.

MacIntyre, C. R., Burgess, M., Isaacs, D., McIntyre, P. B., Menzies, R., & Hull, B. (2007).
Epidemiology of severe hepatitis A in Indigenous Australian children. *Journal of Paediatrics
and Child Health*, 43(5), 383–387. <http://www.ncbi.nlm.nih.gov/pubmed/17489829>
Accessed 14.07.15.

McDermott, R., McCulloch, B. G., Campbell, S. K., & Young, D. M. (2007). Diabetes in the Torres Strait Islands of Australia: better clinical systems but significant increase in weight and other risk conditions among adults, 1999–2005. *Medical Journal of Australia*, 186(10), 505–508. <https://www.mja.com.au/journal/2007/186/10/diabetes-torres-strait-islands -australia-better-clinical-systems-significant?0=ip_login_no_cache%3D4071b6d123372acd33 34cfc8e3bff97c> Accessed 14.07.15.

O'Donoghue, L. (1999). Towards a culture of improving Indigenous health in Australia. *Australian Journal of Rural Health*, 7, 64–69. <http://onlinelibrary.wiley.com/doi/10.1046/ j.1440-1584.1999.00218.x/pdf> Accessed 14.07.15.

O'Grady, K. F., Taylor-Thomson, D. M., Chang, A. B., Torzillo, P. J., Morris, P. S., Mackenzie, G. A., et al. (2010). Rates of radiologically confirmed pneumonia as defined by the World Health Organization in Northern Territory Indigenous children. *Medical Journal of Australia*, 192(10), 592–595. <https://www.mja.com.au/journal/2010/192/10/rates -radiologically-confirmed-pneumonia-defined-world-health-organization> Accessed 14.07.15.

Osborne, B. (2003). Around in circles or expanding spirals? A retrospective look at education in Torres Strait, 1964–2003. *Australian Journal of Indigenous Education*, 32, 61–76. <http://www.atsis.uq.edu.au/ajie/docs/2003326176.pdf> Accessed 14.07.15.

Pearson, N. *The light on the hill, Ben Chifley memorial lecture*. (2000). Bathurst Panthers Leagues Club, Bathurst. <http://capeyorkpartnership.org.au/wp-content/uploads/2000/08/ Ben-Chifley-Memorial-Lecture-2000_Light-on-the-Hill.pdf> Accessed 14.07.15.

Pholeros, P. *TED X Sydney 2013: Housing for health*. (2013). <http://www.healthabitat.com/ big-issues/ted-x-sydney-2013-housing-for-health> Accessed 14.07.15.

Ring, I. T., & Firman, D. (1998). Reducing Indigenous mortality in Australia: lessons from other countries. *Medical Journal of Australia*, 169(10), 528–533. <https://www.mja.com.au/ journal/1998/169/10/reducing-indigenous-mortality-australia-lessons-other-countries> Accessed 14.07.15.

Sarra, C. (2006). Armed for success. In J. Schultz (Ed.), *Griffith Review: Getting smart: The battle for ideas in education* (Vol. autumn ed., pp. 185–194). Brisbane: Griffith University & ABC Books.

Steering Committee for the Review of Government Service Provision. (2014). *Overcoming Indigenous disadvantage key indicators 2014*. Canberra: Commonwealth of Australia. <http:// www.pc.gov.au/research/recurring/overcoming-indigenous-disadvantage/key-indicators -2014/key-indicators-2014-overviewbooklet.pdf> Accessed 14.07.15.

Wild, R., & Anderson, P. (2007). *Ampe akelyernemane meke mekarle : Little children are sacred: Report of the Northern Territory Board of Inquiry into the protection of Aboriginal children from sexual abuse*. Darwin: Northern Territory Government. <http://www .inquirysaac.nt.gov.au/pdf/bipacsa_final_report.pdf> Accessed 14.07.15.

CHAPTER 8

DETERMINING HEALTH

Janie Dade Smith

When we wish upon a star it is often for good health, a long life and happiness. That is, of course, unless we wish for money, which improves all three considerably, as we are about to discover.

There is a direct relationship between health and happiness. As in the Joni Mitchell song of 1970, often 'we don't know what we've got 'til it's gone.' Most people still believe 'it won't happen to me' and that what they eat, drink and smoke will not affect their health, as illness only happens to other people. While this belief may be a comfort to soldiers at war, criminals and racing car drivers, it is also held by those whose behaviour increases their likelihood of sickness, accidents and early death (Lalonde, 1974). People holding these beliefs are found more often in lower socioeconomic groups and in rural and remote areas, where there are open roads, higher levels of unemployment, drinking and smoking, and a 'she'll be right mate' culture that supports these behaviours (Australian Institute of Health and Welfare, 2014).

This chapter explores the concept of health from international, rural and Indigenous perspectives. Using the social determinants of health as a guide, it then examines those factors that determine whether we will be healthy or not, and compares them with the health of Indigenous Australians.

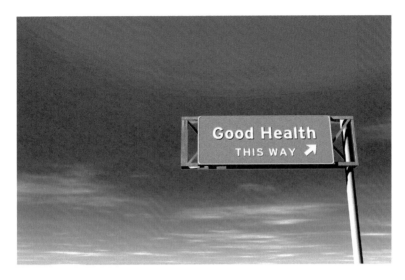

Reproduced with permission from: Shutterstock/eyeidea.

HEALTH PERSPECTIVES

An international perspective

The word 'health' derives from the Old English word *haelth*. It shares the same root as 'whole' (*Australian Concise Oxford Dictionary*, 2000). The derivation implies that to be healthy one needs to be whole, meaning in balance – emotionally, physically and spiritually. There are also some prerequisites for health such as 'peace, shelter, education, food, income, a stable ecosystem, sustainable resources, social justice, and equity' (World Health Organization, 1986, p. 1). Health is intrinsically tied to a person's sense of wellbeing. This was even recognised in the 5th century when the Greek Democritus wrote 'without health nothing is of any use, not money nor anything else', which speaks volumes about its vital importance (cited in Keleher & McDougall, 2009, p. 4).

Today we think of health as 'a balance between the physical, emotional, social and spiritual wellbeing, and not just the absence of disease or infirmity' (World Health Organization, 1974, cited in McMurray, 2003, p. 9). Australian health systems and programs are consequently built upon this understanding of health.

The reason our health is so important is that, as a nation of healthy people, we can do those things that make life worthwhile, such as working with other people towards social progress, raising our children, singing along to music, exercising and enjoying a good night's sleep. Being healthy means being able to work to our full potential as human beings, and it involves being able to make decisions and have control over our own lives in a healthy environment (World Health Organization, 1986). Good health is therefore the bedrock upon which social progress is built

(Lalonde, 1974). And as our level of health increases so does our potential for happiness – the two are intrinsically linked.

Health, like culture, is not static, it changes constantly. For example, one moment a seemingly healthy woman could be driving her car to attend a routine screening procedure, such as a mammogram, and she might walk out shortly afterward diagnosed with breast cancer. Alternatively, she could have a serious car accident on her way home. With either scenario her whole life and her health would have changed in an instant.

An understanding of the meaning of health differs among individuals, cultural groups and even members of the health profession. The way we view our health is important, as it reflects the way in which we approach it. If we see our health as 'the absence of disease' and link it to our daily work and productivity, issues about how to prevent illness take a low priority. This old perception of health has changed over time with the advent of new ways to prevent illness, and prolong and promote good health. However, this old perception still exists within some groups of the Australian community, especially those in rural areas. Yet, when we look at the factors that determine whether we will be healthy or not, they mostly relate to our income and our behaviours such as whether we smoke, drink, exercise, diet and have social support.

PAUSE AND THINK

How would you define health?

What is it that makes us healthy?

What factors impact upon us being unhealthy?

A rural perspective

To be called a 'tough old bastard' in rural or remote Australia is generally taken as a compliment. There are many 'old-timer' stories about farm workers cauterising severed fingers in diesel, methylated spirits or fire to reduce infection so that they can continue working rather than travelling long distances to seek medical help (Elliott-Schmidt & Strong, 1997). The old bush ethos of enduring hardship, being tough and manly and having a 'she'll be right mate' attitude when it comes to illness is seen as the norm in rural Australia. Being sick or injured somehow implies a weakness and a loss of social acceptability (Elliott-Schmidt & Strong, 1997).

This perception is not just held by rural men but also by rural women, who usually take responsibility for the family's health along with their roles as bookkeeper, farm hand, cook, cleaner, home tutor and first-aider. Rural women are also expected to cope with adversity and to be stoical, independent and self-reliant. They are often

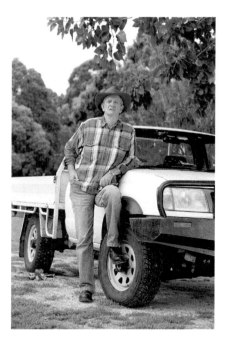

Reproduced with permission from: iStockphoto/John Kirk.

actively discouraged from seeking outside advice, as the family may feel threatened by the intrusion of 'outsiders' or, worse still, by the advice of people they know well, who may threaten the family's confidentiality (Elliott-Schmidt & Strong, 1997). This distrust of strangers is a common feature of rural communities, who are known to be suspicious of 'newcomers', who can often be described as those who were not born in the town (Dempsey, 1990). This may have resulted from the way these communities grew up.

Rural people therefore have a different view of health and wellbeing from that of their city counterparts. Their view of health is based on the absence of disease; they link their wellbeing to productivity and being able to carry on their daily tasks – such as being able to mow the lawn, do their own washing and go for an afternoon stroll (Welch, 2000). It is often only when they cannot carry out their daily tasks because of ill health or disability that they present for health treatment. Rural people are also known to smoke more, drink more and have a much higher incidence of road accidents than city people; in fact, this is described in the first rural health report as 'typical rural behaviour' (Strong, Trickett, Titulaer, & Bhatia, 1998).

Since rural people generally view health as the absence of disease, they see health services as curative services. This means that they will only go to the doctor for curative rather than preventive procedures, such as routine health screening, or will 'make do' for problems that are not visually evident, such as depression and mental health conditions, which often results in outcomes such as higher suicide rates in rural areas

(Australian Institute of Health and Welfare, 2014). These factors impact upon the health of rural Australians, who also tend to present late in the course of a disease, when the problem has often become more complicated (Strasser, Hays, Kamien, & Carson, 2000).

PAUSE AND THINK

What would be the impact of presenting late in the course of a disease?

Why do rural people see health so differently from other Australians?

What different approaches might health professionals use in providing care to a person with a rural background?

An Indigenous perspective

Indigenous Australians – Aboriginal and Torres Strait Islander peoples – say that they have no word in their many languages for 'health' (National Aboriginal Health Strategy Working Party, 1989). They also have a different view from Westerners of what is meant and understood by the word 'health', as it is only one aspect of life. The nearest translation would be a term like 'life is health is life' (National Aboriginal Health Strategy Working Party, 1989). When Aboriginal people have defined the word 'health', they have given much more holistic definitions such as:

> Health is not just the physical well-being of an individual, but refers to the social, emotional, spiritual and cultural well-being of the whole community. This is a whole of life view that includes the cyclical concept of life–death–life.
>
> (NATIONAL ABORIGINAL HEALTH STRATEGY WORKING PARTY, 1989, p. x)

Johnson (1992) found that most Aboriginal groups place heavy emphasis on spiritual aspects, physical appearance, land rights and the absence of alcohol, and relate health to those issues that influence and control their destiny.

> Health to Aboriginal peoples is more a matter of determining all aspects of their lives, including control over their physical environment, dignity, community self-esteem and justice. It is not merely a matter of the provision of doctors, hospitals and medicines or the absence of disease and incapacity.
>
> (NATIONAL ABORIGINAL HEALTH STRATEGY WORKING PARTY, 1989, p. ix)

When we look at this holistic view, it is clear that issues such as Indigenous control over health services are extremely important, since Indigenous Australians work from these definitions of health and provide their health services accordingly.

Houston (2009, p. 104) explains this well: 'culture and identity are central to Aboriginal perceptions of health and ill health. How Aboriginal people view wellness and illness are in part based on their cultural beliefs and values'. This means when Aboriginal people access health services the social interaction surrounding them influences when and why they may or may not accept their treatment, their likelihood of compliance and follow-up and the likely success of prevention and health promotion, as well as their perceptions of the quality of the care provided, the health care providers and personnel (Houston, 2009).

PAUSE AND THINK

Why is it important to understand why different groups have different understandings of health?

What is the relationship between this view of health and community control of health services?

PATIENT-CENTRED CARE

These three different perspectives on the definition of health demonstrate the complexity of developing programs, services and approaches to health care in this diverse and multicultural society. Rural and Indigenous people have their own definitions of health, which differ quite significantly from those used by governments. Governments generally use international definitions of health and wellbeing, as defined by the World Health Organization, and accordingly base their programs on them. This creates a disparity where those who fund health care work base it on different foundations and belief systems from those who are delivering or receiving the services.

PAUSE AND THINK

So, is health a commodity that can be delivered?

If so, how can we deliver health when these three groups are not talking about the same thing?

To be effective, health professionals must work from the world view of the person whose health they are acting upon, whether that is rural, Indigenous or someone from another culture or sexual preference. This care must we well-coordinated and include all those involved in the planning, the delivery and the evaluation of the health care, which is based on mutually beneficial partnerships among health care providers – the doctors, nurses, allied health professionals, the patients and their families (Australian Commission on Safety and Quality in Health Care, 2010). This is called client-centred care or patient-centred care, as the cultural traditions, personal preferences and values of the person and their family are honoured in the decision-making process, and the best evidence is used (Institute for Healthcare Improvement, 2015). It places the patient and their family at the centre of the care, where they are an integral part of the decisions made about their care and are responsible for important aspects of self-care, and gives them the tools and support they need to carry it out. Using a patient-centred approach has been proven to result in increased adherence to care plans, reduced morbidity and improved quality of life for patients, particularly those with chronic illness (World Health Organization, 2005). This is vitally important because of the current growth in care for chronic conditions and the aged.

CASE STUDY

Max is a 55-year-old farmer. He only sees the doctor when something goes wrong and, often, when it is almost too late. It is clear from his notes that Max sees health care as a curative service. Therefore, the doctor or health professional would work from Max's perspective and treat his illness but would also undertake opportunistic health promotion activities while he is there, such as checking his blood pressure, his cholesterol, his PSA, his weight and performing a skin check. The doctor would also talk to him about his smoking and offer a cessation program – this is called a brief intervention. The doctor might also talk to him about how he is managing with the farm in the drought and assess his mental health status, or discuss his diet with Max and his wife, leaving the door open. This is patient-centred care, working from Max's view of health and illness.

CONTEMPORARY VIEWS OF HEALTH

The way we view health in Australia, and indeed in the First World, has changed significantly over the past 30 years. There has been a move away from the hospital with its curative services as the cornerstone of health care, and a push towards a more bottom-up, community-driven process in which people have more control over their own health. These developments have created a shift in thinking whereby Australians now seek more advice from other health professionals, the internet and sources other than their local doctor. They now use complementary medicines far more, and have become more litigious and questioning of their treatment.

With the impact of chronic disease, which can only be controlled not cured, the powerful image of doctors and medicine at the centre of the health care universe in curing diseases, advancing surgical techniques, lowering infant mortality rates and developing new drugs is quickly becoming extinct. These views were found to be an overestimation; conventional medicine was found to account for only 10 per cent of improvements in the health of the population (McMurray, 2003). The other 90 per cent was due to social factors such as lifestyle, improved nutrition, smaller families, social support, better housing, adequate income and education (McMurray, 2003). Despite this, the majority of the annual health budget, estimated to be $140.2 billion between 2011 and 2012, or 9.5 per cent of GDP, continues to be spent on curative services, hospital care, prescription drugs and laboratory tests (Australian Institute of Health and Welfare, 2014). Meanwhile, those things that make better health – the social determinants – are largely not funded from the health budget, as we shall see.

When we think about it we find that, in Australia, we have a bizarre system where the things that very expensive research tells us will affect our health – our income and our level of education – are the responsibility of different government services, such as the Education Department and Centrelink. These government departments have sufficient trouble communicating within their own departments, let alone with other departments, and lip service is often paid to the whole-of-government approach. We then spend 90 per cent of our 'health' money on sickness services, which will only improve the health of Australians by approximately 10 per cent – on a good day. As health professionals we need to be able to focus more of our work on risk factor management, health promotion and behavioural change, as this will bring about improvements in health and positive change. There have been many incidences where a doctor or nurse has advised a patient to stop smoking or lose weight and provides them with tools to do so, and many do. These brief interventions are often the trigger for positive behavioural change.

WHAT MAKES US HEALTHY?

There is a growing body of evidence about what makes people healthy. In 1974 Lalonde set the stage in Canada by establishing a framework for the key factors that seemed to determine how healthy a person would be, or their 'health status'. These included lifestyle, the environment, human biology and health services (Lalonde, 1974). Thinking has progressed further in the past few decades about health and what constitutes it, and how we can measure it and pre-empt problems with it. This has proved to be very useful for health planners and policy makers, who can use this information when planning for future generations. For example, it has been very useful to know that the proportion of Australians 65 years and over is projected to double from around 13 per cent today to 25 per cent by the year 2055, and with enhanced longevity the number of people aged 100 and over is projected to be around 40 000 – well over 300 times the 122 centenarians in 1975 (Australian Government, 2015a). This will have a significant impact on health and aged care services. It has therefore enabled policy makers and planners to re-examine policies for pensions and superannuation schemes, the provision of health care services for the aged, the number of health professionals needed to provide those services and the appropriate infrastructure, such as aged care housing – which are now clearly being articulated in the Australian Government budget.

As this thinking about health changed through a push from international and market forces, so did healthy public policy in Australia. Rather than looking at health from the perspective of illness and disease, we started to look at it from a social perspective and take into consideration those factors that determine whether we will be healthy or not. Then we looked at how, as a nation, we could prevent disease from occurring, and we prioritised Australians' most important health problems and promoted solutions.

Two key initiatives were born from this process, which now feed into all approaches to health care in Australia. The first was the international push, led by Canada in the mid-1970s, to define those factors outside the illness model of health that determine whether we will be healthy or not – the **Social Determinants of Health** (Health Canada, 2011). The second was the push from the Australian Government to determine the nine **National Health Priority Areas** for the Australian population – those diseases and conditions that significantly contribute to the burden of illness and injury in the Australian population (Australian Institute of Health and Welfare, 2015).

Health indicators

There are three main indicators used to measure the health status of a population:

1   life expectancy and mortality (death rates)
2   causes of death
3   morbidity (disease and impairment rates).

These health indicators form the basis of most health information collected. They are used to make health decisions. They also form the basis for determining the National Health Priorities for Australia.

There are two additional measures that are of relevance to rural and remote populations. The first is what is called excess mortality, which is a measure of the number of extra deaths among rural and remote populations if they were compared with urban populations (National Rural Health Alliance, 2011). The second is what is called the burden of disease, which is an estimate of the total amount of illness and injury experienced nationally – it is often measured in years of life lost due to premature death or disability (Australian Institute of Health and Welfare, 2014; National Rural Health Alliance, 2011). For example, in 2010 chronic disease accounted for 85 per cent of the total burden of disease in Australia. Hence, doing something about those factors that cause chronic disease and prevent it would be the best place for policy makers to place their bucks (Australian Institute of Health and Welfare, 2014). However, in the 2014 federal budget the only Australian National Health Preventative Agency, whose role it was to coordinate preventative activities in Australia, was closed.

National health priority areas

The National Health Priority Areas focus on the diseases and conditions that cause the highest morbidity and mortality in the Australian population. These include those chronic diseases that pose a *significant health burden* and those conditions that have potential for health gains and improved outcomes for Australians. In 2015 these were: cancer, cardiovascular disease, injury prevention and control, mental health, asthma, diabetes, arthritis and musculoskeletal conditions, obesity (since 2008) and dementia (since 2012) (see Chapter 9 for an example of how the National Health Priority Areas apply to the health of rural Australians).

In 2005 the Australian Government developed a National Chronic Disease Strategy that provides an overarching framework of national direction for improving chronic disease prevention and care across Australia (National Health Priority Action Council, 2006). It focuses on similar diseases listed in the then national health priorities, though in a more pragmatic way, to encourage a coordinated system-wide action in response to the growing impact of chronic disease on the health of Australians. As we know that chronic disease causes 85 per cent of the burden of disease in Australia, this is an important document (Australian Institute of Health and Welfare, 2014).

THE DETERMINANTS OF HEALTH

So what else determines whether we will be healthy or not? The second key initiative includes addressing those factors that we have little control over, such as our gender, culture and genetic makeup, plus the social factors that can impact upon our health.

1   **Gender** – being male or female determines our predisposition towards certain diseases, our longevity and our relative power in society through our roles, attitudes, behaviours and values that are determined by society (Health Canada, 2011). Attitudes to health also differ between the sexes. For example, to lose weight men are more likely to increase their physical activity as an important healthy behaviour, whereas women tend to focus more on social, environmental and dietary changes (Australian Institute of Health and Welfare, 2014). These gender factors contribute towards determining our health status and programs that might best suit particular groups.

2   **Culture** – a person's culture can contribute to their knowledge, attitudes and belief systems, which influence their health behaviours, such as diet and exercise, and their health status. Culture also contributes towards marginalisation of some groups, stigmatisation and devaluation of their language. These factors can be exacerbated by lack of access to culturally appropriate health care services (Houston, 2009). This is one reason why indigenous groups worldwide prefer community-controlled health services, as indigenous people manage them and work from indigenous understandings of health and wellness.

3   **Genetic makeup** – the basic biology of the human body and our own genetic makeup predispose us to particular diseases or health problems, such as diabetes or haemophilia. Some diseases, such as muscular dystrophy, result entirely from a person's genetic makeup. There is now strong evidence regarding the early origins of chronic disease. Researchers have identified the links between undernutrition and poor foetal growth during pregnancy that can predict the development of hypertension, diabetes, renal disease, hyperlipidemia, 'syndrome X' and

mortality from cardiovascular disease and chronic lung disease in adulthood (Smith, 2006). This is known as the 'Barker hypothesis' – namely, the environmental factors that 'program' particular body systems during critical periods of growth – *in utero* and during infancy – with long-term direct consequences for adult chronic disease (Barker, 1995; Weeramanthri et al., 2003).

4   **Social determinants** – the social determinants of health make up those 'social factors' that can also affect our health, such as our income, diet, level of education, environment and level of social support, and whether we choose to smoke, have 10 children or work in stressful conditions (Wilkinson & Marmot, 2003). Each of these factors is important in its own right. At the same time, they are also interrelated.

For example, if a mother is a smoker, evidence suggests that she is more likely to come from a lower socioeconomic group, that she probably has a lower level of education and that she is more likely to have a child with a low birth weight, which may lead to health problems during childhood and adulthood. Research shows a strong relationship between: 1) the income level of the mother and the baby's birth weight and 2) the mother's level of coping skills and her sense of control over her own life circumstances (Labonte, 1998). Adding these factors to her genetic makeup, culture, level of education and environmental conditions will determine the future health status of the child. We also know that every additional year of education for the mother improves her health literacy and results in better health status for her child (Health Canada, 2011; McMurray, 2003). Therefore, 'educate a woman – educate a nation'.

Figure 8.1 demonstrates the social determinants of health. It includes those factors that we do not have any power over, such as our gender, our biology and our culture,

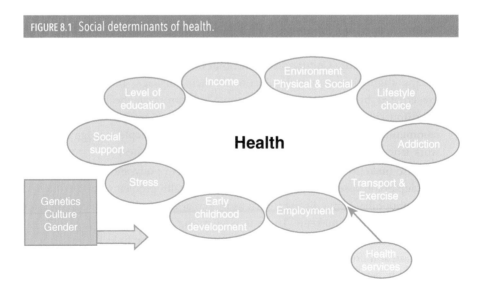

FIGURE 8.1 Social determinants of health.

as well as those factors that we do have power over, such as our income, our level of education and our physical environment including our housing. Note that health care services, which have approximately a 10 per cent impact on health, sit outside this circle as they are affected by our income and our access to health services, which could be due to rurality and private health insurance cover.

DETERMINING INDIGENOUS AUSTRALIANS' HEALTH

The following links the social determinants of health with the health of Indigenous Australians to demonstrate the impact these determinants have on their health.

1   **Income and social status** – income is the most important social determinant of health as it affects all aspects of our lives – our ability to feed our children and live in a good house and the degree to which we feel good about ourselves. Health status improves with each step up the income and social hierarchy (Health Canada, 2013). Being poor means running twice the risk of serious illness and premature death (Australian Institute of Health and Welfare, 2014). There is strong evidence that higher social and economic status is one of the most important determinants of health (Health Canada, 2013). This means that being rich means you will probably live longer and healthier than if you are poor.

    In remote Indigenous Australia many live below the poverty line, receiving a mean income that is 59 per cent that of other Australians (Australian Institute of Health and Welfare, 2014). Some 85 per cent of the remote population live in rented housing, and they pay almost twice the price for their food and have three times the unemployment rate of other Australians (Australian Bureau of Statistics, 2010; 2014a).

2   **Education** – is directly related to employment and income, which in turn affect housing, nutrition and health. Education provides people with skills to access health information; it also assists with problem-solving through improving their health literacy and helps give them a sense of control over their life circumstances (Health Canada, 2013).

    Indigenous Australians in rural and remote areas have much less access to sound educational opportunities, especially in their secondary and tertiary years, unless they are prepared to go to boarding school. Yet the 2015 Prime Minister's Close the Gap Report indicates that there was no overall improvement in Indigenous reading and numeracy in the previous decade and progress was not on track (Australian Government, 2015b).

3   **Social support networks** – support from families, friends and communities helps people solve problems, deal with adversity and maintain a sense of mastery and control over their life circumstances (Health Canada, 2013). The caring and respect that occurs in social relationships seem to act as a buffer against health problems (Health Canada, 2013). Indigenous Australians often have very strong social support and family networks. These social networks have a powerful protective effect on their health because they make people feel cared for, loved,

respected and valued (Wilkinson & Marmot, 2003). However, decades of discriminatory policies and practices have created distrust and have resulted in a fracturing of knowledge lines, some family support structures, traditional laws and customs as well as loss of language and social roles.

4   **Stress** – social and psychological circumstances can cause long-term stress. Continuing anxiety, insecurity, low self-esteem, social isolation and lack of control over work and home life have a powerful effect on health (Wilkinson & Marmot, 2003). The biological stress response can cause depression, susceptibility to infection, diabetes, high blood pressure and the risk of heart attack or stroke (Wilkinson & Marmot, 2003).

Indigenous Australians were dispossessed of their land and traditions; thousands were stolen as children and suffer an enormous burden of disease, low self-esteem, lack of control over their lives, enduring discrimination, high detention rates and traumatisation as a result (Human Rights and Equal Opportunity Commission, 1997). These factors accumulate during life and increase the chances of poor mental health, suicide and premature death, cardiovascular disease, hypertension and diabetes, all of which are much higher in the Indigenous population (Australian Institute of Health and Welfare, 2014).

5   **Early childhood development** – the important foundations of adulthood are laid in prenatal life and early childhood (Wilkinson & Marmot, 2003). Poor maternal diet, smoking and parental poverty can reduce prenatal and infant development. Slow early growth is associated with reduced renal, respiratory and cardiovascular functioning (Wilkinson & Marmot, 2003). Indigenous Australians have a higher incidence of premature births and low birth weight babies, and a higher incidence of hearing problems, slower early growth, malnutrition, juvenile diabetes and communicable disease in early life (Australian Bureau of Statistics & Australian Institute of Health and Welfare, 2005). In rural areas Indigenous women have a higher incidence of smoking and poverty, and poorer access to prenatal care and nutritious food (Australian Bureau of Statistics, 2014c). These factors during early life raise the risk of poor physical health and reduce physical, cognitive and emotional functioning in adulthood (Wilkinson & Marmot, 2003).

6   **Employment and work conditions** – unemployment, stressful or unsafe work and underemployment are associated with poorer health (Health Canada, 2013). Healthier people have more control over their work and often live longer than those in more stressful or riskier work situations. Having less control over one's work is associated with low back pain and cardiovascular disease (Wilkinson & Marmot, 2003).

The unemployment rate of Indigenous Australians is about 17.2 per cent – three times the national average of 5.5 per cent (Australian Bureau of Statistics, 2014b). The 2018 Closing the Gap target of halving the gap in employment for Indigenous Australians is not on track and has not improved in the past decade (Australian Government, 2015b). Those in remote areas have much less access to employment due to distance, lack of opportunities and low levels of education, and most work for the dole program. Lack of employment perpetuates the cycle of poverty and limits access to food, housing and education, resulting in a lack of control over one's life circumstances and higher stress levels. These factors, in turn, increase the risks of premature death and cardiovascular disease (Wilkinson & Marmot, 2003), which are higher in the Indigenous population (Australian Bureau of Statistics & Australian Institute of Health and Welfare 2005).

7 **Addiction** – alcohol dependence, illicit drug use and cigarette smoking are all closely associated with markers of social and economic disadvantage and worsening inequalities in health (Wilkinson & Marmot, 2003). Indigenous people are less likely to drink alcohol than non-Indigenous people; however, of those who do drink, they are more inclined to drink to dangerous levels (Australian Indigenous HealthInfoNet, 2014). Forty-one per cent of Indigenous Australians aged 15 years and over smoke on a daily basis, which is double the non-Indigenous rate (Australian Bureau of Statistics, 2014c). This rate is significantly higher among those in remote areas where 50 per cent of Indigenous people smoke compared with 38 per cent in non-remote areas, which is attributed to the significantly higher incidence in young Indigenous people (Australian Bureau of Statistics, 2014c).

8 **Physical environment – housing, food, air, water** – access to good affordable food makes more difference to what people eat than health education. People on low incomes – the elderly and unemployed – are least able to eat well (Wilkinson & Marmot, 2003). Factors related to housing, and the design of communities, can significantly affect physical and psychological wellbeing. Waste disposal, clean water and access to a shower and healthy sewerage systems help prevent disease (Healthhabitat, 2015b). Remote Indigenous community houses are affected by considerable issues including overcrowding, poor maintenance, unreliable electricity supply, inadequate access to clean water and problems with functioning sewerage and waste disposal systems (Healthhabitat, 2015b).

9 **Transport and exercise** – healthy transport means less driving, more walking or cycling, backed by better public transport; it also reduces pollution and increases social contact with others (Wilkinson & Marmot, 2003). Rural and remote people exercise less than those in the city (Australian Institute of Health and Welfare, 2014). They have much less access to services and often need to travel great distances for basic supplies, health services and education facilities. Indigenous Australians use health transport services five times more frequently than other Australians (Australian Bureau of Statistics & Australian Institute of Health and Welfare, 2005). In 2013, 62 per cent of Indigenous adults reported being physically inactive (Australian Indigenous HealthInfoNet, 2014). Exercise is strongly linked with obesity, which causes diabetes and cardiovascular disease, which are of much higher incidence in the Indigenous population (Australian Indigenous HealthInfoNet, 2014).

10 **Lifestyle choices and coping skills** – our lifestyle choices can prevent disease and help us cope with challenges, solve problems and make choices that enhance health and develop self-reliance (Health Canada, 2013). These may not just be our individual choices, but also the influences of social, economic and environmental factors on the decisions people make about their health. These can include 'personal life skills, stress, culture, social relationships and belonging, and a sense of control' (Health Canada, 2013).

You can see from the above comparison between the social determinants of health and the health of rural and remote Indigenous peoples that, on every determinant, Indigenous Australians are much worse off – occupying the lowest rung on the health care ladder. Another factor we need to consider here is the history of colonisation and the impact it has had on health, to better understand it.

Australian colonial determinants of health

Another viewpoint is found in what are called the colonial determinants of health, which particularly pertain to Indigenous peoples worldwide – those who have been colonised. The poor state of Indigenous health is widely attributed to colonisation and its ongoing manifestations such as racism (Kowal & Paradies, 2005). In Australia, Indigenous health is a highly politicised and contested arena. Ramsden (2002) calls this lower standard of health, educational achievement and socioeconomic status 'normalised, obvious, and grossly unfair', yet it has been this way for many generations. Therefore the 'colonial determinants of health' could be described as the 'cause and the effect' of the colonisation process.

The 2005 Social Justice Report draws out the relationship between the common socioeconomic and environmental factors that affect poor Indigenous health in Australia (Human Rights and Equal Opportunity Commission, 2005). These social determinants of health include:

- how poor education and literacy are linked to poor health status – they affect the capacity of people to use and find information about their health
- how having a lesser income reduces the accessibility of health care services and medicines
- how overcrowded and run-down housing is associated with poverty and contributes to the spread of communicable diseases
- how poor infant diet is associated with poverty and chronic diseases later in life
- how smoking and high-risk behaviour are associated with lower socioeconomic status.

The colonial determinants of health provide recognition that colonisation has caused many of the poor health indicators linked to lifestyle and socioeconomic status, and that these are associated with historical and present experiences of Australia's Indigenous peoples (Human Rights and Equal Opportunity Commission, 2005).

Now let us look at one determinant that affects health – our physical environment. Paul Pholeros, an architect, and Paul Torzillo, a doctor from Healthhabitat, have worked for several decades to improve the physical environments of people living in poverty in some of the poorest, most remote parts of the world, especially remote Australia. They work on those areas that most of us take for granted such as having clean water, a running shower, working taps and electrics, healthy sewerage systems, areas to prepare and cook food and appropriate architecture that reduces overcrowding (Healthhabitat, 2015a). An important part of their work is that they employ local people and train them to undertake the work, though this has recently been stopped by government in Australia. Over the years they found that, in remote Australia, only 35 per cent of houses had a working shower, 10 per cent had safe electrics and 18 per cent could remove waste water; and 70 per cent of necessary maintenance was routine maintenance, 21 per cent was due to faults and poor construction and only 9 per cent was due to resident damage (Healthhabitat, 2015b). We know that being able to have a shower every day is important for our skin, our wellbeing and our health, especially where people live in overcrowded conditions, surrounded by dogs in hot

Presentation link from Paul Pholeros. Video access through Student Consult.

desert or tropical conditions. So, having a daily shower will have more impact upon the health of the people than anything we can do as health professionals to fix skin sores or provide medication. We need 'upstream' models of care where illness is prevented in the first place – see Chapter 10.

THE CYCLE OF POVERTY

Research tells us that to be poor means means also to be unhealthy (World Health Organization, 2007). Poverty is linked with all aspects of people's lives. It is linked with our ability to access a good education, which affects our ability to find a good job, which affects the type of housing we can live in and the quality of food we can put on the table for our children. Being unemployed does not make us feel good about ourselves – it does not allow us to have 'real control' over our lives. This often makes us depressed, and we drink more alcohol and smoke more in order to feel momentarily happy. We then worry about how we are going to pay the mortgage and feed our kids – this in turn affects our family relationships and our social support systems and restricts what we can do socially. This whole process of being unemployed becomes a vicious cycle that places us in a certain social class – the 'unemployed'. And this can turn into the 'cycle of poverty', which can be passed down from generation to generation, because we know nothing different (see Figure 8.2). What this basically means for our health is that, 'if you are rich, you will live longer and be healthier than if you are poor'.

Now let us add two more contributing factors to this cycle of poverty. The first is geographical location. The second is culture, which is compounded by issues such as racism. They are the two things that differentiate Indigenous and rural Australians

FIGURE 8.2 Cycle of poverty.

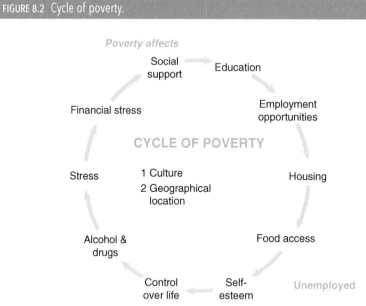

from the rest of Australian society. When we combine these two factors with the social determinants of health they form what might be called the 'triple whammy' – Indigeneity, remoteness and the social determinants of health.

CONCLUSION

The way we define health differs for different groups and different cultures. Rural people view their health as the absence of disease and their ability to be productive, which is evidenced in their behaviours. They present later for treatment and consequently have poorer health outcomes than city-dwelling Australians, as they see health services as curative services. Indigenous Australians also view their health differently from other Australians. They see health holistically – as including the social, emotional, spiritual and cultural wellbeing of the whole community –and place heavy emphasis on the land, dignity and community self-esteem (National Aboriginal Health Strategy Working Party Evaluation Committee, 1994). Nevertheless, they also come off second best when we compare their health with all the social determinants of health. These factors all increase with geographical remoteness.

It is of concern that government-funded health services use and are based on international definitions of health, not these definitions used by Australian rural and Indigenous peoples. These factors contribute significantly to the way in which health services are provided to rural, remote and Indigenous communities, yet they work from different foundations and value systems. Hence, many health promotion initiatives are not taken up, or are rejected by, rural and Indigenous people as they are inappropriate and the cycle of ill health continues.

We know that more doctors, nurses and hospitals do not make better health; they only provide health services and infrastructure, which contribute only 10 per cent towards health outcomes (McMurray, 2003). Nonetheless, rural health dollars are largely spent on providing workforce incentives and running innovative programs for health professionals rather than on those factors that make for better health, such as access to education, nutritious food, adequate income, control over one's life, clean water and suitable housing. Additionally, the key factors that make for better health are funded from other government departments – housing, education and employment – outside the health department. A lack of coordination exists between the Commonwealth, state and regional health departments. Therefore, attempts to impact upon these other departments compound the problem.

To find a way forward it is necessary to develop a national approach, based on the social determinants of health, which views health from a social and economic justice perspective and incorporates health promotion and behaviour change. And, while this is being mooted in the background of health (Social Determinants of Health Alliance, 2015), we need to look to other countries that use the social

Discussion Points

1   Develop your own definition of health. Does your definition fit into the international, rural or Indigenous definitions found in this chapter? Discuss.

2   How can the rural definition of health affect rural people's health outcomes?

3   When working with rural people, what other factors might you need to consider in their long-term care? Discuss.

4   Think of a patient in your care. Do you take a social history? Using the social determinants of health as a guide, write down the factors that you know about them – their level of education, income, social support and so on.

   - What factors are missing?

   - Discuss how you would have changed the care you provided as a result of knowing about these factors.

   - Discuss the concept of patient-centred care.

   - How does the explanation of patient-centred care fit with the care you provide to this patient?

   - Discuss the issues that you would need to consider to change your practice into a patient-centred approach.

   - Using the cycle of poverty as a guide, what impact has this patient's socioeconomic status had on their health? Discuss.

determinants as the basis for organising their health care systems and ensure that government departments collaborate with each other to bring about change. This will assist in reducing the gap that exists between research, policy development and implementation at the local level. This may then reassure Australians, irrespective of their culture or geographical location, that they can reach retirement age in good health.

References

Australian Bureau of Statistics (ABS). (2010). 4714.0 – *National Aboriginal and Torres Strait Islander social survey, 2008*. Canberra: ABS. <http://www.abs.gov.au/AUSSTATS/abs@.nsf/ Latestproducts/4714.0Main%20Features102008?opendocument&tabname=Summary &prodno=4714.0&issue=2008&num=&view#PARALINK1> Accessed 27.07.15.

Australian Bureau of Statistics. (2014a). *Estimates and projections, Aboriginal and Torres Strait Islander Australians, 2001 to 2026*. Canberra: ABS. <http://www.abs.gov.au/ AUSSTATS/abs@.nsf/DetailsPage/3238.02001%20to%202026> Accessed 03.03.15.

Australian Bureau of Statistics. (2014b). 4102.0 – *Australian social trends, November 2013*. Canberra: ABS. <http://www.abs.gov.au/ausstats/abs@.nsf/Lookup/4102.0Main +Features20Nov+2013#PARTICIPATIONANDUNEMPLOYMENT> Accessed 27.07.15.

Australian Bureau of Statistics. (2014c). 4727.0.55.001 – *Australian Aboriginal and Torres Strait Islander health survey: First results, Australia, 2012–13*. Canberra: ABS. <http:// www.abs.gov.au/ausstats/abs@.nsf/Lookup/39E15DC7E770A144CA257C2F00145A66 ?opendocument> Accessed 27.07.15.

Australian Bureau of Statistics & Australian Institute of Health and Welfare. (2005). *The health and welfare of Australia's Aboriginal and Torres Strait Islander peoples*, 4704.0. Canberra: ABS & AIHW.

Australian Commission on Safety and Quality in Health Care (ACSQHC). (2010). *Patient -centred care: Improving quality and safety by focussing care on patients and consumers*. Canberra: ACSQHC.

Australian Concise Oxford Dictionary. (2000). *The Australian concise Oxford dictionary* (3rd ed.). Melbourne: Oxford University Press.

Australian Government. (2015a). *2015 Intergenerational report: Australia in 2055*. Canberra: Australian Government.

Australian Government. (2015b). *Closing the Gap Prime Minister's report 2015*. Canberra: Department of the Prime Minister and Cabinet, Australian Government.

Australian Indigenous HealthInfoNet. (2014). *Overview of Australian Indigenous health status, 2013*. Perth: Australian Indigenous HealthInfoNet, Edith Cowan University. <http:// www.healthinfonet.ecu.edu.au/uploads/docs/overview_of_indigenous_health_2013.pdf> Accessed 27.07.15.

Australian Institute of Health and Welfare (AIHW). (2014). *Australia's health 2014*. Canberra: AIHW.

Australian Institute of Health and Welfare. (2015). *National health priority areas*. Canberra: AIHW. <http://www.aihw.gov.au/national-health-priority-areas/> Accessed 16.05.15.

Barker, D. (1995). Fetal origins of coronary heart disease. *British Medical Journal*, 311, 171–174.

Dempsey, K. (1990). *Smalltown: A study of social inequality, cohesion and belonging*. Melbourne: Oxford University Press.

Elliott-Schmidt, R., & Strong, J. (1997). The concept of well-being in a rural setting: understanding health and illnesses. *Australian Journal of Rural Health*, 5, 59–63.

Health Canada. (2011). *Population health approach: What determines health*. Ottawa: Public Health Agency of Canada. <http://www.phac-aspc.gc.ca/ph-sp/determinants/index-eng.php> Accessed 27.07.15.

Health Canada. (2013). *What makes Canadians healthy and unhealthy?* Montreal: Public Health Agency of Canada. <http://www.phac-aspc.gc.ca/ph-sp/determinants/determinants -eng.php#income> Accessed 27.07.15.

Healthhabitat. (2015a). *The healthy living practices: Safety and the nine healthy living practices*. Sydney: Healthhabitat. <http://www.healthabitat.com/what-we-do/the-healthy -living-practices-hlps> Accessed 19.05.15.

Healthhabitat. (2015b). *Housing for health guide*. Sydney: Healthhabitat. <http://www .housingforhealth.com/about/> Accessed 27.07.15.

Houston, S. (2009). Cultural security as a determinant of Aboriginal health. In H. Keleher & C. McDougall (Eds.), *Understanding health*. Melbourne: Oxford University Press.

Human Rights and Equal Opportunity Commission (HREOC). (1997). *Bringing them home report: Report of the national inquiry into the separation of Aboriginal and Torres Strait Islander children from their families*. Canberra: HREOC.

Human Rights and Equal Opportunity Commission. (2005). *Social justice report 2005*. Sydney: HREOC.

Institute for Healthcare Improvement (IHI). (2015). *Person and family centred care*. Cambridge USA: IHI. <http://www.ihi.org/Topics/PFCC/Pages/Overview.aspx> Accessed 18.05.15.

Johnson, S. (1992). Aboriginal health through primary health care. In R. Pratt (Ed.), *Issues in Australian Nursing 3* (3rd ed., pp. 151–170). South Melbourne: Churchill Livingstone.

Keleher, H., & McDougall, C. (Eds.), (2009). *Understanding health*. Sydney: Oxford University Press.

Kowal, E., & Paradies, Y. (2005). Ambivalent helpers and unhealthy choices: public health practitioners' narratives of Indigenous ill-health. *Social Science & Medicine*, 60, 1347–1357.

Labonte, R. (1998). *Changing cultures within health care systems: an international perspective*. Paper presented at the Cultures in Caring: 4th Biennial Australian Rural and Remote Health Scientific Conference, Toowoomba, Qld.

Lalonde, M. (1974). *A new perspective on the health of Canadians: A working document* (pp. 1–75). Ottawa: Government of Canada.

McMurray, A. (2003). *Community health and wellness: A sociological approach* (2nd ed.). Marrickville NSW: Mosby.

National Aboriginal Health Strategy Working Party. (1989). *National Aboriginal health strategy*. Canberra: Commonwealth of Australia, Australian Government Printing Service.

National Aboriginal Health Strategy Working Party Evaluation Committee. (1994). *The national Aboriginal health strategy: An evaluation* (pp. 1–78). Canberra: Aboriginal and Torres Strait Islander Commission.

National Health Priority Action Council (NHPAC). (2006). *National chronic disease strategy*. Canberra: NHPAC, Australian Government Department of Health and Ageing.

National Rural Health Alliance (NRHA). (2011). *Fact Sheet: The determinants of health in rural and remote Australia*. Canberra: NRHA. <http://ruralhealth.org.au/sites/default/files/ publications/factsheet-determinants-health-rural-australia.pdf> Accessed 27.07.15.

Ramsden, I. (2002). *Cultural safety and nursing education in Aotearoa and Te Waipounamu.* Wellington: Victoria University.

Smith, J. D. (2006). *Educating to improve population health outcomes in chronic disease* (2nd ed.). Darwin: Menzies School of Health Research.

Social Determinants of Health Alliance (SDHA). (2015). *The social determinants of health alliance.* Canberra: SDHA. <http://www.socialdeterminants.org.au/> Accessed 19.05.15.

Strasser, R., Hays, R., Kamien, M., & Carson, D. (2000). Is Australian rural practice changing? Findings from the national rural general practice study. *Australian Journal of Rural Health*, 8, 222–226.

Strong, K., Trickett, P., Titulaer, I., & Bhatia, K. (1998). *Health in rural and remote Australia: The first report of the Australian Institute of Health and Welfare on rural health*, Cat No PHE 6 (pp. 1–131). Canberra: Australian Institute of Health and Welfare.

Weeramanthri, T., Hendy, S., Connors, C., Ashbridge, D., Rae, C., Dunn, M., et al. (2003). The Northern Territory preventable chronic disease strategy: promoting an integrated and life course approach to chronic disease in Australia. *Australian Health Review*, 26(3), 31–42.

Welch, N. (2000). *Toward an understanding of the determinants of rural health* (pp. 1–9). Canberra: National Rural Health Alliance.

Wilkinson, R., & Marmot, M. (Eds.), (2003). *Social determinants of health: The solid facts* (2nd ed.). Geneva: World Health Organization. <http://www.euro.who.int/document/e81384.pdf> Accessed 27.07.15.

World Health Organization (WHO). (1986). *Ottawa charter for health promotion.* Paper presented at the 1st International Conference on Health Promotion, Ottawa, Canada. Geneva: WHO.

World Health Organization. (2005). *Preventing chronic diseases: A vital investment.* Geneva: WHO. <http://www.who.int/chp/chronic_disease_report/full_report.pdf> Accessed 27.07.15.

World Health Organization. (2007). *Everybody's business: Strengthening health systems to improve health outcomes, WHO's framework for action.* Geneva: WHO.

CHAPTER 9

RURAL PEOPLE'S HEALTH

Janie Dade Smith

Mologa
What became of the bakery,
the Mechanics Hall,
where fiddlers played
farm families danced
and kids skidded on the floor?
The general store, with yarns on the step,
a school house, where ponies drowsed till
the door flew open like a hen-house coop
as the clock on the wall struck four.
Dusty roads, dry creek beds,
sere paddocks where harsh boxthorn
sports its berries and vicious spikes,
and the country folk we knew have long departed.

(JEAN RINGLAND, 2005)

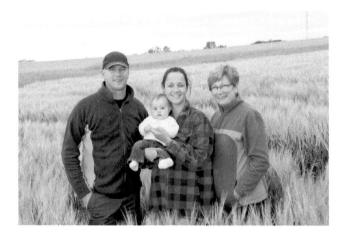

Reproduced with permission from: iStockphoto/Living Images.

HEALTHY AUSTRALIANS

Australians are one of the healthiest groups of people in the world. We enjoy a life expectancy for men that is the third highest in the world after Iceland and Switzerland. Australian women have a life expectancy of 84.3 years and men can expect to live to 80 years (Australian Institute of Health and Welfare, 2014c). The number of Australians who are 65 years and older is projected to double by the year 2055, with an escalating number of centenarians from approximately 5000 in 2015 to 40 000 by 2055 (Australian Government, 2015). There is also a trend among these ageing populations to retire to regional and coastal areas in search of cleaner air, fresher food and a healthier lifestyle. Australians can therefore generally expect to live out their long and healthy lives walking by the seaside and carrying their thongs in their hands. However, not all members of the Australian community can have this expectation.

Many inequalities exist, depending upon where we choose to live and our cultural grouping. Those who have lived their lives in rural areas die about four years younger than other Australians, and this increases with greater remoteness and lower socio-economic status (Australian Bureau of Statistics, 2011a). When we add Indigenous to the equation this increases dramatically. Consequently, the average remotely living

---

PAUSE AND THINK

Why are rural and remote Australians dying younger than their city counterparts?

Why are Indigenous Australians dying a decade younger than other Australians?

Why does the area where we live and our cultural grouping have such an impact upon our health?

Indigenous Australian may never reach the age of retirement, nor draw on their superannuation, as old age is considered to start at about 45 years.

In this chapter I will examine the health status of rural Australians, using data mainly from the Australian Bureau of Statistics and the Australian Institute of Health and Welfare. I will then draw out the marked inequalities by comparing the health status of rural Australians with the National Health Priorities for Australia. It should be noted that the first report on the health of rural and remote Australians was only produced in 1998 (Strong, Trickett, Titulaer, & Bhatia), and few national rural-specific reports have been produced since that time, apart from those found on state government websites. Hence, it is difficult to draw a national picture.

THE HEALTH OF RURAL AUSTRALIANS

When imagining rural Australians one automatically thinks of a farmer or, these days, a miner. However, most workers in rural and remote Australia are in the retail, health, education, government, manufacturing, processing and transport sectors (Phillips, 2009). They make up about seven million people or about 31 per cent of the overall Australian population, when we include those in outer regional, remote and very remote communities (Australian Institute of Health and Welfare, 2014b). And while some live on farms most live in regional cities and rural towns.

The current picture of a rural Australian is typically someone who is overweight, more likely to smoke and drink alcohol, has high blood cholesterol and who is not very active (Phillips, 2009). These rural Australians have unique health concerns that relate directly to their living conditions, social isolation, socioeconomic disadvantage and distance from health services. They have neonatal death rates that are double the urban rate, four times the death rate due to injury and road accidents, and double the death rates due to diabetes (National Rural Health Alliance, 2011; Australian Institute of Health and Welfare, 2014b). Yet rural people have poorer access to health care compared with their metropolitan counterparts because of distance, time factors, costs and transport availability. This is compounded by shortages of health facilities and health professionals, and rural people's perceptions of health. Figure 9.1 describes the significant differences in death rates by remoteness.

THE TRIPLE WHAMMY

There are three major factors that impact upon a person's health – their age, their culture and their geographical location. When we add the three together it is like the 'triple whammy', as we will see in the following section.

PAUSE AND THINK

What does it mean for rural Australians when we put these three factors together?

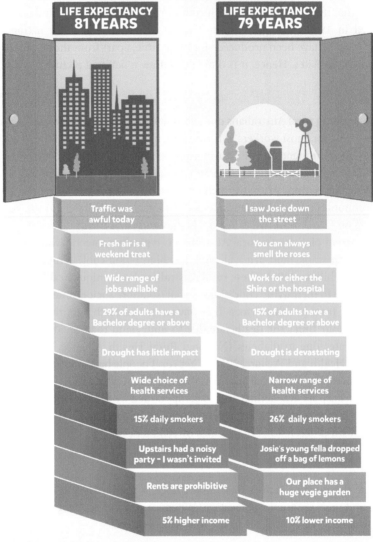

Discover all the facts at www.ruralhealth.org.au/factsheets

Adapted with permission from: National Rural Health Alliance. <http://www.ruralhealth.org.au/content/spot-your-community>.

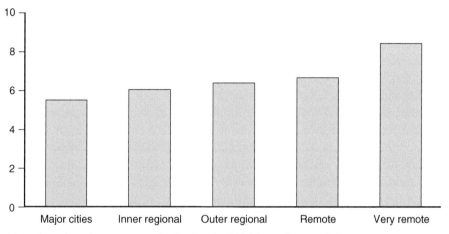

FIGURE 9.1 Age standardised death rates by remoteness area, 2012.

Deaths per 1,000 population

Note: Rates have been age-standardised to the 2001 Australian population.

Adapted with permission from: Australian Institute of Health and Welfare. (2015). *Australia's health, health behaviours and other risks to health*. <http://www.aihw.gov.au/australias-health/2014/health -behaviours/#t6>.

Age discrimination
Older people

Australia's population generally is ageing. Just over half of those who are over 65 years of age have some form of chronic disease or disability. Older people are less likely to live in major cities, though the two-thirds who do experience a longer life expectancy than those who live rurally (Australian Institute of Health and Welfare & Department of Health and Ageing, 2007). The remaining third of Australia's older population have taken a sea change or tree change. About a quarter live in inner regional areas and 11 per cent live in outer regional areas. The remaining 2 per cent live in remote and very remote areas (Australian Institute of Health and Welfare & Department of Health and Ageing, 2007). This varies by state and region with just over 17 per cent of all older Australians living in Tasmania and only 6 per cent living in the Northern Territory (Australian Institute of Health and Welfare, 2014b). On the mid-north coast of New South Wales one-quarter of the population are over 65 years of age; hence there is a greater need for aged care services in that region. However, there is some anecdotal evidence that many are moving back to the city of Canberra in their 70s as their health care needs change. Additionally, dementia is now seen as a national health priority due to its increased incidence (Australian Institute of Health and Welfare, 2015a).

Young people

Lower health status also discriminates for young rural people. Infant mortality rates in remote centres are double those found in city areas and 3–5 times the rate for very remote areas (Australian Bureau of Statistics, 2011c). Young rural and remote people aged between 12 and 24 years also have considerably worse health compared to their city counterparts. The death rates of young rural and remote people are double the urban rates and injury rates are 3 times the national rate (National Rural Health Alliance, 2011). The rates for hospital separations for transport accidents were 3.2 times higher and the rates for assault were 5.7 times higher for remote areas (Australian Institute of Health and Welfare, 2011). Rural and remote young people are more likely to experience violence, have higher rates of alcohol and substance abuse, are less likely to meet the minimum standards for reading, writing and numeracy, are more likely to have dental decay and are less likely to access a GP (Australian Institute of Health and Welfare, 2011). The leading cause of death for young Indigenous people is suicide, which is 4–6 times the non-Indigenous rate, and the assault rate is 6 times the non-Indigenous rate (Australian Institute of Health and Welfare, 2011). Same sex attracted young people in rural and remote areas experience much higher rates of isolation, discrimination and suicide (Rosenstreich, 2013). All of these factors multiply with socioeconomic disadvantage and remoteness.

An important factor, which we must examine here, is the age structure of Australia's youth due to the links between age and culture in rural and remote communities. In 2009 there were four million young people in Australia and they represented 20 per cent of the total Australian population (Australian Institute of Health and Welfare, 2011). Of these young people, a little over 3 per cent were Indigenous. These 3 per cent, however, make up 27 per cent of the total Australian Indigenous population, which has a much younger age profile generally (Australian Institute of Health and Welfare, 2011). Health factors such as obesity incidence have a greater impact upon this population group. What this means is that, when resources are distributed and programs are developed for Australia's young people, governments need to consider the much higher young Indigenous population and develop programs based on the age and cultural distribution that target these groups, and not apply the urban models to remote Indigenous populations.

Figure 9.2 demonstrates the age structure and population distribution between Indigenous and non-Indigenous Australians. It illustrates the much higher proportions of Indigenous babies, children and young people, and the much lower population of Indigenous older people.

Cultural discrimination

Health status also discriminates according to culture. Indigenous Australians have the worst health status in this country, and on some health indicators they rank worst in the world (Australian Institute of Health and Welfare, 2014a). The life expectancy of an Indigenous boy born in 2011 was 69 years and 73 years for an Indigenous girl,

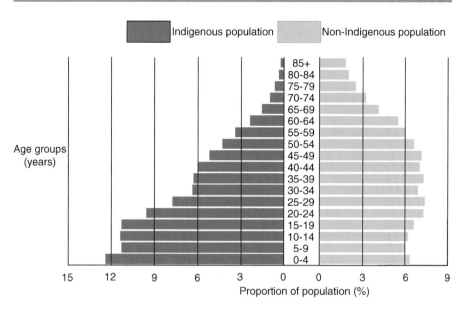

FIGURE 9.2 Population pyramid of Indigenous and non-Indigenous populations, 2011.

Adapted with permission from: Australian Bureau of Statistics. (2012). *Australian demographic statistics, March quarter 2012.* Canberra: ABS. <http://www.healthinfonet.ecu.edu.au/health-facts/health-faqs/aboriginal-population>.

which is about 11 years less than non-Indigenous Australians, hence the lower number of older people seen in Figure 9.2 (Australian Institute of Health and Welfare, 2014b).

On almost every indicator, Indigenous Australians are disadvantaged compared with all Australians. The largest differences are in smoking status, psychological distress and cardiovascular conditions, which affect one in eight (Australian Institute of Health and Welfare, 2014a). Infant mortality rates are double the non-Indigenous rate; ischaemic heart disease is double for men and four times higher for women; and the incidence of diabetes doubles with remoteness, and is up to 30 per cent of the population in some remote communities (Australian Institute of Health and Welfare, 2014b). While recent research indicates some improvement in health status, there are significant state differences, and evidence of improved health outcomes was found where systematic chronic disease monitoring and prevention strategies and measures were being implemented (McDermott, Tulip, & Schmidt, 2004).

Geographical discrimination

Seventy per cent of the total Indigenous population live outside major cities, and those living in remote and very remote communities make up over a quarter of the total Indigenous Australian population (Australian Bureau of Statistics, 2011a). We know that health status worsens significantly with remoteness; therefore the health

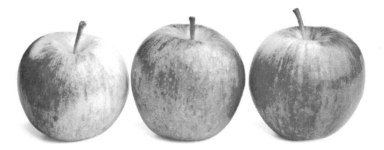

Reproduced with permission from: iStockphoto/expertm1973.

concerns raised have a much greater significance for young Aboriginal and Torres Strait Islander peoples as one population group, for they make up 18 per cent of the total remote population.

Diabetes and the triple whammy

Let us examine what happens when we put the triple whammy together – age, culture and geographical location – with a chronic health condition such as diabetes.

- **Diabetes incidence:** diabetes has doubled in the Australian population over the past two decades. Today over 4.6 per cent of the total Australian population suffer from diabetes, mostly type 2 diabetes (Australian Bureau of Statistics, 2011b). Diabetes is associated with long-term circulatory and eye conditions, and it significantly increases the risk of developing coronary heart disease, stroke and peripheral vascular disease. Diabetes mellitus, or type 2 diabetes, is strongly linked with obesity, diet and exercise.

- **Now let's add age:** diabetes mellitus was often called maturity onset diabetes as it was usually only found in those over 40 years of age. However, it is now escalating in younger people due to the increase in obesity in the Australian population and other First World populations.

- **Now let's add culture:** Indigenous Australians were more than four times as likely as non-Indigenous Australians to report some form of diabetes and have one the highest incidences in the world (Diabetes Australia, 2013; Indigenous HealthInfoNet, 2013). Diabetes affects up to 39 per cent of those aged over 55 years (Indigenous HealthInfoNet, 2013). Diabetes hospitalisation rates are 3–5 times higher for Indigenous Australians than other Australians (Diabetes Australia, 2013). Indigenous Australians are almost 7 times more likely to die from diabetes than other Australians (Diabetes Australia, 2013).

- **Now let's add geographical location:** almost one-third of all diabetics live in the most disadvantaged areas. Young females in regional areas were 30 per cent more likely to be overweight or obese than those in the city. Indigenous Australians living in remote areas are almost twice as likely to have diabetes – 9 per cent in remote areas, 5 per cent in non-remote areas (Australian Institute of Health and Welfare, 2014a).

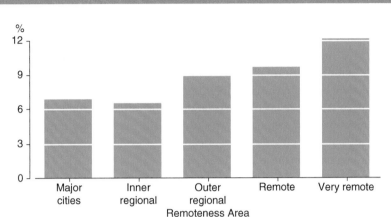

FIGURE 9.3 Diabetes/high sugar levels, Aboriginal and Torres Strait Islander people by remoteness – 2012–13.

Adapted with permission from: Australian Bureau of Statistics. (2013). *Australian Aboriginal and Torres Strait Islander Health Survey: First results, Australia, 2012–13.* Cat. no. 4727.0.55.001.

What these figures tell us is that being young and living rurally is a health disadvantage. An even greater health disadvantage is being young and living in a remote area, as demonstrated in Figure 9.3 above. The greatest health disadvantage of all is to be young, to live remotely and to be Indigenous. I examine this more closely in Chapter 7.

RURAL CULTURE

There is a strong feeling in rural communities that they are different from, and have special qualities not found in, city communities. Rural people see themselves as having a different world view and a different set of values and priorities from city-living Australians. Rural people are generally close-knit, supportive of one another, fiercely independent and self-reliant; their emphasis is on getting their work done and being productive. Ironically, they are also renowned for their higher levels of risk-taking behaviours, such as smoking, drinking and driving for long distances after a night out on the town. These factors have consequently added to their perception of health as 'the absence of disease' and their 'she'll be right mate' attitude to minor health ailments; as a result they tend to delay attending to their health issues (Strasser, Hays, Kamien, & Carson, 2000).

Providing rural health services

In this rural culture of self-reliance and independence, rural GPs reportedly see more patients than do their metropolitan counterparts, but see them less often because their patients' primary concerns are those of illness, not of wellness, and because of their limited ability to access a doctor (Strasser, 2002).

Many Australians, especially those living and working in rural and remote areas, would agree that 'it's different in the bush' compared with urban areas. Those who provide health care services also understand that their roles differ compared with those of their metropolitan counterparts, and know that they need advanced and additional skills to work rurally. This, however, is not generally recognised by those who fund rural health, research it, lobby for it and govern it.

It is fair to say that many outsiders question the validity of some of the rural and remote initiatives, and cannot see why rural health services are not just a part of mainstream services. Of course, these people are working from their own urban understanding of 'mainstream'. For example, researchers might ask: *'How different is rural health?'* and *'Where is your evidence?'* Economic rationalists might say: *'Is it different enough to demand a separate policy, separate budgets and separate training?'* and *'Why does it cost more than if we ran it in Sydney?'* Health care providers would want to know: *'Are the people sick enough to warrant special attention?'* and *'Just how sick are they?'* Humanists would argue: *'The people, irrespective of where they live, should have equal access to health care services – it's a matter of equity.'* The Australian Government would say: *'That's a state responsibility.'* And the state government would respond: *'But the Australian Government doesn't give us enough money to adequately support these programs.'* In the meantime, the rural and remote people would probably shout: *'Fair go mate, I've got a family to support and a business to run. Just sort this bloody mess out!'* A number of reviews and initiatives have occurred over the past decade to do just that (National Heath and Hospital Reform Commission, 2009).

Government blame-shifting processes

A factor that specifically impacts upon rural health services is our peculiar, inherited three-tier system of government with its Commonwealth, state and regional levels, which jointly provide funding for health services. This poorly coordinated system creates a situation whereby many rural and remote programs are conducted using a cost-splitting device, with investment from both the state and Commonwealth governments. Frequently, in rural areas, where the costs for travel, recruiting or providing services are considerably higher than the base amount allocated, there is a discrepancy between the state and Commonwealth government contributions. Yet the Commonwealth often sees the discrepancy as a state responsibility, and the states see it as insufficient provision of funds by the Commonwealth. One only has to read the paper or watch the news on television to hear the blame shifting going on between the state and federal governments, particularly to do with health and education (National Heath and Hospital Reform Commission, 2008). This blame-shifting syndrome has a direct impact on the provision of health care services and has led to many recruitment exercises for rural medical trainee positions not being filled, leaving those communities most in need without services. An example is the rural specialist trainee workforce in the Kimberley region of Western Australia, where the state and Commonwealth governments jointly fund rural specialist training positions. Attracting a specialist to this area will cost more than placing someone in, say, Bunbury in the south-west corner's wine-growing country, which is another rural specialist training post. The additional cost lies in the extensive travel a doctor has to undertake to provide clinical services across thousands of square kilometres, the additional specialist resources needed and the usual necessary incentives such as housing, study leave, adequate locum relief and a car. However, the Commonwealth Government provides the same amount for this rural training position as it does to support a specialist in Bunbury, which is a two-hour drive from Perth. Therefore, many training positions in areas of workforce need are not being filled; and rural people are not being provided with adequate specialist services.

Let us examine the health of rural Australians using Australia's National Health Priorities, both as a basis for determining the health status of rural and remote people and in an attempt to answer some of the questions above.

PRIORITISING RURAL PEOPLE'S HEALTH

The National Health Priority Areas (NHPA) initiative focuses on the nine biggest causes of morbidity* and mortality† in the Australian population. These include those chronic diseases that pose *a significant health burden* and those conditions that have a *potential for health gains* and improved outcomes for Australians – asthma, arthritis, cardiovascular health, cancer control, dementia, diabetes mellitus, mental health, obesity and injury prevention and control (Australian Institute of Health and Welfare, 2015a). It is interesting to note that obesity was only added in 2008 and dementia was only added in 2012, due to their increasing incidence in the population. Table 9.1 compares, for the nine National Health Priority Areas, the morbidity and mortality experienced by rural and remote Australians to that of all Australians.

Note: Many people may believe that the reported health status of rural people is due to the poorer health of Indigenous Australians, who largely live in rural and remote areas. This is not the case, for two reasons. First, there continues to be limited data about the health status of rural and remote Australians. The Australian Institute of Health and Welfare published the first and only national report in 1998 (Strong et al.). Second, the Indigenous data sets are incomplete in most reports. What Indigenous data that do exist are taken from usually only four or five Australian states. Rural health disadvantage is therefore not a result of poorer Indigenous health; it reflects the health disadvantage of all rural Australians.

---

*Morbidity is the rate of incidences of disease or impairment.
†Mortality is the rate of deaths.

TABLE 9.1 National Health Priority Areas: Health status for all Australians compared with rural and remote Australians

	ALL AUSTRALIANS	RURAL AND REMOTE AUSTRALIANS
Asthma	• Over 2 million (10%) of Australians have asthma – that is 14–16% of children and 10–12% of adults. This rate has plateaued recently, although 37 500 Australians are still admitted to hospital each year due to asthma (Australian Institute of Health and Welfare [AIHW], 2015a) • The prevalence of asthma in the Indigenous population is almost double (18%) compared with the non-Indigenous population (AIHW, 2015d) • The risk of dying from asthma increases with age. Up to 60% of asthma deaths may be avoidable (AIHW, 2015a)	• The prevalence of asthma is highest in inner regional areas. The urban and rural incidences of asthma are about the same (AIHW, 2015d) • Asthma mortality rates are higher for people living in more remote areas and those of lower socioeconomic status (AIHW, 2015d) • Asthma is higher in the Indigenous population and their death rates from asthma are more than double those of non-Indigenous people (AIHW, 2015a)
Cancer control	• Cancer accounts for 30% of all deaths registered in Australia. One in two men and one in three women could be directly affected by cancer by their 85th birthday (AIHW, 2015a) • The five most common cancers are prostate cancer, bowel cancer, breast cancer, melanoma of the skin and lung cancer (AIHW, 2014d, 2015a) • Indigenous people have 2.8 times the liver cancer rate, 2.3 times the cervical cancer rate and 1.7 times the lung and uterine cancer rates of other Australians (AIHW, 2014b). Aboriginal men are 50% more likely to die from prostate cancer (Cancer Council, 2015)	• The incidence of cancer is highest in inner regional areas and lowest in very remote areas (AIHW, 2014b). Remote areas have the highest incidence for cancer of unknown primary site and bladder cancer (AIHW, 2014b). However, death rates from all cancers combined were highest in very remote and remote areas, with the highest incidences being lung cancer, prostate cancer and kidney cancer (AIHW, 2014b) • Men living in rural NSW were found to be 32% more likely to die from prostate cancer than urban men (Yu, Luo, Smith, O'Connell, & Baade, 2014). Rural and remote people have to travel to major centres for cancer treatment and often chose surgery over radiation so that they could return home earlier

TABLE 9.1 National Health Priority Areas: health status for all Australians compared with rural and remote Australians—cont'd

	ALL AUSTRALIANS	RURAL AND REMOTE AUSTRALIANS
Cardiovascular health	• Cardiovascular disease causes more deaths annually than any other disease, accounting for 33% of all deaths in 2009 (AIHW, 2015a). Males have higher death rates from cardiovascular disease than women and this reduces with improved socioeconomic status • Indigenous death rates from coronary heart disease are 1.8 times higher than in the non-Indigenous population • Much of the burden caused by cardiovascular disease is preventable. The main risk factors are obesity, poor diet, smoking, excessive alcohol consumption, hypertension and high blood cholesterol	• Rural people experience higher levels of cardiovascular disease and it is higher again for remote males. Death rates from cardiovascular disease in remote and very remote areas were 1.4 times as high as in cities (AIHW, 2015a, 2015c) • Rural and remote people are more likely to be smokers, drink to dangerous levels, be obese and have much higher blood pressure than city people (AIHW, 2015a)
Dementia	• Dementia was added as a National Health Priority in 2012 due to the increased incidence in the population. In 2011 1 in 10 Australians aged over 65 years had dementia and 3 in 10 over age 85 years. It is estimated that the number of affected people will double by 2050 (AIHW, 2015a)	• No specific data on rural or remote distribution could be found
Diabetes mellitus	• Diabetes has doubled in the past 2 decades. In 2012 about 1 million Australians had diabetes, of whom 84% had type 2 diabetes. Northern Territorians experience twice the rate of diabetes (excluding remote) (AIHW, 2015b) • Diabetes is more prevalent in overseas born people and is increasing in younger people. Over three-quarters of people with diabetes were aged over 45 years with a higher incidence in men than women (Australian Bureau of Statistics [ABS], 2011b)	• Rural and remote people experience almost 2–3 times the incidence of diabetes and twice the hospitalisation and death rates. Indigenous Australians suffer 3 times the incidence of diabetes and were 7 times more likely to die from diabetes (AIHW, 2015a) • The incidence of Indigenous people with diabetes in very remote areas is twice the incidence of those living in cities (AIHW, 2014a)

Continued

TABLE 9.1 National Health Priority Areas: health status for all Australians compared with rural and remote Australians–cont'd

	ALL AUSTRALIANS	RURAL AND REMOTE AUSTRALIANS
	• Diabetes is the second most common cause of kidney failure, eye damage, ulceration and gangrene; its complications contribute significantly to ill health, cardiovascular disease, disability and premature death in Australia (AIHW, 2015b)	• Indigenous Australians have one of the highest prevalences of diabetes in the world, which is up to 30% of the population in some remote communities (Diabetes Australia, 2013)
Injury prevention and control	• Injury is the fifth leading cause of death in Australia and is more common in men. The main causes of injury in Australia are falls, half of which occur in the 65+ age group, followed by transport accidents and self-harm (AIHW, 2015a) • Indigenous people are twice as likely to be admitted to hospital for injury and have twice the rate of self-harm as other Australians (AIHW, 2013) • Men die from suicide at 4–5 times the rate of women (ABS, 2012)	• The rates of hospitalised injury and transport injury are double in remote and very remote areas (AIHW, 2013) • Rates of assault and intentional self-harm increased with remoteness and were highest in very remote areas (AIHW, 2013). Men in remote areas are 3 times more likely to suicide than urban men, most commonly by hanging. Rural men also have better access to guns and are less likely to seek support for depression and financial issues. Two-thirds were older farm owners or managers (Alston, 2012)
Mental health	• 45% of Australians aged between 16 and 85 years have experienced a mental disorder at some time in their life (AIHW, 2014e). One in 5 Australians experienced a mental disorder in the previous year. These are mostly anxiety disorders (14.4%), mood disorders (6.2%) or substance abuse disorders (5.1%) (AIHW, 2014e) • Females are more likely to suffer from mental disorders, particularly anxiety, and men are twice as likely to experience substance abuse disorders (Slade et al., 2009) • Mental ill health is the fourth most common reason for seeing a GP, and depressive illness is the fifth most common	• The stress associated with drought, unemployment and poverty contribute towards the health and wellbeing of rural and remote people. Rural and remote people were slightly more likely to have a mental disorder at some point in their life than urban people (ABS, 2013) • However, they were 34% less likely to report *very* high levels of psychological distress (ABS, 2013) • Suicide rates are almost double in rural areas and up to 6 times higher in very remote areas (National Rural Health Alliance [NRHA], 2009) • Younger rural Australians are almost twice as likely to suicide as their urban counterparts (NRHA, 2009)

TABLE 9.1 National Health Priority Areas: health status for all Australians compared with rural and remote Australians—cont'd		
	ALL AUSTRALIANS	RURAL AND REMOTE AUSTRALIANS
	• Same sex attracted Australians are 4 times more likely to experience major depressive illness and twice as likely to experience very high levels of psychological distress (Rosenstreich, 2013) • The death rate due to mental disorder has increased significantly over the past decade. Expenditure on mental health services has increased by 5.7% over the 5 years to 2011 (AIHW, 2014e) • Mental disorders accounted for 7% of the disability adjusted life-years lost worldwide in 2013	• Rural and remote same sex attracted Australians are estimated to have suicide rates of up to 14 times those of other Australians (Rosenstreich, 2013). They also have less access to the internet to access health information and were more likely to report feeling unsafe, isolated and discriminated against (Hillier et al., 2010)
Arthritis and musculoskeletal conditions	• Arthritis and musculoskeletal conditions are the most prevalent diseases and conditions among the National Health Priority Areas, with almost 6.1 million, or 28%, of Australians estimated to have arthritis and musculoskeletal conditions long term (AIHW, 2015a) • Back problems (14%), osteoarthritis (8%), osteoporosis (3%) and rheumatoid arthritis (2%) are the most prevalent forms in Australia (AIHW, 2015a) • Arthritis and musculoskeletal conditions mostly affect women and are a significant cause of disability • Between 2003 and 2013 there was a 47% increase in knee replacements and a 17% increase in total hip replacements (AIHW, 2015a)	• The prevalence of arthritis is highest for those living outside cities, particularly for males, Indigenous Australians and those of lower socioeconomic status • Indigenous Australians in rural and remote areas are 1.45 times more likely to have osteoarthritis and 1.92 times more likely to have rheumatoid arthritis (NRHA, 2014) • Rural and remote Australians have limited access to preventative, diagnostic and specialised care services (NRHA, 2014)

Continued

TABLE 9.1 National Health Priority Areas: health status for all Australians compared with rural and remote Australians–cont'd		
	ALL AUSTRALIANS	**RURAL AND REMOTE AUSTRALIANS**
Obesity	• Three out of every 5 Australians is overweight or obese – over 12 million people. One in 4 children are overweight (AIHW, 2015e). This is a fourfold increase in the past 30 years • Obesity is a risk factor for diabetes, cardiovascular disease, kidney disease and other chronic diseases (Obesity Australia, 2013)	• Over 30% more people living in rural and remote areas are obese than their city counterparts (AIHW, 2015e) • Indigenous Australians are twice as likely to be obese as non-Indigenous Australians (Obesity Australia, 2013)

CONCLUSION

Australians generally have exceptional levels of health based on world standards. Rural Australians have unique health concerns that relate to their culture, their living conditions, socioeconomic disadvantage and social isolation. They also relate health to their ability to be productive, and see themselves as dissimilar to their urban counterparts. This concept of difference places them in a different category from other Australians where health is concerned. Compounding this situation is their limited access to health care and transport, shortages of health facilities and professionals, and poorly coordinated government processes.

Rural health is not an issue that can be addressed in one government portfolio. It crosses into many other areas such as employment, education, housing, transport, social security and reconciliation. Yet governments continue to maintain narrowly defined departments, even when the issues require a whole-of-government response (Humphreys, Hegney, Lipscombe, Gregory, & Chater, 2002). While there has been some improvement in the past decade there is a need for a consistent, nationally coordinated approach that considers the uniqueness of our country and the needs and diversity of its populations.

The above snapshot, showing a comparison of health status between urban and rural Australians, demonstrates marked inequalities in almost every National Health Priority Area based on geographical location, age and culture. It shows why different health approaches, based on rural understandings of health, are needed. While this picture provides an image of inequity and social disadvantage, it also raises an important question. Should rural people expect the same level of health as their metropolitan counterparts?

With the increasing trend in the baby-boomer generation to move to smaller regional areas to retire, where does this leave this higher health maintenance population, who are used to immediate quality health care, when there are fewer services and people to provide them? Can they still expect to live out their long lives, walking on a level playing field, carrying their thongs in their hands?

Discussion Points

1   Discuss the different value systems operating in rural communities that contribute towards rural people viewing their health differently from city people.

2   Using the National Health Priorities as a guide discuss the differences in health status between rural, remote and city-living Australians. Why do these differences exist?

3   Should rural people expect the same level of health as their metropolitan counterparts? If so, why? If not, why not? Discuss.

4   How do you think health services could be changed to better meet the needs of rural and remote people? Discuss.

5   If rural people are living in environments where there are open spaces and where food is grown, why are they not leading the way in giving up smoking, decreasing alcohol consumption, increasing exercise and eating healthily? Discuss.

References

Alston, M. (2012). Rural male suicide in Australia. *Social Science & Medicine*, 74(4), 515–522.

Australian Bureau of Statistics (ABS). (2011a). *Australian social trends. 4102.0 – Health outside major cities.* Canberra: ABS. <http://www.abs.gov.au/AUSSTATS/abs@.nsf/Lookup/4102.0Main+Features50Mar+2011> Accessed 28.07.15.

Australian Bureau of Statistics. (2011b). *Diabetes in Australia: A snapshot 2007–08.* Canberra: ABS. <http://www.abs.gov.au/ausstats/abs@.nsf/Lookup/4820.0.55.001main+features32007-08> Accessed 28.07.15.

Australian Bureau of Statistics. (2011c). *Mortality rates by remoteness.* Canberra: ABS. <http://www.abs.gov.au/ausstats/abs@.nsf/0/6BF83C1213FEDA97CA257943000CF105> Accessed 28.07.15.

Australian Bureau of Statistics. (2012). *Suicides, Australia, 2010 – 3309.0.* Canberra: ABS. <http://www.abs.gov.au/ausstats/abs@.nsf/Products/3309.0~2010~Chapter~Suicide+in+Australia> Accessed 28.07.15.

Australian Bureau of Statistics. (2013). *Australian Social Trends, April 2013. 4102.0 – The average Australian.* Canberra: ABS. <http://www.abs.gov.au/AUSSTATS/abs@.nsf/Lookup/4102.0Main+Features30April+2013#back7> Accessed 28.07.15.

Australian Government. (2015). *2015 Intergenerational report, Australia in 2055.* Canberra: Treasury, Australian Government. <http://www.treasury.gov.au/PublicationsAndMedia/Publications/2015/2015-Intergenerational-Report> Accessed 28.07.15.

Australian Institute of Health and Welfare. (2011). *Young Australians: Their health and wellbeing 2011*. Cat. no. PHE 140. Canberra: AIHW. <http://www.aihw.gov.au/publication-detail/?id=10737419261> Accessed 28.07.15. Alter depending on above ref.

Australian Institute of Health and Welfare. (2013). *Trends in hospital injury Australia 1990–00 to 2010–11*. Injury research and statistics series Number 86. Canberra: AIHW. <www.aihw.gov.au/WorkArea/DownloadAsset.aspx?id=60129544396> Accessed 28.07.15.

Australian Institute of Health and Welfare. (2014a). Chapter 7: Indigenous health. In AIHW (Ed.), *Australia's health 2014*. Canberra: AIHW.

Australian Institute of Health and Welfare. (2014b). *Australia's health 2014*. Canberra: AIHW. <http://www.aihw.gov.au/australias-health/2014/indigenous-health/> Accessed 28.07.15.

Australian Institute of Health and Welfare. (2014c). *Life expectancy*. Canberra: AIHW. <http://www.aihw.gov.au/deaths/life-expectancy/> Accessed 28.07.15.

Australian Institute of Health and Welfare. (2014d). *Cancer in Australia: An overview 2014*. Cancer series Number 90. Canberra: AIHW. <www.aihw.gov.au/WorkArea/DownloadAsset.aspx?id=60129550202> Accessed 28.07.15.

Australian Institute of Health and Welfare. (2014e). *Mental health services, in brief*. Canberra: AIHW. <www.aihw.gov.au/WorkArea/DownloadAsset.aspx?id=60129549620> Accessed 27.07.15.

Australian Institute of Health and Welfare. (2015a). *National Health Priority Areas*. Canberra: AIHW. <https://www.aihw.gov.au/national-health-priority-areas> Accessed 28.07.15.

Australian Institute of Health and Welfare. (2015b). *How common is diabetes?* Canberra: AIHW. <http://www.aihw.gov.au/how-common-is-diabetes/> Accessed 28.07.15.

Australian Institute of Health and Welfare. (2015c). *Cardiovascular disease by populations of interest*. Canberra: AIHW. <https://www.aihw.gov.au/cardiovascular-health/populations-of-interest> Accessed 28.07.15.

Australian Institute of Health and Welfare. (2015d). *Who gets asthma?* Canberra: AIHW. <www.aihw.gov.au/asthma/prevalence> Accessed 28.07.15.

Australian Institute of Health and Welfare. (2015e). *Overweight and obesity*. Canberra: AIHW. <www.aihw.gov.au/overweight-and-obesity> Accessed 28.07.15.

Australian Institute of Health and Welfare & Department of Health and Ageing (DHA). (2007). *Older Australians at a glance* (4th ed.). Canberra: AIHW & DHA. <http://www.aihw.gov.au/publication-detail/?id=6442468045> Accessed 28.07.15.

Cancer Council. (2015). *Aboriginal men are 50 per cent more likely to die of prostate cancer*. NSW: Cancer Council. <http://www.cancercouncil.com.au/media-release/aboriginal-men-are-50-per-cent-more-likely-to-die-of-prostate-cancer> Accessed 28.07.15.

Diabetes Australia. (2013). *Aboriginal and Torres Strait Islanders and diabetes, Action plan*. Canberra: Diabetes Australia.

Hillier, L., Jones, T., Monagle, M., Overton, N., Gahan, L., Blackman, J., et al. (2010). *Writing themselves in 3. The third national study on the sexual health and wellbeing of same sex attracted and gender questioning young people*. Melbourne: La Trobe University.

Humphreys, J., Hegney, D., Lipscombe, J., Gregory, G., & Chater, B. (2002). Whither rural health? Reviewing a decade of progress in rural health. *Australian Journal of Rural Health*, 10, 2–14.

Indigenous HealthInfoNet. (2013). *Overview of Australian Indigenous health status, Diabetes.* Perth: Indigenous HealthInfoNet, Edith Cowan University. <http://www.healthinfonet.ecu .edu.au/health-facts/overviews/selected-health-conditions/diabetes> Accessed 28.07.15.

McDermott, R., Tulip, F., & Schmidt, B. (2004). Diabetes care in remote northern Australians Indigenous communities. *Medical Journal of Australia*, 180(10), 512–516.

National Heath and Hospital Reform Commission (NHHRC). (2008). *Beyond the blame game: Accountability and performance benchmarks for the next Australian Health Care Agreements.* Canberra: NHHRC.

National Heath and Hospital Reform Commission. (2009). *A healthier future for all Australians: Final report June 2009.* Canberra: NHHRC.

National Rural Health Alliance (NRHA). (2009). *Suicide in rural Australia*, Fact sheet 14. Canberra: NRHA. <ruralhealth.org.au/sites/default/files/fact-sheets/fact-sheet-14> Accessed 28.07.15.

National Rural Health Alliance. (2011). *Diabetes in rural Australia*, Fact sheet 21. Canberra: NRHA. <ruralhealth.org.au/.../fact-sheet-21-diabetes-rural-australia.pdf> Accessed 28.07.15.

National Rural Health Alliance. (2014). *Arthritis and rural and remote Australia*, Fact sheet. <ruralhealth.org.au/.../files/publications/nrha-factsheet-arthritis.pdf> Accessed 28.07.15.

Obesity Australia. (2013). *Obesity Australia action agenda.* Sydney: Obesity Australia. <www.obesityaustralia.org> Accessed 28.07.15.

Phillips, A. (2009). Health status differentials across rural and remote Australia. *Australian Journal of Rural Health*, 17, 2–9.

Rosenstreich, G. (2013). *LGBTI people mental health and suicide* (2nd ed.). Sydney: National LGBTI Health Alliance.

Slade, T., Johnston, A., Teesson, M., Whiteford, H., Burgess, P., Pirkis, J., et al. (2009). *The mental health of Australians 2. Report on the 2007 National Survey of Mental Health and Wellbeing.* Canberra: Department of Health and Ageing.

Strasser, R. (2002). *Preparation for rural practice. The new rural health. I. Blue* (pp. 204–220). South Melbourne: Oxford University Press.

Strasser, R., Hays, R., Kamien, M., & Carson, D. (2000). Is Australian rural practice changing? Findings from the national rural general practice study. *Australian Journal of Rural Health*, 8, 222–226.

Strong, K., Trickett, P., Titulaer, I., & Bhatia, K. (1998). *Health in rural and remote Australia: The first report of the Australian Institute of Health and Welfare on rural health*, Cat No PHE 6 (pp. 1–131). Canberra: AIHW.

Yu, X. Q., Luo, Q., Smith, D. P., O'Connell, D. L., & Baade, P. D. (2014). Geographic variation in prostate cancer survival in New South Wales. *Medical Journal of Australia*, 200(10), 586–590.

CHAPTER 10

CARING FOR THE POPULATION

Janie Dade Smith

This old but good story describes how different people and groups approach health in Australia.

> Once upon a time a woman strolling along a riverbank hears a cry for help and, seeing a drowning person she rescues him. She no sooner finishes administering artificial respiration when another cry requires another rescue. Again, she has only just helped the second person when a third call for help is heard. After a number of rescues, the woman begins to realise that she is pulling some people out of the river more than once. By this time the rescuer is exhausted and resentful, feeling that if people are stupid and careless enough to keep landing in the river, they can rescue themselves. She is too annoyed, tired and frustrated to look around her. Shortly, another woman walking along the river hears the cries for help

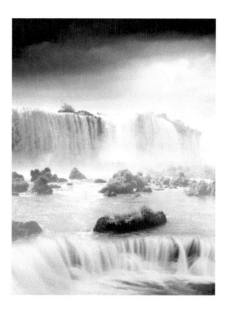

Reproduced with permission from: Shutterstock/PlusONE.

and begins rescuing people. She, however, wonders why so many people are drowning in this river. Looking around her, she sees a hill where something seems to be pushing people off. Realising this is a source of the drowning problems, she is faced with a difficult dilemma – if she rushes uphill, people presently in the river will drown, and if she stays at the river pulling them out, more people will be pushed in.

(DERMAN-SPARKS & BRUNSON, 1997)

This story offers a way in which to examine different approaches to rural and remote health, as the woman described as the rescuer portrays many health professionals working in rural and especially remote Australia, as that is the way they were educated to do so.

PAUSE AND THINK

How do you approach health care?

Are you a rescuer?

Have you ever wondered why so many people are drowning in the river?

UPSTREAM, MIDSTREAM AND DOWNSTREAM APPROACHES TO HEALTH

The above story offers several possible solutions. These solutions are often labelled 'upstream', 'midstream' or 'downstream' approaches to health (Keleher & McDougall, 2009).

The **downstream approach** refers to dealing on a one-to-one basis with an individual who is sick or injured. In the above scenario the woman would rescue the drowning people, give them artificial respiration and return them home to their normal conditions – often those that caused the problem. This could be labelled as the '*biomedical model*' approach. It deals with the presenting problem or disease and uses individual treatment systems and drug therapies based on scientific evidence, which are often the result of considerable investment in scientific research. The biomedical model regards health as the 'absence of disease' and its focus is on disease and its cure. Within this definition, health is understood only as a 'state of being where no abnormalities in physical functioning exist, as defined and measured against accepted norms and standards of bodily functions and an intervention is required to restore health', for example by medication (Lloyd, 2012). However, we also know that cure is often not available for many chronic diseases, which can only be managed – one can only manage diabetes as it is not curable. Therefore, a different approach is required with these patients.

The **midstream approach** refers to dealing with the lifestyle and behaviours of the individual. Using the midstream approach, the woman would rescue the people and tell them how to manage their own problems so that, if they 'get pushed in the river' again, at least they would not drown. This could be labelled the '*behavioural, health promotion and prevention*' approach, which focuses on individual behaviours, lifestyle and prevention programs. In the above scenario this would include promoting swimming programs that prevent drowning. Other types of behavioural approaches include stop smoking programs, which assist people in changing their behaviour. They may also include providing drug and alcohol education programs in primary schools with the hope that it will prevent children from using drugs – on the basis that they are educated about possible side effects.

The **upstream approach** refers to dealing with the big picture, or macro level, which prevents illness from occurring across the population, and dealing with the causes of ill health and disability from the social, political, economic or cultural aspects (Smith, 2006b). Using the upstream approach, the woman would organise with the people to destroy the source of the problem through identifying the cause. This might mean that, instead of saving lives at the riverbank, she would actually travel upstream to find out who was pushing the people in the water. This could be labelled the '*population health*' and/or the '*public health*' approach, as it focuses on the entire population and the eradication of the source of the problem. Examples can include developing government policy that affects the whole population; public health measures that eradicate the source of the problem, such as the eradication of smallpox and diphtheria; plus other political measures, such as global trade agreements and funding population health research, to identify the sources of the problem (Keleher & McDougall, 2009). It could also be labelled the *'socioenvironmental'* approach, as it focuses on how social issues such as unemployment, stress, the environment and income affect the health of the people. In this case the woman would travel upstream and find out why the people are jumping in rather than being pushed in.

PAUSE AND THINK

Which approach do you think you would use?

Why would you use this approach?

In fact, most people use a combination of approaches without even realising it. There are also many other approaches, none of which are mutually exclusive. They are usually combined in various ways. For example, a doctor is treating a patient for diabetes mellitus. The treatment is based on the scientific evidence available. The patient and his wife are smokers. Medical evidence tells the doctor that diabetes can also cause cardiovascular disease, eye damage, poor circulation, ulceration and gangrene, and that smoking affects the circulatory system (Australian Institute of Health and Welfare, 2008). Using the scientific evidence available, the doctor can focus on the patient's individual behaviours to help him stop smoking, while also considering how social issues such as the home environment and stress impact upon his condition. The doctor is combining all three of the above approaches – downstream, midstream and upstream.

In this chapter I will discuss four key approaches that are particularly relevant to rural, remote and Indigenous health services:

- public health
- population health
- primary health care
- community-controlled health services.

The story 'Yvonne and Ken live in Homesville' will then demonstrate the biomedical and primary health care approaches to health in a rural setting, and will also show how health outcomes can differ depending on the approach used.

PUBLIC HEALTH APPROACH

In the early 1900s the public health approach focused on eradicating communicable diseases that killed whole communities of people, such as smallpox, tuberculosis, typhoid and diphtheria. This was achieved by establishing good sanitation systems, a clean water supply, pest control, food preparation standards and infectious disease control methods. The public health approach 'focuses on prevention, promotion and protection rather than on treatment; on populations, rather than individuals, and on factors and behaviours that affect health and cause illness and injury' (Australian Institute of Health and Welfare, 2014).

These days the public health approach also addresses non-infectious diseases, such as injury prevention, environmental exposure and chronic diseases that affect the whole community. This is particularly true for obesity, which has doubled in Australia over the past 20 years. Obesity contributes towards the development of type 2 diabetes, which is expected to double in Australia by 2031 to 3.3 million Australians being affected (Diabetes Australia, 2013). Diabetes Australia tells us that approximately 280 Australians develop diabetes every day, which is 100 000 per year. The problem is so severe, led in the first world by the USA, that the World Health Organization (WHO) listed obesity among the top 10 enemies of health globally (World Health Organization, 2013). They list childhood obesity as one of the most serious public health challenges of the 21st century with an estimated 42 million preschool children being overweight in 2013 (World Health Organization, 2013). Ironically, WHO also lists underweight as one of the third world's greatest killers – especially in Southern Asia and Africa (World Health Organization, 2013). The public health approach has had a significant impact on our life expectancy, which has increased by approximately 30 years in the past century (Australian Institute of Health and Welfare, 2014).

POPULATION HEALTH APPROACH

The term 'population health' is a fairly recent arrival in Australia. It overlaps significantly with public health and originated in Canada. Population health is the organised response by society to reduce, *protect* and *promote* health and *prevent* illness, injury, disability and early mortality across the entire population (Department of Health, 2014). This is done through a reduction in the incidence of preventable mortality and morbidity, such as through national public health initiatives including national bowel cancer screening for over 55s; the promotion of healthy lifestyles and disease prevention (e.g. the National Diabetes Strategy); as well as health screening and immunisation programs (Department of Health, 2014).

The population health approach is based on strong evidence that health care systems for chronic conditions, for example cardiovascular disease, are most effective when they prioritise the health of a defined population rather than a single unit of patient seeking care (Epping-Jordan, 2005). What this means is that using a systematic approach across the entire population will have a greater long-term impact upon the health of the people than individual care, and it will also be far more financially efficient in the long run (Wagner, 1998; Wagner et al., 2001).

In the population health approach there is:

- a focus on upstream issues of the entire population and specific population groups – pregnant women, primary school children and cultural groups – as opposed to a focus on the individuals who make up the population (Smith, 2006a)

- an emphasis on health promotion and disease prevention strategies at the particular population level

- a concern with the underlying social, economic, biological, genetic, environmental and cultural determinants of the health of the whole population (Baum et al., 2004).

This is done in Australia through leadership from the Australian Government, which coordinates a range of national initiatives aimed at understanding and controlling the determinants of disease – those factors that cause illness or improve health, such as smoking or exercise. It is based on the effective use of health information, the application of research evidence in the design of programs to improve health and the knowledge of factors that affect the health of the population and specific at-risk groups such as Aboriginal and Torres Strait Islander peoples and rural and remote populations (Department of Health, 2015).

Examples of these programs include:

- **prevention of disease:** the Quit Now Campaign – smoking; the Hepatitis C Strategy 2005–2008; the National Drug Strategy: Australia's Integrated Framework 2004–2009; the National Chronic Disease Strategy (Department of Health 2015)

- **promotion of wellness:** Environmental Health Program; National Mental Health Strategy; A National Healthy Weight Guide, posters, brochures, fridge magnets, an app and guidelines to promote health and wellbeing and reduce the risk of chronic disease (National Health and Medical Research Council, 2013).

- **protection of particular groups:** Immunise Australia Program – children; Breast-Screen Australia – women; bowel cancer screening program – over 55s; National Aboriginal and Torres Strait Islander Nutrition Strategy and Action Plan 2000–2010 – specific at-risk populations (Department of Health, 2015).

The above programs target the behaviours and diseases that cause the highest morbidity and mortality in the population. It is therefore easy to see the relationship between population health and both the national health priorities and the social determinants of health.

For example, Australia is leading the world in tobacco control of its population, as we know from research that smoking harms health and causes cardiovascular disease and cancer (National Health Priority Action Council, 2006). Between 1991 and 2013 daily smoking rates of Australians halved. In 2013 the smoking rates were about 12.8 per cent of the Australian population (Australian Institute of Health and Welfare, 2013). This policy was something that the then Health Minister, the Honourable Nicola Roxon, continued between 2011 and 2013, which resulted in plain cigarette packaging and lockable cupboards in shops that sold them (Australian Associated Press, 2011).

We can see that combining scientifically based national policy with stop smoking and prevention programs as well as a tax increase on cigarettes has been very successful in stopping many in the Australian population from smoking. The exception has been the specific at-risk groups of Aboriginal and Torres Strait Islanders, who have double the smoking rates of other Australians (Australian Institute of Health and Welfare, 2013). This tells the government that the program has been successful, though they will still need to develop specific prevention and stop smoking programs to target this particular population group.

What does this mean for the rural and remote primary health care practitioner?

To have a greater impact on the health status of rural and remote communities, which experience extremely high levels of chronic illness, it will be essential for primary health care practitioners to shift their view from a downstream individual clinical focus to an upstream focus (Smith, 2006a). The critical distinction between the individual approach and the population health approach is the difference between considering sick individuals and sick populations.

PAUSE AND THINK

When working from a **population health approach**, one might ask:

1   *'Why does this particular population have a high incidence of diabetes or renal disease?'*

Whereas, when working from an individual **biomedical approach**, one might ask:

2   *'Why did this person develop diabetes or renal disease? Is there a family history?'*

Source: Baum et al., 2004.

Population health approaches are typically concerned with interventions that address the first question. They typically go upstream to consider causes of ill health and disability that are fundamental aspects of the social, political, economic and/or cultural aspects of the society (Baum et al., 2004). Most other health service provision focuses on downstream approaches or dealing with individuals who have become sick or injured. This does not mean individual service provision operates in isolation from population health strategies, but that it informs and may be a means of delivering population health strategies. This is often identified when monitoring systems are in place, which pick up trends in the population's health (Baum et al., 2004).

'Acute' model versus 'chronic' model of care

It is important that rural and remote practitioners refocus their approach when they are working with clients with chronic conditions, the incidence of which rapidly increases with remoteness.

Historically, the workforce has been structured to be reactive and to provide health care services to communities based largely on an acute medical model of care. The acute model of care was originally developed to address infectious diseases such as typhoid and diphtheria in the early 19th century – where there was an acute onset, accurate prognosis, short-term treatment and a cure was usually likely (World Health Organization, 2002). This acute care model of practice emphasises:

- triage, patient flow
- short appointments
- diagnosis and treatment of symptoms
- reliance on laboratory tests and prescriptions
- didactic patient education
- patient-initiated follow-up (Wagner, 2014).

The deficiencies of this model include rushed practitioners, lack of coordination of care, lack of active follow-up and patients being inadequately educated to care for themselves (Wagner, 2014). The majority of the workforce has been, and continues to be, trained in large tertiary teaching hospitals and universities that promote this acute model of care, and the graduating workforce has become comfortable working this way (Smith, 2006a).

Yet what is required in rural and remote areas is a workforce that can work in the different ways required to prevent, detect and manage the current epidemic of chronic disease, rather than dealing with the acute results of chronic illness (Smith, O'Dea, McDermott, Schmidt, & Connors, 2006). As chronic illness often has a gradual onset with multiple causes, uncertain prognosis and a lifelong duration with cure a rarity, it is easy to see that a new way of working is required. Figure 10.1 demonstrates the difference between the two models of care when we compare an acute problem like influenza with a chronic problem like diabetes. What is needed is a paradigm shift away from the single disease model towards a comprehensive population-based approach.

FIGURE 10.1 Comparing the acute model of care with the chronic model of care.

Acute vs chronic care approach

Acute illness e.g. influenza

- Acute onset
- Single cause
- Accurate prognosis
- Short term treatment
- Cure is likely

Chronic illness e.g. diabetes

- Gradual onset
- Multiple causes
- Uncertain prognosis
- Lifelong duration
- Cure unlikely

Chronic care

Patients and families struggling with chronic conditions have different needs. They require planned, regular interactions with their caregivers, with a focus on function and prevention of exacerbations and complications. This includes:

- systematic assessment
- attention to treatment guidelines
- behaviourally sophisticated support for the patient's role as a self-manager
- clinically relevant information systems
- continuing follow-up initiated by the provider (Wagner, 2014).

Overcoming these deficiencies will require nothing less than a transformation of health care, from a system that is essentially 'reactive' – responding to a person who is sick – to one that is 'proactive' and focused on keeping a person as healthy as possible (Wagner, 2014).

The chronic care model developed by Wagner et al. at the MacColl Institute of Healthcare Innovation in the USA is being widely used in Australia. It identifies the essential elements of a health care system that encourage high-quality chronic disease care. These elements include:

- **reorientation of the health service** – creating a culture, organisation and mechanisms that promote safe, high-quality, organised and planned care with strong leadership and support from management
- **evidence-based practice** – relying on a high-grade evidence base and protocols to improve daily practice and outcomes
- **patient-centred support** – meeting the patient's needs for confidence and skills in self-management of their condition through education
- **clinical information systems** – organising patient and population data to facilitate efficient and effective care and teamwork
- **the community** – mobilising community resources to meet the needs of patients – partnerships, policies and programs, plus cultural sensitivity and awareness (Wagner, 2014).

This model (see Figure 10.2) aims to result in informed, activated self-managing patients and prepared, proactive teams of health professionals. It is reportedly working well in some Australian health services (McDermott, McCulloch, Campbell, & Young, 2007).

PAUSE AND THINK

What do you think needs to happen in the education of health professionals to get them to provide more appropriate care for those with chronic conditions?

How can you be assured you have an informed and activated patient?

What do you need to change about your own practice to be able to provide more appropriate chronic care?

FIGURE 10.2 The chronic care model.

Chronic care model

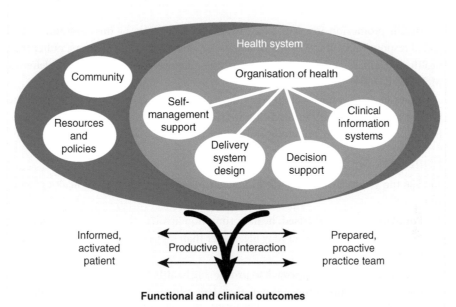

Reproduced with permission from: Wagner E. H. (1998). Chronic disease management: what will it take to improve care for chronic illness? *Effective Clinical Practice, 1,* 2–4.

HEALTH PROMOTION

One thing all health professionals need to do well is health promotion. Health promotion is the provision of education to individuals or groups that can promote healthy ideas and concepts to motivate people to adopt healthy behaviours. One recent initiative is the Fitbit (an electronic pedometer) that we all wear on our wrists to ensure we do our 10 000 steps per day, thereby promoting a healthy behaviour – walking.

Health promotion is one approach to population health that involves a process of enabling people to increase control over, and to improve, their health (World Health Organization, 1986, p. 1). It focuses on achieving health equity by reducing any health status differences and ensuring that equal opportunities and resources are available to all people to achieve their fullest health potential (World Health Organization, 1986, p. 1). This includes:

- creating a supportive environment
- providing access to information

- building healthy public policy
- developing life skills
- strengthening community action
- increasing opportunities for making healthy choices (World Health Organization, 1986).

Health promotion involves participation by all sectors of the community as a global responsibility. It is where individuals are viewed as health creators, rather than health consumers, knowing that the people themselves win health (Keleher & McDougall, 2009).

Many health professionals see health promotion as 'only' using pamphlets and posters to provide health information to patients. While these tools have their uses, health promotion is far broader (Smith, 2006a).

Principles for health promotion

In 1986 the World Health Organization determined the principles for health promotion as:

1 **Population-health focused:** health promotion involves the population as a whole in the context of their everyday life, rather than focusing on the individual at risk of specific diseases.

2 **Social determinants approach to promoting health:** health promotion is directed towards acting upon those things that determine whether we will be healthy or not – the determinants or causes of health. For example, smoking, alcohol intake, exercise, nutrition, food supply, sewerage, water supply, social support and education.

3 **Combining a variety of methods:** health promotion combines diverse, but complementary, methods or approaches, including communication, education, legislation, fiscal measures, organisational change, community development and spontaneous local activities against health hazards.

4 **Building collaborative partnerships:** health promotion aims particularly at effective and concrete public participation.

5 **Health workforce role:** primary health care professionals have an important role in nurturing and enabling health promotion. They should therefore work towards developing their special contributions in education and health advocacy – this is especially so for those working in remote cross-cultural environments (World Health Organization, 1984 cited in Catford, 2004).

All members of the rural and remote health workforce must be able to provide prevention, early interventions and curative care for their clients. This requires a good understanding of health promotion, the social determinants of health and population health strategies, as well as what they can do in their role to improve health outcomes for all people, particularly those who suffer a high burden of chronic disease. Table 10.1 provides practical examples of health promotion in action and what rural and remote health professionals can do.

TABLE 10.1 Examples of health promotion in action and what the rural and remote health professional can do	
PROBLEM	WHAT CAN THE RURAL AND REMOTE HEALTH PROFESSIONAL DO?
Lack of physical activity	Advocate for: • shaded walkways to encourage people to walk • swimming pool installation to encourage physical activity, social interaction, improved self-esteem and prevention of otitis media and skin infections • community daily 'walking drop-offs groups'
Obesity	*Community* – work with the store to improve healthy food options: • promote healthy take-away food at the store • 'shelf talkers' in the store • educate the community about healthy food options and physical activity • target at risk groups – diabetics, school children, older people *Individual* – use brief interventions in each consultation regarding food intake and the importance of physical activity: • run videos in the clinic waiting room about nutrition
Spread of disease	Work *with* the community to identify the environmental factors that cause disease in the community, and advocate for change – disposal of rubbish, nappies, electricity supply to refrigerate food and sewerage and maintenance systems Work *with* the community council to develop an environmental policy
Diabetes	*Support group* – assist in establishing a support group for diabetics in the community *Community* – provide community education about prevention of diabetes – food supply, exercise, early origins of disease to school children, nutrition etc
Smoking	*Individual* – incorporate brief interventions in each consultation *Community* – provide smoke-free zones in public buildings: • conduct education to school kids about smoking • run smoking education programs as part of healthy heart week • encourage smoke-free houses and no smoking around little kids

Adapted with permission from Judd, *cited in:*

Baum, F., Putland, C., Lawless, A., Swerissen, H., Lewis, V., & Weeks, A. (2004). *Thinking populations: Population health and the primary health care workforce.* Adelaide: Flinders University.

Smith, J. D. (2006). *Educating to improve population health outcomes in chronic disease* (2nd ed.). Darwin: Menzies School of Health Research.

Health promotion should be everyone's business

The key to working effectively in the prevention, early detection and management of disease involves health promotion being seen as 'everyone's business' (World Health Organization, 2007). Excellent approaches to improving health outcomes can include working with groups and communities. They require innovative methods of organising remote and rural community health centres and better ways of utilising the skills of the health workforce. A good example includes using appropriate community consultation to negotiate an afternoon where Aboriginal health practitioners and others go out of the clinic and conduct activities on identified health issues, such as healthy food choices, cooking classes and exercise programs (Smith, 2006a).

Most health professionals may find that their work falls into the downstream primary care approach. The important thing to remember is that infrastructure and systems change can be made at the local level, and this will assist in improving health outcomes for all. Examples of this might include having specific men's and women's areas in the clinic or better access for young people or gay and lesbian people. It is also important to recognise that integrated multi-level strategies and interventions require health and other sectors to work in partnership with the community to enhance health (Smith, 2006a, p. 41).

PRIMARY HEALTH CARE APPROACH

So far in this chapter we have discussed the biomedical, public health and population health approaches, which are interlinked and are about *what* we do. The primary health care approach is about *how* we do it – how we approach health – within the whole health care system, as opposed to what we do. The way we approach health will have a greater impact upon a person's health than what we actually do, as we have seen in Chapter 6.

Primary health care is a social approach to health that is about ensuring that everyone in the Australian community, irrespective of their culture, environment, ethnic background or place of residence, has a right to *affordable*, *accessible* and *appropriate* health care. It is based on the principle of human rights, in that it conceptualises health as a fundamental right and an individual and community responsibility (McMurray & Clendon, 2010). Primary health care is a holistic approach to health development. It is based on social justice, equity, community participation, social acceptability, cultural safety and trust (Johnson cited in Eckermann et al., 2006). It is a broad approach that links strongly with the social determinants of health and results in empowerment and self-reliance that enable people to lead equitable, socially productive and economically viable lives (Keleher & McDougall, 2009).

The primary health care approach was endorsed by the World Health Organization in 1978 and formed part of the Alma Ata Declaration. It reflects the way in which health care should ideally be delivered.

The World Health Organization defines primary health care as:

… an essential health care based on practical, scientifically sound and socially acceptable methods and technology, made universally accessible to individuals and families in the community through their full participation, and at a cost that the community and country can afford to maintain, at every stage of their development in the spirit of self-reliance and self-determination. It forms an integral part both of the country's health system, of which it is the central function and main focus, and of the overall social and economic development of the community. It is the first level of contact of individuals, the family and community with the national health system, bringing health care as close as possible to where people live and work, and constitutes the first element of a continuing health care process.

(WORLD HEALTH ORGANIZATION, 1978, p. 1)

This declaration represented a watershed in public health, as its focus was on empowering people to have control over decisions that affect their families' and their communities' health, rather than on allowing health professionals to decide what is best for them (McMurray & Clendon, 2010). For health professionals it is about *how* you do it, rather than *what* you do.

As a result the primary health care approach to health has the potential to revolutionise the entire health system through a strategy of organising health care in such a way that the right level of care is provided (World Health Organization, 1978).

Johnson (cited in Eckermann et al., 2012, p. 173) words it well when she states: 'in a "nutshell" primary health care is health for the people, by the people… it involves turning the pyramid of health of the health bureaucracy upside down, so that the people are the starting point for any health endeavour. It is about altering the power structure of health care'. This places the health professional 'on tap' and not 'on top' (Werner, 1978, cited in Johnson, 1992). As a result, many people today take charge of their own health by accessing health information from the internet, seeking advice from other health professionals, self-managing their conditions and choosing to use alternative health remedies.

Primary care is a part of primary health care and is the first line of care provided, as opposed to secondary or tertiary care, which are provided by a hospital, a doctor or a specialist. It also includes the primary management of the person's condition, which may be ongoing: 'but it is still primary, in that it is aimed at helping people with whatever health problem required care in the first place' (McMurray, 2003, p. 35).

Applying the principles of primary health care

Health professionals can use a variety of different approaches to health care in a rural community and the approach chosen can impact upon the people's health. The following story demonstrates how this can happen. It compares two different approaches to health – the biomedical and primary health care approach. This story could be used as a teaching resource in a lecture or tutorial, or as part of an individual assignment.

Story 4: Yvonne and Ken live in Homesville

Yvonne was born and bred in a small town in South Australia. Her father was a miner and her mother a housewife. In 1984, while she was training as a nurse at the local hospital, she met Ken, the local bank teller, at a party. Ken was different from the other local boys in town; he was from the city and he seemed so smooth and sophisticated. She knew he was the man she would marry; she loved him, and he would get her out of this town.

Over the past 20 years Yvonne and Ken have moved five times as the regional bank branches progressively closed and they were transferred to another town. Today they live in Homesville with their two lovely daughters, aged 12 and 15. They have been there for the past eight years and own their own home by the river. Ken is the local bank manager, a Rotary member and a generally respected man about town. Yvonne used to work part-time at the local hospital but has recently started working full-time as the community nurse at the local community health centre. She plays basketball on Tuesdays and likes to read and cook.

Homesville is a nice little town built on a river in northern New South Wales. It has a population of about 5000 people and up to about 10 000 if the outlying cane, fruit and hobby farms are included. There is a big new supermarket and the town council has recently upgraded the streets with nice terracotta footpaths, a children's play area and lighting around the new road that now cuts off the town from the freeway traffic. It's much quieter now, and several of the local stores have had to close as many of the locals now shop at Freshville, the regional town, about an hour's drive away. There used to be seven banks, but now there are only three.

The community seems a little suspicious of Ken, who has had to foreclose on some of the locals' bank loans. He and Yvonne are still seen as the 'newcomers' in the town and the community assumes they will eventually move on, like all the other outsiders who appear. Yvonne knew this meant she would have to become involved in the local tuck shop, church and sporting club, otherwise the town would ignore her. The town consists of many established families who have lived in Homesville for generations. Ken envies the values these old families share, as they seem to have a tremendous bond with the town – something more solid than what someone like himself, who has moved around a lot, has.

Yvonne's nursing role is to coordinate the diabetes and cardiac programs at the community health centre. She has taken this on with great enthusiasm. Having worked at the hospital, she knows that the diabetics will need to be able to take their blood glucose accurately, exercise regularly and eat wholemeal bread and spaghetti, and lots of fresh fruit and vegetables. Yvonne runs a couple of the fortnightly local diabetes meetings over morning tea. She presents great over-heads of the pancreas beautifully coloured in; she talks about how the insulin works and the importance of exercise and good foot care, as they all nibble on the healthy snacks she has prepared. After two months she is dismayed to see that numbers are dropping off and that all the diabetics are about the same as they were when she started – reasonably uncontrolled – and that all they really want to do is talk to each other about their week's events.

Julie, the other community nurse who has worked there for four years, takes Yvonne on some of her home visits. During the first week Yvonne thinks Julie is really slack, as all she seems to do is have cups of tea, drive people around in the health vehicle and talk to the patients, whom she calls 'clients'. Yet, she seems to know so much about them and their relationships with everyone in the town. Many are old school friends who still call each other by their maiden names, although they have been married for 50 years. She seems to know how the social system works in the town and who is related to whom. She knows their families and how they fit into the town, who likes who, who is pregnant, who has babies and who are seen as the 'no-hopers' and, of course, Julie even knows them by name. Julie knows that the old lady who has been religiously coming to Yvonne's diabetics' class cannot read. She knows that old Tom has never cooked for himself since his wife died, so that Yvonne's great lecture about wholemeal spaghetti was wasted on him. Julie knows when pension day is and who is broke that week. She knows the president of the local Probis club, the ladies from Meals on Wheels and members of the choral and arts society. She knows the social worker, the doctors, the pharmacists, the visiting physio, the podiatrist and the community workers. She also knows all the locals: the fruiterer who reduces his prices on Thursdays, the priests and counsellors, the council workers and even the strange guy from the Unemployment Bureau.

Yvonne finds that Julie rarely talks to her clients about their disease. Instead, she talks to them from their own perceptions of wellness, which they often relate to their ability to be productive and useful. One client they visit says: '*What use is a man if he can't even mow his own lawn?*'. After which Julie, instead of seeing everyone else on her list for that day, spends most of the day talking to the occupational therapist on the phone to see if she can send down special handles for a lawnmower. Julie talks to her clients about their families and friends, and their activities for the day. Yet she always seems to weave in subtle health messages in an empowering way, approaching the subject from their understanding of health and wellness. The final decision is always their own.

Ah ha moment

Yvonne has begun to realise that Julie works within a different framework from hers: one that sees the community as a whole first. This framework takes into account the environmental problems associated with the sugar mill, the availability and costs of food and resources and how these factors work within this community. Then she looks at how her individual clients fit in, from their own perception of health.

Yvonne's and Julie's different approaches to health

These two community health nurses work from two different approaches to health. Yvonne works from a biomedical approach and Julie works from a primary health care approach. Let us look at old Tom's situation as an example of how these two community nurses approach his health care.

Yvonne – The biomedical approach

Yvonne sees Tom as a diabetic who lives alone. From a biomedical approach, Tom needs to follow a certain diet, exercise regularly, look after his feet, stop smoking, test his blood glucose twice daily, take his tablets daily, visit his doctor regularly and see the diabetic specialist from the city every six months for more blood tests. She regards it as Tom's responsibility to take his doctor's advice; otherwise he will develop gangrene in his feet, renal problems and eye disease.

The biomedical approach to health, illustrated in Figure 10.3, puts the focus on the individual, who requires treatment for a disease that has been diagnosed and biochemically measured quantitatively. The biomedical model places the doctor in control and measures success in terms of blood tests and the patient's compliance with the doctor's evidence-based treatment.

The effectiveness of biomedical approaches to health in eradicating disease has generally been overestimated; in the last three centuries they have accounted for only 10 per cent of improvements in the health of the population (McMurray, 1999). The remaining 90 per cent are attributed 'to public health efforts, improved nutrition and better quality of life' (McMurray, 1999, p. 10). It was these factors that prompted the determination of the new international approaches and the endorsement of the Alma Ata Declaration on Primary Health Care by the United Nations in the 1970s.

FIGURE 10.3 Biomedical approach.

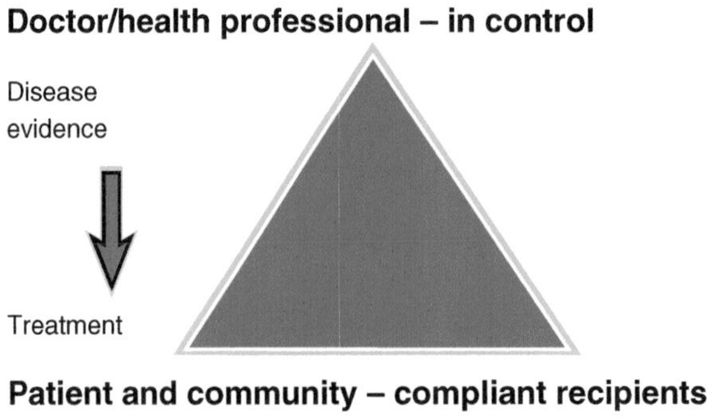

Doctor/health professional – in control

Disease
evidence

Treatment

Patient and community – compliant recipients

Julie – The primary health care approach

Julie sees Homesville as a friendly little rural town built on a river around a sugar mill that creates some environmental and health problems for its residents during the sugar season. She sees a town where there are an ageing population, high unemployment levels and kids who often have to leave home to get a job in the city. She sees a town with a whole range of sporting, artistic and recreational pursuits, good levels of social trust and people who know your name and have a strong sense of belonging. She sees a proud town where mateship, holding your head high even though you went broke in the drought, being part of a traditional family structure and having old-fashioned values are held in high esteem.

In Homesville Julie found that there are numerous old families, and Tom's is one of them. After talking to Tom one day she found out that his father Mario and Mario's younger brother emigrated from Italy in the early 1900s to cut cane and to build a new life in the 'lucky country'. They eventually bought 100 acres just outside Homesville and established their own cane farm. Tom was born there and is the last one of the family's six boys. He married Agnes, against his mother's wishes, 40 years ago. Tom and Agnes moved into the retirement home in town two years ago after Tom handed over the running of the farm to his eldest son. Agnes died of cancer three months ago; she was just 66. 'She was a good wife and mother,' Tom says with tears in his eyes, 'hardworking, never complained and could always make something out of nothing.' Tom misses her dreadfully. Tom has four sons; two live locally. Apart from the sons checking in on him once a week and occasionally bringing him a meal, he mixes with few people in town. He cannot cook and does not know what to do with himself now he has retired. He still drives around town in his car, though the locals call him a 'bloody old menace'. He plays bocce on Thursday mornings, but apart from that he rarely goes out. He sits at home, fiddles with his lawnmower, enjoys another smoke, watches the TV and waits for his grandson to call in after school some afternoons. Tom is also a diabetic. He doesn't see it as a big problem – just that he needs to give up sugar in his tea. However, Tom has noticed that his diabetes is more stable since Julie has been coming to visit him to check his blood sugar every day. He has also noticed that, when she takes him for a walk along the river in the afternoons, he sleeps a little better without needing sleeping tablets. He thinks he may start playing bocce twice a week now that he is feeling a bit better.

Julie, who uses a primary health care approach as illustrated in Figure 10.4, works from the social context of health within the whole community, whereby the power structures of health care delivery and the health triangle are turned upside down. She sees her role as part of the wider health team, which is multidisciplinary and involves community development, advocacy, liaison, public health, education, research, evaluation and personal care services. Julie's focus is on prevention and social and economic justice. It emphasises greater self-reliance and responsibility on the part of both the client and the community. This makes them feel empowered to improve their own health at a cost that they, and the community, can afford.

FIGURE 10.4 Primary health care approach.

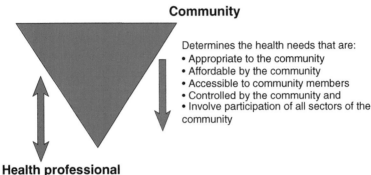

Community

Determines the health needs that are:
• Appropriate to the community
• Affordable by the community
• Accessible to community members
• Controlled by the community and
• Involve participation of all sectors of the community

Health professional
Acts as a health resource and advocate using: practical, scientifically sound, socially acceptable, and locally accessible methods, which are based on equality, and social and economic justice. including: prevention, advice, public health, education, promotion, research, evaluation and community development – delivered in an empowering multidisciplinary way that helps people to help themselves

Julie's role is supported by, and she has input into, a good range of health services and support systems that are based on the community's local needs and involve members of the local community in their planning and implementation. The services she provides are based on the effective and efficient use of the available resources, the use of visiting specialist services as required and the goodwill of many volunteers.

We can see from the above story that the way in which we approach health can affect the outcome for the patient, the community and the nation, and may even be more rewarding for the health professional.

There is one further model, also based on primary health care, that deserves particular mention, as it relates to those Australians who suffer the worst health status in this country – Aboriginal and Torres Strait Islander peoples.

COMMUNITY-CONTROLLED HEALTH SERVICE APPROACH

Integral to the primary health care philosophy is our ability to have control over our own health. This is due to the fact that 'people cannot achieve their fullest health potential as human beings, unless they are able to take control of those things which determine their health' (World Health Organization, 1986, p. 2).

As discussed in Chapter 6, Indigenous Australians view health quite differently from mainstream Western society. They have different definitions of health that are more holistic. They have developed a model of primary health care that reflects this holistic view and a process whereby they have control over it.

In the Sydney suburb of Redfern in 1971 the first Aboriginal Community Controlled Health Service (ACCHS) was established, in response to the aspirations of Aboriginal people as well as their urgent need to provide decent, accessible health services for the Redfern population (National Aboriginal Community Controlled Health

Organisation, 2015). This holistic ACCHS model of primary health care combines illness care with disease prevention, advocacy for social justice and the full participation of all players (Couzos & Murray, 2003). The World Health Organization endorsed this model of health care in 1978. There are over 150 Aboriginal Medical Services in Australia today. The main difference is that, under community control, the people who use the health service control the health service. They decide what programs are appropriate, and how, when and where to deliver them. Programs are initiated by the community, based in the local community needs, governed by an Aboriginal body, which is elected by the local Aboriginal community. Holistic and culturally appropriate services are delivered by employees using both Aboriginal and non-Aboriginal people with expertise who work under the direction of the Aboriginal community (National Aboriginal Community Controlled Health Organisation, 2015).

An example of the types of programs ACCHSs offer can be seen in the Central Australian Aboriginal Congress in Alice Springs, which provides a wide range of comprehensive primary health care services to Aboriginal people living within a 100-kilometre radius of Alice Springs. These include:

- medical clinics in Alice Springs and five remote sites
- a women's health clinic and a men's health clinic in Alice Springs
- a children and families program – providing childcare, child health, immunisation, outreach, a family partnership program, family support services, a preschool readiness program and a youth outreach program
- a women's health and birthing centre – Congress Alukura by the Grandmother's Law
- wellbeing services – community wellbeing, lifestyle and tobacco cessation program, renal primary health program for those on haemodialysis and a safe and sober support program
- Aboriginal health practitioner education and a community health education program
- transport services
- public health and political advocacy
- health promotion and community-controlled research (Central Australian Aboriginal Congress, 2015).

Many other ACCHSs provide similar services such as the Apunipima Cape York Health Council (2015) in North Queensland, which provides health services to eleven Cape York communities. They also run health promotion programs via their healthy lifestyles and family health teams who work in areas such as diabetes care, tackling smoking, eating well and keeping active, and through their mums and bubs, men's health, women's health and child health programs. Others, such as Nguiu in the Northern Territory and Kimberley Aboriginal Medical Service in Western Australia, also provide dialysis services for the high number of Aboriginal people with renal disease.

Aboriginal Medical Services provide an excellent example of primary health care in action based on the individual community's needs in the provision of accessible, affordable and appropriate health care services. These services are preferred, and well used by, Indigenous Australians, as well as by many non-Indigenous Australians who often attend them because of the holistic approaches used.

CONCLUSION

There are many different ways in which we approach health care in Australia. We have seen in the story that *how* we approach health and provide health services, as opposed to *what* we actually do, can have a significant impact on the health of the people. This social view of health, which is founded in the philosophy of primary health care, suggests the way forward. Genuine approaches that invite communities to take the lead in defining their health needs and give them more control over their health in a socially and economically just manner, which are endorsed and supported by government, provide an avenue for change.

For a true primary health care approach to be successful in rural and remote Australia there is a need for an attitudinal shift by all players. This needs to be one where governments see themselves as investing in health, where the people become the 'change agents' and health professionals view themselves as the tools that communities use to achieve their goals. This will then provide rural and remote people with health services that are affordable, accessible and appropriate. It will also contribute to an Australian health care system that is founded on social and economic justice, equality and equity, and will fulfil one of our most basic human rights: our right to health.

Discussion Points

1 Write your own definition of public health and population health.

2 Describe the differences between the four approaches to health discussed in this chapter. Extract and discuss the differences and the strengths and weaknesses of these approaches to health.

3 Read the story 'Yvonne and Ken Live in Homesville' and discuss the two different approaches to health care described. List the different values of rural people that you observed in this story. What were the different outcomes for the patients? Discuss *how* we approach health can have an impact on the health of the people.

4 What examples of primary health care in action have you seen in your own practice settings? Discuss.

5 Reflect upon your own practice. What could you change as a result of this discussion? Discuss with the group.

6 What do you think are the main barriers in our current health care system to the primary health care approach being successfully used? Discuss.

References

Australian Associated Press. (2011). Cigarette packaging war gets dirty. Brisbane: *Courier Mail.*

Australian Institute of Health and Welfare (AIHW). (2008). *Australia's Health 2008.* Canberra: AIHW.

Australian Institute of Health and Welfare. (2013). *National drugs strategy household survey.* Canberra: AIHW. <http://www.nationaldrugstrategy.gov.au/> Accessed 28.07.15.

Australian Institute of Health and Welfare. (2014). *Australia's health.* Canberra: AIHW.

Apunipima Cape York Health Council. (2015). *Services.* Cairns: Apunipima Cape York Health Council. <http://www.apunipima.org.au/services> Accessed 16.05.15.

Baum, F., Putland, C., Lawless, A., Swerissen, H., Lewis, V., & Weeks, A. (2004). *Thinking populations: Population health and the primary health care workforce.* Adelaide: Flinders University.

Catford, J. (2004). Health promotion: origins, obstacles, and opportunities. In H. Keleher & B. Murphy (Eds.), *Understanding health: A determinants approach* (pp. 134–151). South Melbourne: Oxford University Press.

Central Australian Aboriginal Congress. (2015). *How we help.* Alice Springs: Central Australian Aboriginal Congress. <http://www.caac.org.au/how-we-help/health-clinics/> Accessed 16.05.15.

Couzos, S., & Murray, R. (2003). *Aboriginal primary health care: An evidence based approach* (2nd ed.). Melbourne: Oxford University Press.

Department of Health. (2014). *Budget statements: Section 2 Department outcomes: Population health.* Canberra: Department of Health, Australian Government. <http://www.health.gov.au/internet/budget/publishing.nsf/Content/2014-2015_Health_PBS_sup1/$File/2014-15_Health_PBS_2.01_Outcome_1.pdf> Accessed 28.07.15.

Department of Health. (2015). *Population Health Division.* Canberra: Department of Health, Australian Government. <http://www.health.gov.au/internet/main/publishing.nsf/Content/health-pubhlth-index.htm> Accessed 13.05.15.

Derman-Sparks, L., & Brunson, C. (1997). *Teaching/learning anti-racism: A developmental approach.* New York: Teachers College Press, Columbia University.

Diabetes Australia. (2013). *Diabetes in Australia.* Canberra: Diabetes Australia. <http://www.diabetesaustralia.com.au/Understanding-Diabetes/Diabetes-in-Australia/> Accessed 28.07.15.

Eckermann, A. K., Dowd, T., Chong, E., Nixon, L., Gray, R., & Johnson, S. (2006). *Binan Goonj: Bridging cultures in Aboriginal health* (2nd ed.). Sydney: Churchill Livingstone, Elsevier.

Eckermann, A. K., Dowd, T., Chong, E., Nixon, L., Gray, R., & Johnson, S. (2012). *Binan Goonj: Bridging cultures in Aboriginal health.* Chatswood NSW: Elsevier International.

Epping-Jordan, J. (2005). Integrated approaches to prevention and control of chronic conditions. *Kidney International,* 68, S86–S88.

Johnson, S. (1992). Aboriginal health through primary health care. In G. Gray & R. Pratt (Eds.), *Issues in Australian Nursing 3* (pp. 151–170). South Melbourne: Churchill Livingstone.

Keleher, H., & McDougall, C. (Eds.), (2009). *Understanding health: A determinants approach.* Sydney: Oxford University Press.

Lloyd, L. (2012). *Health and care in ageing societies: A new international approach.* Bristol: Policy Press.

McDermott, R. A., McCulloch, B. G., Campbell, S. K., & Young, D. M. (2007). Diabetes in the Torres Strait Islands of Australia: better clinical systems but significant increase in weight and other risk conditions among adults, 1999–2005. *Medical Journal of Australia*, 186(10), 505–508.

McMurray, A. (1999). *Community health and wellness: A sociological approach* (pp. 5–14). Sydney: Mosby Publishers Australia Ltd.

McMurray, A. (2003). *Community health and wellness: A sociological approach*. Sydney: Mosby.

McMurray, A., & Clendon, J. (Eds.), (2010). *Community health and wellness: A primary health care in practice* (4th ed.). Sydney: Elsevier International.

National Aboriginal Community Controlled Health Organisation (NACCHO). (2015). *NACCHO history*. Canberra: NACCHO. <http://www.naccho.org.au/about-us/naccho -history/> Accessed 16.05.15.

National Health and Medical Research Council (NHMRC). (2013). *Australian dietary guidelines*. Canberrra: NHMRC. <https://www.nhmrc.gov.au/guidelines-publications/n55> Accessed 03.05.15.

National Health Priority Action Council (NHPAC). (2006). *National chronic disease strategy*. Canberra: NHPAC, Australian Government Department of Health and Ageing.

Smith, J. D. (2006a). *Educating to improve population health outcomes in chronic disease* (2nd ed.). Darwin: Menzies School of Health Research.

Smith, J. D. (2006b). Start the revolution in thinking. *The Rural Nurse, Association for Australian Rural Nurses*, 14(1), 8–9.

Smith, J. D., O'Dea, K., McDermott, R., Schmidt, B., & Connors, C. (2006). Educating to improve population health outcomes in chronic disease: an innovative workforce initiative across remote, rural and Indigenous communities in northern Australia. *Rural and Remote Health*, 6, 606.

Wagner, E. H. (1998). Chronic disease management: what will it take to improve care for chronic illness? *Effective Clinical Practice*, 1, 2–4.

Wagner, E. H. (2014). *Overview of the chronic care model*. Seattle, WA: Improving chronic illness care. <www.improvingchroniccare.org/change/model/components.html> Accessed 13.05.15.

Wagner, E. H., Glasgow, R. E., Davis, C., Bonomi, A. E., Provost, L., McCulloch, D., et al. (2001). Quality improvement in chronic illness care: a collaborative approach. *Journal on Quality Improvement*, 27(1), 63–79.

World Health Organization (WHO). (1978). *Declaration of Alma Ata*. International conference on primary health care, USSR, 6–12 September. Geneva: WHO. <www.who.int/ publications/almaata_declaration_en.pdf> Accessed 28.07.15.

World Health Organization. (1986). *Ottawa charter for health promotion*. 1st International Conference on Health Promotion, Ottawa, Canada. Geneva: WHO.

World Health Organization. (2002). *Innovative care for chronic conditions: Building blocks for action*. Geneva: WHO.

World Health Organization. (2007). *Everybody's business: Strengthening health systems to improve health outcomes, WHO's framework for action*. Geneva: WHO. <www.who.int/ healthsystems/strategy/everybodys_business.pdf> Accessed 28.07.15.

World Health Organization. (2013). *10 facts on obesity*. Geneva: WHO. <http://www.who.int/ features/factfiles/obesity/facts/en/index2.html> Accessed 14.05.15.

CHAPTER 11

PROVIDING HEALTH SERVICES – THE WORKFORCE

Janie Dade Smith

Imagine a perfect rural Australia, where wheat grows in the sunshine with just enough rain for bumper crops and where people breathe fresh air, glow with good health and eat their own freshly grown food or buy it at the local supermarket at reasonable prices. In this world all people are equal, no child lives in poverty and children go off to school each morning with their multicultural friends to learn, so that they can contribute to a rural Australia that they love and have no intentions of ever leaving. This is a place where all the people trust and respect one another for the

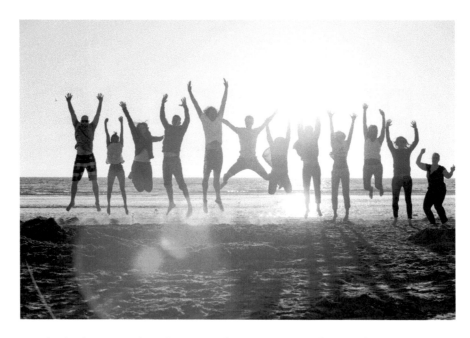

Reproduced with permission from: <http://www.nrhsn.org.au/>. Group of students from the RNHSN.

contribution each one makes. Here people can access their primary health care centre to see a health professional for their ailments; deliver their babies supported by their partners and friends; and never have to leave home to see a specialist, nor wait for an appointment at those times when they are not well. Ah, the perfect world – the land of the 'fair go'.

Earlier we discussed the two key factors that differentiate between the health status of rural and remote Australians and that of their city counterparts: their culture and their geography – where they live. A third key factor that impacts upon the health of rural and remote Australians is their access to affordable and appropriate health services.

The picture of the rural and remote health workforce in Australia has changed over the past decade. There are higher numbers of fly-in fly-out services, drive-in drive-out specialty services, agency nurses providing remote services, the shifting of service to Aboriginal community control and an increase in health services to mining sites where miners are splattered in their fluorescent orange vests across the landscape.

In this chapter, I provide a national picture of the health workforce who provide the health care services in rural and remote Australia and discuss their distribution, their different and common roles and their workforce trends. I then examine the reasons why they go rural, why they stay and why they leave and question whether we are in the right forest.

INTERNATIONAL WORKFORCE PERSPECTIVES

As we entered the 21st century, the health care needs of people were changing. In 2012, non-communicable diseases, such as chronic conditions, were responsible for 67.8 per cent of global deaths – this is expected to rise to 80 per cent by the year 2020 (World Health Organization, 2002, 2015). First World populations were getting older and fatter and, by 2031, nearly 20 per cent of the population in Australia will be over 65 years of age (Australian Bureau of Statistics, 2013a). These factors of ageing populations and increasing chronic disease require a differently prepared workforce, one that will face the greatest challenges for health care systems throughout the world.

In the past two decades, there have been many changes in the way in which we organise health care services. These changes affect the way in which we need to prepare the workforce (Health Workforce Australia, 2012a; World Health Organization, 2005). There has been a shift away from the hospital as the centre of the 'health care universe' towards a community and client-orientated approach. There have been rapid advances in technology, leaving hospitals looking more like mini intensive care units and e-health connecting patients from afar. The public are also more extensively informed by the media and the internet, resulting in an increase in health literacy across the community and a need for an up-to-date, well-informed and technologically savvy workforce to meet these needs (World Health Organization, 2005). With advances in surgical practices and increased community care there are now shorter-term acute care hospital stays and a greater emphasis on the provision of home and community care (Bachelor of Nursing Redevelopment Working Group, 2005). While these international factors call for the need for systematic reform throughout our entire health care system, they also greatly impact upon the way in which the health workforce is prepared to meet the needs of the population in the 21st century (Health Workforce Australia, 2012a; World Health Organization, 2005).

THE AUSTRALIAN HEALTH WORKFORCE

There have been many changes in the Australian health workforce over the past decade. We have seen major initiatives undertaken to identify what is required for health workforce reform in this country (Health Workforce Australia, 2012a). This has resulted in the establishment of a national registration and accreditation scheme to improve quality and public safety (Australian Health Practitioner Regulation Agency, 2015), plus national taskforces and reform commissions into the workforce issues and student scholarships. There has also been significant investment from government into infrastructure to explore clinical supervision requirements and data collection sets to predict what is required in the future (Health Workforce Australia, 2012a, 2012b, 2014; Productivity Commission, 2005). These are all very positive changes that aim to tackle the challenges of the past.

There are several things that we all know as health professionals working in Australia. The first is that we are an ageing population, and this will increase the demand for skilled health professionals in the near future. We know that, due to the huge increase in chronic conditions, we require a significant shift in practice from acute focused care to chronic focused care and self-management. This will also require a shift in how we educate health professionals. We know that we can barely meet our current population's health care needs due to workforce demand and supply issues, and that many areas are severely undersupplied, especially remote and rural areas (Health Workforce Australia, 2013). We know that these problems exist mostly in inland areas and not coastal areas, which are seen as more attractive by the workforce.

Most importantly, we also know that the major 'stuff-ups' we make in health care are often due to poor communication between the health professions, and that these are compounded by reporting structures that prevent equal role recognition when it comes to reporting incompetent practice. The Dr Death scenario in Bundaberg, Queensland, in 2005 is one such example (Sandhill, 2005). We also know, if we have ever stopped to think about it, that the way in which we work in our disciplinary silos is a way of the past if we want to have an impact upon the workforce supply issues in this country (Smith, 2006b).

To try to address these issues, in 2005 the Productivity Commission released a position paper called *Australia's Health Workforce*. They recommended that radical change was required to attempt to 'fix' the problem. Their recommendations included: broad health policy reform to ensure workforce innovation; more responsive education and training arrangements; a consolidated national accreditation regime and registration system; and more effective approaches to improving outcomes in rural and remote areas (Productivity Commission, 2005).

Since that time many positive changes have occurred in the way we organise, educate and register health professionals to work in Australia. In 2010, national registration and accreditation was established and, by 2015, they were registering the top 15 health professions (Australian Health Practitioner Regulation Agency, 2015). There has also been a national refocus of the workforce and planning to take us to 2025 (Health Workforce Australia, 2012a). A report by Health Workforce Australia tells us that there is likely to be a continuation of health workforce changes out to 2025 with highly significant shortages of nurses and less so for doctors (Health Workforce Australia, 2012a).

There is much to do to turn the workforce around to meet the needs of the next generation. We could learn from the United Kingdom, which had similar workforce problems resulting from their Bristol and other inquiries. They have turned their workforce around through the New Generation Project by restructuring the scope of health professional practice by using horizontal, rather than siloed, approaches to education (National Health Service, 2001). They have done this through interprofessional learning that occurs from the first undergraduate year across the health professions (Humphris, 2005). They are finding that cross-disciplinary communication has greatly increased as a result, which will ultimately improve the quality of health care provided to the population. The most important thing for government and for us to remember is that the greatest resource we have in health is a human one – our workforce (Smith, 2006a).

THE RURAL AND REMOTE HEALTH WORKFORCE

In spite of the attractions of a rural practice, such as the lifestyle and the fascinating medicine, governments and employers have had great difficulty in recruiting health professionals to live and work in the country, and in retaining them. There have been serious workforce shortages and a maldistribution of most workforce groups. While an extensive range of initiatives to address these issues has been put into place, and some of these initiatives are having an impact, this continues to be one of the more complex problems facing government, policy makers, health professionals and rural and remote populations.

The rural and remote health workforce is those health professionals who work in rural and remote practice in Australia. They include: Indigenous health practitioners, doctors, medical specialists, rural nurses, remote area nurses, pharmacists, occupational therapists, social workers, physiotherapists, psychologists, dentists, radiographers, radiotherapists, optometrists, speech pathologists, dietitians and numerous other allied health professionals who work in a growing number of fields, such as podiatrists, and a full range therapists from all disciplines. The more remotely located these professionals are, the fewer of them there are, and the more diverse and advanced their scope of practice will be. Many also perform additional roles with increasing remoteness, which can include those of ambulance driver, social worker, community liaison officer, veterinarian and pharmacist.

Despite the fact that there are numerous health professionals working in rural and remote practice, there is limited national literature available about their roles and their turnover rates, except for reports on general practitioners, which could fill a semi-trailer. For example, the first national report on allied health professionals in Australia was only undertaken in 2012 (Australian Institute of Health and Welfare, 2013a). Consequently, the following workforce information will only cover those disciplines that make up the majority of the rural and remote workforce, and about which sufficient reliable information can be found.

THE NURSING WORKFORCE

> 87 per cent of all health care across the world is provided by nurses and nurse-midwives.
>
> (JOHN HOPKINS JHPIEGO)

More than 50 per cent of the entire Australian health workforce are nurses and midwives (Australian Institute of Health and Welfare, 2015a). In 2013 there were 296 029 employed registered nurses and midwives in Australia, of whom 90 per cent worked in clinical practice (Australian Institute of Health and Welfare, 2015c). The picture of nursing in Australia is predominantly one of an ageing female profession, who make up almost 90 per cent of the nursing workforce (Australian Institute of Health and Welfare, 2013c). The average age of a nurse in 2013 in Australia was 44 years, with the proportion aged 50 and over slowly increasing, and this is particularly so in very remote Australia (Australian Institute of Health and Welfare, 2013c; Lenthall et al., 2011). The majority of nurses work in aged care, followed by medical and surgical wards in the urban hospital setting, although those working in the private sector are increasing. Those working in the Northern Territory, and those working in very remote areas, had the greatest number of hours worked per week, 41.5 hours, compared with the national average of 34.3 hours (Australian Institute of Health and Welfare, 2013c).

The picture of midwifery has also changed, with the recent establishment of midwifery as a separate profession from nursing as new direct entry midwifery training arrangements come into place. Concerningly, there has been a significant decrease in the number of registered midwives in Australia from 52 273 in 2009 to 33 969 in 2013, which is thought to be due to new registration requirements (Australian Institute of Health and Welfare, 2015f). This is having a major impact in remote areas where there has been a reported drop in midwives from 65 per cent to 29 per cent, which affects the whole continuum of care for women, from antenatal to postnatal care, as well as the care of the infant (Lenthall et al., 2011). They also note a drop in nurses with child health qualifications.

Geographical nursing distribution

Nursing makes up the largest and best-distributed rural and remote health workforce in Australia. While rural and remote nurses are relatively evenly distributed across remoteness areas, the *Health Workforce 2025* report warns that 'this should not be taken to imply sufficiency' (Health Workforce Australia, 2012a). Workforce shortages in some areas are high with significant turnover rates, which are reportedly seasonal and age-related and increase with remoteness (Garnett et al., 2008). However, there is a scarcity of retention information nationally. A number of initiatives have been put into place to replace existing staff including short-term agency staff, short-term locums and fly-in fly-out nursing, midwifery and dialysis staff.

Table 11.1 describes the employed nurses and midwives by remoteness. It is clear to see that younger nurses work in cities, those in remote areas are the elders and there are more men in very remote Australia where nurses work longer hours in clinical roles (Australian Institute of Health and Welfare, 2013b).

Rural and remote nurses

There are two specific groups of nurses working in rural and remote areas and, as their geographical titles suggest, they are 'rural nurses' and 'remote area nurses', and since 2000 there has been a splattering of nurse practitioners who specialise in particular areas of nursing, some in remote practice. So what is it that rural and remote nurses do that is so different and has caused them to establish their own professional organisations?

Rural nurses

Rural nurses and midwives are those who practise outside metropolitan areas, often in the hospital and community setting. This differs between inner and outer regional

TABLE 11.1 Employed nurses and midwives: selected characteristics, remoteness areas, 2013[a]							
	REMOTENESS AREA						
CHARACTERISTIC	Major cities	Inner regional	Outer regional	Remote	Very remote[b]	Not stated	AUSTRALIA
Number	209 925	53 813	25 093	4103	2426	669	296 029
Average age (years)	43.8	46.6	46.1	44.6	46.8	45.3	44.5
Aged 50 and over (per cent)	36.6	46.6	45.0	40.1	48.3	41.7	39.3
Men (per cent)	10.8	9.7	8.6	10.6	15.4	11.2	10.4
Registered nurses (per cent)[c,g]	85.1	77.4	75.5	79.8	85.5	87.7	82.8
Clinical nurses (per cent)[d]	89.7	90.7	91.4	89.8	92.9	86.3	90.0
Average weekly hours worked[e,h]	34.3	33.3	34.8	37.5	41.5	36.0	34.3
FTE rate[f,h]	1161	1119	1111	1255	1265	–	1155

[a]Derived from remoteness area of main job where available; otherwise, remoteness area of principal practice is used as a proxy. If remoteness area details are unavailable, remoteness area of residence is used. For records with no information on all three locations, they are coded to 'not stated'.

[b]Includes Migratory areas.

[c]Includes direct entry midwives.

[d]Clinical nurses include those whose role in their main job was 'clinical nursing' or 'clinical management and/or nurse/midwifery administration'.

[e]Care should be taken in interpreting change in the estimates on hours worked due to changes in the question on hours worked from 2009 to 2013.

[f]Full-time equivalent (FTE) number per 100 000 population. FTE is based on total weekly hours worked (see **Glossary**).

[g]Data for registered nurses include people registered with dual registrations and as a 'midwife only' in 2013.

[h]In 2012, the survey design changed so that the hours reported were split by nursing and midwifery. In 2013, a total of 9414 nurses and midwives reported working the same number of hours in both nursing and midwifery, so the total hours worked in each may be a duplication. This may result in an overestimate of the total hours worked by 0.3%.

Adapted from: AIHW Nursing and Midwifery Labour Force Survey 2009; National Health Workforce Data Set: nurses and midwives 2013.

areas. In 2013 there were 53 813 nurses working in inner regional areas and 25 093 working in outer regional areas (Australian Institute of Health and Welfare, 2013b). In total, they make up approximately 26.6 per cent of all nurses in the Australian workforce. Rural nurses fit the same profile as nurses nationally in that they are predominantly female but older, with an average age of 46.6 years (Australian Institute of Health and Welfare, 2013b). They are more inclined to work where they live, and remain in the same work location for a long period. Most were trained in the hospital-based model, though this is gradually changing as a new breed of university educated nurses take on these roles.

Rural nurses historically have a rich heritage of resilience, resourcefulness, adaptability and creativity and have previously been seen as 'expert generalists' in their specialty areas of practice (Bushy, 2002). These features are common descriptors across the medical, nursing and allied health literature for all practitioners working in these settings (Bushy, 2002; Humphreys et al., 2009; Lenthall et al., 2011; Liaw & Kilpatrick, 2008). In Australia the tradition of 'rural nursing has long been associated with images of quiet achievement, constancy and stoicism' – the same attributes that typify rural cultural values (Dempsey, 1990; Knight, 1997). However, things are 'a-changing' on the rural nursing landscape as a new breed of Generation Y nurses enter the workforce and bring with them improved technology and ways of working.

While there is no agreed definition of a rural nurse, common factors relate to the advanced and extended roles for which they have not necessarily been trained, geographical distance, accessibility to a doctor, diversity and population size (Blue, 2002). These are the same factors that differentiate the roles of the rural nurse and the remote area nurse. For example, a rural nurse is more likely to work in hospital-based practice in a larger rural town as part of a multidisciplinary team that includes a readily accessible doctor. In contrast, a remote area nurse is more likely to work in a smaller isolated community in a primary health care centre without ready access to a doctor, other than through telephone contact.

Australian rural nurses were once represented by their own professional association – the Association for Australian Rural Nurses (AARN). However, this was transferred in the mid-2000s to the Australian College of Nursing and Midwifery, who now have a rural 'community of interest' for rural nurses. Many rural nurses have therefore joined CRANAplus, the peak body for remote health, who may understand their context better.

Remote area nurses

Remote area nurses and midwives are those who practise in geographically remote and very remote areas of Australia. In 2013 there were 4103 nurses working in remote areas and 2426 in very remote areas, making up 2.2 per cent of the total Australian nursing workforce (Australian Institute of Health and Welfare, 2013b). The profile of remote area nurses is similar to that of rural nurses, except for a slightly larger proportion of men, especially in the Northern Territory, and an older population in very

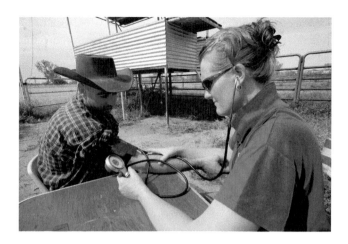

Reproduced with permission from: CRANAplus.

remote areas where the average age is 46.7 years (Australian Institute of Health and Welfare, 2013b).

CRANAplus is the peak body for all remote health in Australia; they set the standards for remote nursing and provide education, support and representation on all issues to do with remote health across the health disciplines (CRANAplus, 2015). They were previously the Council of Remote Area Nursing of Australia for 25 years prior to expanding their scope in 2007 to include all remote and isolated health professionals in Australia and her territories. They define a remote area nurse/midwife as:

> … a registered nurse whose day-to-day scope of practice encompasses broad aspects of primary health care and requires a generalist approach. This practice most often occurs in an isolated or geographically remote location. The remote area nurse/midwife is responsible, in collaboration with others, for the continuous, coordinated and comprehensive health care for individuals and their community.
>
> (CRANAPLUS, 2014, p. 32)

Remote area nursing is a unique field of health care where nurses work with both advanced and extended skills. The majority, 85 per cent, of remote area nurses work in very remote primary health care clinics in largely remote Indigenous communities where there is usually no immediate access to a doctor, or in very remote hospitals with inpatient facilities (Lenthall et al., 2011). They can be employed in a wide range of settings, including government health services, community controlled health services, Aboriginal medical services, primary health care clinics, multi-purpose centres, private general practices, mining and other industries, mobile and fly-in fly-out services, detention centres, on islands and tourist resorts, as well as private and non-governmental organisation (NGO) health services (CRANAplus, 2014). They are typically considered to be 'hard-working', flexible, adaptable, resourceful and passionate about their work (CRANAplus, 2014).

Despite the fact that remote area nurses work in social and professional isolation, in geographically and culturally challenging areas, and perform extended roles that are normally performed by doctors and allied health professionals, there is no requirement for them to undertake educational preparation for their role. This varies between states and regions. In 2011, Lenthall et al. found that only 5 per cent of remote area nurses in very remote Australia had specific qualifications in rural or remote health, despite numerous tertiary programs being available for many years. They also found that there had been a reduction in child health qualifications from 18 per cent in 1995 to 11 per cent in 2008, and, concerningly, a large reduction in midwifery qualifications from 65 per cent in 1995 to 29 per cent in 2008 (Lenthall et al., 2011). This is thought to be due to the new registrations requirements. However, this is an important point as these nurses are responsible for the antenatal and postnatal care of the mother and infant in these vulnerable remote communities, which experience high levels of infant and maternal mortality.

The adequate preparation, orientation and ongoing professional development of remote area nurses are extremely important to ensure they can provide quality health care to the sickest population in Australia. Most educational opportunities come through CRANAplus, who deliver short education courses in remote communities and online modules (CRANAplus, 2015). Previous remote programs were found to have a significant impact on retention of the workforce, renowned for high turnover rates, but they seem to change at the whim of remote managers with funding priorities (Jones, Blue, Adams, & Walker-Jeffreys, 2003).

PAUSE AND THINK

Given the advanced and extended roles remote areas nurses perform on the sickest people in this country, why are they not required to have specific qualifications for the advanced roles they perform?

Why is there no national educational benchmark for remote nursing practice in Australia?

NURSING WORKFORCE TRENDS

While the distribution of nurses equates well with the overall population, there are major concerns regarding the supply and ageing of the existing nursing workforce that have implications for the profession as a whole, but particularly for those in rural and remote practice.

Nursing workforce shortages

Nurses make up the largest group of health professionals in the world. They also constitute a global shortage in all fields (International Council of Nurses, 2005).

While there has been an increase in nursing numbers in the past ten years, there has also been an increase in the population, and nursing has the highest number of predicted shortages of all the health professions (Health Workforce Australia, 2012a).

In 2012 Health Workforce Australia undertook a study to project the requirements of the Australian health workforce in 2025 (Health Workforce Australia, 2012a). They found that nursing workforce shortages were in the order of 109 000 or 27 per cent of nurses and that there was a shortage of only 3 per cent for doctors though they are less evenly distributed. This is of huge concern given the global shortage of nurses. In their rural and remote workforce reform strategy Health Workforce Australia recommend the redesign and better use of existing roles, better education and clinical training, leadership support and enhancing the industrial and legislative framework to promote reform and build the rural and remote workforce (Health Workforce Australia, 2013).

Yet, we see nurses leaving nursing and graduates are not entering the profession. This, combined with insufficient numbers being educated, is a major factor in the nursing shortage. Graduates are reportedly not staying in nursing because of a lack of perceived confidence in areas other than medicine and surgery, or in locations other than city or regional hospitals (Department of Education, Science and Training, 2002). Many states are looking overseas for solutions rather than better educating the nurses knocking at their front doors. Additionally, employers are not 'growing their own' and are looking outside their own state for graduate nurses despite insufficient graduate places and interstate nurses who often do not stay in the long term (Smith, Wolfe, & Croker, 2010). Others report that universities are turning out graduates who are not 'job-ready' and who become increasingly disillusioned over the context in which they are expected to work (Wells, 2005). This often results in them leaving and going to other sectors to find work. It seems time to reflect about how we are approaching this issue rather than just using immigration from other countries to deal with shortages.

These numerous factors have resulted in changes in community expectations of a new type of nurse. The nurse for the 21st century needs to be well prepared to meet the needs of a diverse and ageing population, regardless of where they are employed. This will mean a shift from the principal focus of the registered nurse as the provider of care, to the nurse as the knowledge broker and the organiser of care in a variety of settings (Wells, 2005). These factors will change the face of nursing as their scope of practice changes. We are already seeing new and broader roles as programs for nurse practitioners and practice nurses are accredited. These trends will have a major impact upon the role of the rural and remote nurse.

Ageing workforce

Over the past 20 years the age structure of the nursing workforce has undergone significant change. Nurses are now an ageing population; the average age of a nurse is 44.5 years and the proportion of those over 50 years has increased to make up 38.6 per cent of the nursing workforce in 2011 (Australian Institute of Health and Welfare,

2012). Twenty years ago a quarter of the nursing workforce was under 25 years old, whereas today this age group represents less than 8 per cent of the entire nursing workforce (Australian Institute of Health and Welfare 2001). While this trend may be a good thing for rural practice, as what is required is a more experienced nurse, it will become a problem in the next decade when nurses try to retire and there are few younger nurses to take on their roles.

THE MEDICAL WORKFORCE

There were 82 498 employed registered medical practitioners in Australia in 2013 (Australian Institute of Health and Welfare, 2015b). Thirty-nine per cent were women, 25 per cent were aged over 55 years, and they work an average of 42.8 hours per week mostly in a clinical role (Australian Institute of Health and Welfare, 2015e). The medical profession make up a total of 16 per cent of the total health workforce in Australia (Australian Institute of Health and Welfare, 2015a). In 2014 only 221 of these doctors were Indigenous, and they make up only 0.3 per cent of all employed medical practitioners in Australia, despite the Indigenous population being 3 per cent (Australian Institute of Health and Welfare, 2014b). While the number of doctors has increased significantly by 44 per cent over the past decade, the distribution across the workforce has stayed about the same (Health Workforce Australia, 2012b).

In 2014 the Australian Capital Territory had the highest number of doctors, 474 per 100 000 population, followed by the Northern Territory (443), and NSW had the lowest number of doctors (309), followed by Victoria (333) (Australian Institute of

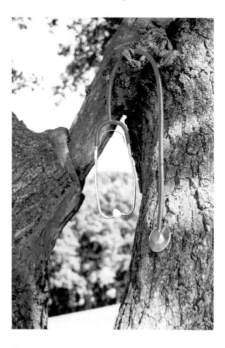

Reproduced with permission from: iStockphoto/Herzstaub.

Health and Welfare, 2015e). Those in remote and very remote areas worked the longest hours, 44.6 and 45.8 hours, respectively (Rural Health Workforce Australia, 2015).

Geographical distribution

In 2011, the geographical proportions of employed doctors per 100 000 population were 372 in major cities, 212 in inner regional areas, 188 in outer regional areas and 216 in remote and very remote areas (Health Workforce Australia, 2012b). (However HWA warn that the remote and very remote numbers should be viewed with caution due to very small numbers.) Hence, geographical distribution of the workforce continues to be a serious workforce problem despite a positive shift over the past decade (Rural Health Workforce Australia, 2015).

In 2010 the Rural Doctors Association of Australia calculated that rural Australia was short of at least 1800 doctors (Rural Doctors Association of Australia, 2010). They also noted that the rural and remote medical workforce is ageing with the average age of rural GPs being 50.5 years for men and 45.7 years for women. International medical graduates on restricted provider numbers now make up more than 41 per cent of the rural medical workforce to relieve the problem (Rural Doctors Association of Australia, 2010). The workforce modelling undertaken by Health Workforce Australia suggests that, for Australia's medical workforce to be self-sufficient by 2025, the geographical distribution of our doctors would need to improve by 100 per cent over the 2012 numbers (Health Workforce Australia, 2012a).

Many significant initiatives to improve the distribution of doctors have occurred. In 2003, the Australian Government felt the geographical distribution problem was so great they initiated a 'More doctors for outer metropolitan areas' program, which provided relocation incentives and training places for over 200 doctors (Australian Medical Workforce Advisory Committee, 2005). Since that time, there have been a number of initiatives including: significant increases in general practice places and medical student numbers, significant scholarships for students, training reforms and significant rural practice incentives for general practitioners and specialists. They came with recommended reforms to include changed models of practice, changes to scope of practice and reduced demand through improved preventative health measures (Health Workforce Australia, 2012a). However, the two major coordinating organisations for health workforce data, educational innovations and the organisation of general practice education and training in Australia – Health Workforce Australia and Australian General Practice Education and Training – were both closed down in the 2014 federal budget. Their activities were returned to the Health Department, along with a major reduction in rural scholarships for students to experience rural practice.

We wait to see the impacts of these initiatives, in particular those affecting our future – medical students. In 2012, Health Workforce Australia listed as a matter of significant concern the projected growth in graduates as being unlikely to make significant inroads to relative geographical equity under the current policy settings (Health Workforce Australia, 2012a). Concerningly, the Rural Doctors Association of Australia reports that less than 5 per cent of medical school graduates have taken up rural practice during the past 15 years, and the majority of doctors in rural practice are international medical graduates on restricted provider numbers (cited in Teo, Lockardt, Pushparajah, Waynforth, & Smith, 2015). This is not so in north Queensland where James Cook University report good geographical distribution of their first seven cohorts of medical students to rural and remote areas (Sen Gupta, Woolley, Murray, Hays, & McCloskey, 2014). So, one wonders if we can rely on Generation Y, as well as our universities, who select and educate students and our policy makers to find the solutions to this geographical distribution.

Medical specialists

The maldistribution is worse in the medical specialties. In 2011, there were 25 400 practising medical specialists in Australia. Over 85 per cent work in major cities despite the fact that 31 per cent of the Australian population lives in rural and remote Australia (Australian Bureau of Statistics, 2013b). The proportion of specialists working in regional areas was around half (61.1 per 100 000) that of the proportion in major cities (144.1 per 100 000), while in remote areas the proportion was particularly low (15.5 per 100 000) (Australian Bureau of Statistics, 2013b). While specialists are usually based in urban settings, some do travel to rural and remote areas providing fly-in fly-out or drive-in drive-out services via the Medical Specialist Outreach Assistance Program.

Rural medical generalism

Over the past decade a new type of rural and remote medical practitioner has arisen – the rural medical generalist – as what is required is not sub-specialisation but generalist specialists. This initiative commenced in Queensland and there are now training pathways in every state. The rural generalist provides a broad scope of medical care that includes primary care, emergency care, procedural practice, a population health approach, working as part of a multi-professional team both local and distant within a system of care that is responsive to community needs (Australian College of Rural and Remote Medicine, 2013). Rural generalism was endorsed as a distinct scope of medical practice and the Australian College of Rural and Remote Medicine now has a training pathway for rural generalist medicine that commences prior to medical school and extends throughout life on to lifelong learning (Australian College of Rural and Remote Medicine, 2013).

Remote medical practice

In 2008 a group of remote doctors set about defining the eight key features of remote medical practice (Smith et al., 2008). They also developed a definition of remote medical practice as follows:

> Remote medical practice is strongly multidisciplinary extended practice that includes the provision of diagnostic and management advice via telehealth; fly-in and fly-out service models; innovative methods of practice; limited clinical diagnostic support and specialist services; different

treatment protocols; primary, secondary and tertiary levels of care that require a higher level of clinical acumen; public health knowledge; cross-cultural understanding; resourcefulness; and increased responsibility.

(SMITH et al., 2008, p. 160)

The other key features of remote medical practice are that most remote doctors are usually employed, as opposed to private practice; they have highly geographically mobile roles, and a high community profile. They often work with marginalised populations with poorer health status, different world views and cultural understandings of health that result in a different mindset (Smith et al., 2008). This might include those doctors working in remote mainland Australian communities as well as those in Antarctica, in detention centres, internationally with the Defence Forces and in other public health settings.

There has been a pleasing and slow increase in the number of doctors working in remote and very remote areas over the past decade, which has historically been provided by fly-in fly-out medical services. This has largely been due to the establishment of the Remote Vocational Training Scheme, whereby registrars in training are placed in a remote, very remote, isolated or Aboriginal and Torres Strait Islander community and supported by government to undertake their vocational general practice training for periods of up to four years (Remote Vocational Training Scheme, 2015). They are supervised and educated remotely by medical educators. This is resulting in improved retention in these remote areas where doctors are staying for prolonged periods of time (Mitchell, Wellman, & Gullo, 2015).

MEDICAL WORKFORCE TRENDS

Several significant workforce trends in the United Kingdom, New Zealand and Canada are also being experienced in Australia.

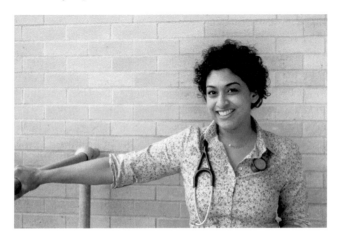

Reproduced with permission from: Rural Health Workforce Australia <http://www.rhwa.org.au/site/index.cfm?display=288847>.

Cultural change

A cultural change has also occurred in the Australian medical workforce in the past 20 years. There has been a greater proportion of women entering medical schools; a tripling of medical sub-specialisation due to technological developments; and a greater focus on quality of care and patient safety, which has resulted in a push from junior doctors for safe working hours (Smith & Hays, 2004). This has created a situation whereby general specialists, like general surgeons or general physicians who 30 years ago made up 80 per cent of all surgeons or physicians, now make up less than 20 per cent as the push towards sub-specialisation continues (Smith & Hays, 2004). This factor has huge implications for rural and remote people who require general surgeons and physicians.

Urban general practice has also moved towards increasing corporatisation. GP superclinics are multiplying and provide an expanded range of services through the employment of general practitioners as well as pharmacists, radiologists, pathologists, podiatrists, psychiatrists, nutritionists, psychotherapists, practice nurses, nurse practitioners and travel medicine specialists. Despite an oversupply in some inner city areas, general practitioners have also used a variety of strategies to resist market pressures to move, such as sub-specialising in areas such as nutrition, weight loss and sports medicine; and they are more inclined to bulk bill and provide more follow-up than their rural counterparts.

Medical indemnity insurance

A second significant cultural shift results from the impact of medical indemnity insurance upon the medical workforce. This is particularly the case with obstetric services that are usually provided by rural doctors and general practitioners. Today, most rural doctors refer their obstetric patients to larger regional centres, or cities, to have their babies under shared care arrangements. This is due to the unaffordable professional indemnity insurance cover required for the limited number of deliveries that they perform annually. This has resulted in a lose–lose situation for both families and doctors. The backlash has resulted in many women having to drive for hours in labour to get to major towns – and families being greatly inconvenienced as they are forced to pay for accommodation and arrange childcare. Additionally, rural doctors and midwives are being deskilled and are dissatisfied with the care they can provide; and caesarian rates are rising. There are many stories now emerging about parents delivering their babies on the side of the road when they cannot make it to larger centres (Koch, 2006). It would seem that the quality of health care provided to rural and remote women is being compromised greatly by financial disincentives, hence putting the needs of the provider above the needs of the consumer.

Feminisation of the medical workforce

The third significant trend is the feminisation, or equalisation, of the medical workforce. For the first time in Australian medical history, the 1999 national medical student intake saw a majority (53 per cent) of women being selected (McEwan, 2001). Today the number of women entering medical schools is about the same: 53.4 per cent (Teo et al., 2015). However, despite this significant increase in females entering the medical workforce during the past 20 years, the total employed medical workforce remains strongly male – over 61 per cent – as does the rural medical workforce, with only 29.7 per cent of female general practitioners in rural and remote practice (Australian Institute of Health and Welfare, 2015e). In the specialties only 26.8 per cent of specialist clinicians were female in 2012 (Australian Institute of Health and Welfare, 2014b), and these are largely represented in nonprocedural practice, such as psychiatry.

Female medical distribution is a significant factor for both rural women and the medical profession. First, it leaves rural and remote women without the choice of accessing a female doctor in important areas like obstetrics, gynaecology, psychiatry and paediatrics. Additionally, rural women have been found to make different treatment choices from city women, as they are less likely to access services that take them away from home for long periods, such as radiation oncology treatment (Royal Australian and New Zealand College of Radiologists, 2012).

Secondly, the current models for recruiting and retaining rural practitioners were developed from the perspective of a predominantly male workforce. Yet we know that women practise differently from men in that they see a greater number of problems per consultation and do more prevention and more counselling (Wainer, Bryant, Strasser, Carson, & Stringer, 1999). This means that, if the initiatives are to attract more female practitioners, these models will need to be recreated and incentives and support programs targeted to allow for gender differences and increased female participation (Wainer, 2001). Issues such as long hours, on-call responsibilities, inflexible work practices, lack of part-time opportunities for women in their child-rearing years and lack of professional development opportunities remain the key disincentives for female medical practitioners (McEwan, 2001; Wainer, 2001).

International medical graduates

The fourth trend, which is particularly relevant to the rural and remote workforce, is the number of international medical graduates (IMGs) working in Australia. IMGs now make up 25 per cent of the overall medical workforce, and more than 41 per cent of the rural medical workforce, where they largely work on restricted provider numbers while undertaking vocational training (Health Workforce Australia, 2012b; Rural Doctors Association of Australia, 2010). While they are providing increased services to those areas of designated workforce need – particularly rural and remote areas – they also provide a cultural shift in the thinking of rural people who seek their care.

The impact of Australia draining the overseas doctor pool has been raised as a serious ethical and global concern. Van Der Weyden and Chew (2004) argue that the 'brain drain' of health care professionals from many developing countries compromises their health care systems and demoralises their health care workforces that are already struggling to cope with major public health problems such as HIV and malaria. This leaves recruiting countries such as Australia faced with particular challenges to develop creative solutions so as not to broaden the gulf between developed and underdeveloped countries (Van Der Weyden & Chew, 2004). However, IMGs are being seen as a long-term solution for another decade in the workforce 2025 report (Health Workforce Australia, 2012a).

INDIGENOUS HEALTH PRACTITIONER WORKFORCE

In 2011, it was estimated that there were approximately 1256 Aboriginal and Torres Strait Islander Health Workers/Practitioners employed in Australia, 36 per cent of whom work in remote and very remote areas (Health Workforce Australia, 2014). There has previously been little data on the Indigenous health workforce due to a lack of clear role definitions, the absence of a recognised career structure or state registration and a multitude of different state and territory training requirements. The first national study for 15 years found that the Aboriginal and Torres Strait Islander workforce has almost doubled from an estimated 672 in 1996 to 1256 in 2011 (Health Workforce Australia, 2014). It is a predominantly female profession with women making up 72 per cent of the workforce with an average age of 41 years. The majority, 56 per cent, are qualified to certificate, diploma or advanced diploma level; and 15 per cent had a bachelor degree or higher (Health Workforce Australia, 2014). Approximately two-thirds work in the private sector, mostly Aboriginal Community Controlled Health Services or not-for-profit organisations, and 88 per cent are employed in health care and the social assistance industry; only one-third worked in hospitals, which may include Aboriginal Liaison Officer roles (Health Workforce Australia, 2014).

Historically, Indigenous health workers/practitioners have generally worked in their own community, selected by their peers to undertake training and work as

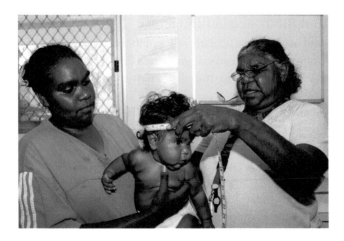

Courtesy of: CRANAplus.

health workers, though this is slowly changing as many travel to other states to work. They are usually viewed by the Indigenous community as the most appropriate people to provide health services, as they see health holistically and work from a philosophy of primary health care within their own cultural and community context.

While there is an undersupply, this is the only health discipline with few retention problems. Yet Indigenous health workers often live in the communities where the greatest health workforce recruitment and retention problems exist, and where the worst health status in the nation is found, which many of them also suffer (Australian Bureau of Statistics, 2014).

Role of the Indigenous health worker

Historically, indigenous health workers throughout the world have worked in various positions and under various titles. In China they were trained in both traditional and Western medicine and were called barefoot doctors; in South America they were called village health workers; in Canada Native Indians and Inuit people were trained as community health workers; and in Australia they are called primary health care workers and liaison officers (Werner & Martens, cited in Curtin Indigenous Research Centre, 2000). Traditionally, health workers were used for their cultural brokerage skills between Indigenous and non-Indigenous cultures, based on on-the-job experience. Their roles were diverse and included clinical, curative, preventive, environmental and traditional medicine, as well as agricultural extension, public health, mental health, cultural brokerage and community education work (Werner, 1997, Willis, 1984, cited in Curtin Indigenous Research Centre, 2000).

In Australia, the health worker role was largely developed in the Northern Territory with the employment of women as leprosarium workers in the 1950s and later as medical assistants in the 1960s (Johnston, 1991, cited in Curtin Indigenous Research Centre, 2000). With the advent of Community Controlled Health Services in the 1970s Indigenous health worker roles were further developed within an Indigenous primary health care framework. However, health workers were almost always educated and directed by nurses and doctors. This was because there was no structured disciplinary path for them to follow until the early 1990s, when accredited training programs were developed in Queensland, the Northern Territory and later in Western Australia. Today there is a National Strategic Framework for Indigenous health workers, a set of core competencies, a national health worker association, a career structure, a core curriculum and registration requirements.

With national registration of health professionals in 2012, Aboriginal and Torres Strait Islander health workers/practitioners are now required to be registered (Health Workforce Australia, 2014). Those in the Northern Territory had been required to be registered since 1985; however, this was not the case in other states. In 2013 there were only 310 registered.

The National Aboriginal and Torres Strait Islander Health Worker Association (2015) defines an Aboriginal and/or Torres Strait Islander Health Worker as an

Aboriginal and/or Torres Strait Islander person who is in possession of a minimum qualification within the fields of primary health care work or clinical practice. This includes Aboriginal and Torres Strait Islander Health Practitioners who are one specialty stream of health workers. They define their scope of practice as being able to perform a broad range of tasks including:

- the treatment of disease or injuries; maintaining health records and statistics
- acting as communicator and interpreter on behalf of clients and other health workers
- taking part in case management and follow-up, either independently or with other health care providers
- providing health education to individual clients and health staff
- providing cultural education to people outside the cultural community
- providing life skills education, counselling and referral for crisis intervention in the community they serve
- providing input into the planning, development, implementation, monitoring and evaluation of all health programs in the community
- carrying out administrative duties including budgeting and correspondence
- managing projects and programs at a senior level' (National Aboriginal and Torres Strait Islander Health Worker Association, 2015).

While doctors teach doctors, nurses teach nurses and physiotherapists teach physiotherapists, it is rare to see Indigenous health practitioners formally responsible for teaching Indigenous health workers, even though their profession has existed for decades. Why is this so?

It should be acknowledged that 'the dominance of the medical model of health in Australia has been influential in how the status and role of the Indigenous health worker is variously interpreted' (Curtin Indigenous Research Centre, 2000, p. 15). This dominance leaves a basic conflict between a community-driven primary health care model and the attempts of Indigenous health professionals to attain status, recognition and clear role definitions. It also reduces Indigenous ability to control the health services they provide, which in turn affects the health of the people who receive the services. Perhaps with these new pathways and systems the education of Aboriginal and Torres Strait Islander Health Practitioners will be firmly placed back into the hands of the people.

ALLIED HEALTH WORKFORCE

It is estimated that the allied health workforce makes up 25 per cent of the total Australian health workforce (Australian Institute of Health and Welfare, 2014a). There is no nationally or internationally accepted definition of allied health. Common descriptions include: all other university-trained health professionals except nurses and doctors who provide clinical, investigative, diagnostic or resource services and direct patient care to the community (Hodgson et al., cited in Fitzgerald, Hornsby, &

Hudson, 2000). Interestingly, Aboriginal and Torres Strait Islander Health Practitioners have recently been placed in this domain.

In 2012, the total number of allied health practitioners registered in Australia was 126 788, of whom almost a quarter were 29 387 psychologists, some 23.2 per cent. The next largest group were the 27 025 pharmacists making up 21.3 per cent, followed by physiotherapists at 19 per cent, occupational therapists at 11 per cent, medical radiation practitioners at 10.5 per cent, optometrists at 3.6 per cent, chiropractors at 3.6 per cent, 3885 Chinese medicine practitioners and podiatrists (both 3.1 per cent) and osteopaths making up 1.4 per cent of the total allied health workforce (Australian Institute of Health and Welfare, 2013a).

Common features of the allied health workforce are they are predominantly female, especially occupational therapists and psychologists at 91.5 per cent and 76.5 per cent, respectively, with the exception of chiropractors and optometrists at 34.8 per cent and 48.2 per cent, respectively (Australian Institute of Health and Welfare, 2013a). They are also generally younger than nurses and doctors and largely work in private practice in major cities – between 76 and 87.5 per cent (Australian Institute of Health and Welfare, 2013a).

The Department of Health tell us that there are no problems with recruitment of allied health practitioners in metropolitan areas but in rural, and especially in inland, areas there can be recruitment difficulties to long-term vacancies (Australian Government, 2015). Yet there are few data at the national level, and there is a well-recognised maldistribution of allied health professionals in rural and remote areas, in both the private and public sectors.

RURAL PHARMACY WORKFORCE

The pharmacy workforce deserves a special mention due to the trends that relate directly to rural pharmacy practice. There has been a significant increase in the

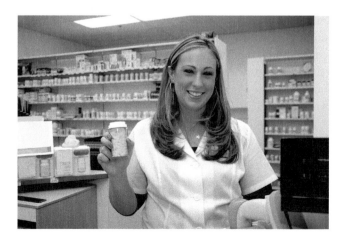

Reproduced with permission from: iStockphoto/ftwitty.

number of pharmacy students and the number of registered pharmacists in the past decade. In 2006 there were 15 539 registered pharmacists in Australia compared with 27 972 registered pharmacists in 2012, a 55 per cent increase (Australian Institute of Health and Welfare, 2013a; Department of Health and Ageing, 2008).

Geographical distribution

Despite their increase in numbers they remain unevenly distributed between the various states and geographical areas (Australian Institute of Health and Welfare, 2015d). Even though a third of Australians live in outer regional, remote and very remote areas, 91.5 per cent of pharmacists live in metropolitan or inner regional areas, leaving outer regional and remote and very remote areas to be serviced by only 8.5 per cent of the workforce (Australian Institute of Health and Welfare, 2013a).

Age and gender profile

Pharmacists are mostly younger women, some 60 per cent, whose average age is about 39.7 years, with many looking for part-time work (Australian Institute of Health and Welfare, 2013a). There has also been a significant shift in the age profile over the past decade whereby the average age of a male pharmacist in 2003 was 50 years, whereas today only 16 per cent are aged over 55 years (Australian Institute of Health and Welfare, 2003). However, age differs with rurality. In 2011, a national study found that rural pharmacists were older than the national average, with an average age of 55.8 years (Smith et al., 2013). They also found shortages of pharmacists in remote areas and in inland areas, whereas they noted a 'ripple effect' being experienced, as new graduates had to move to outer metropolitan and inner regional areas to find jobs.

Pharmacist rural roles

They also reported the rural hospital pharmacist role as a very generalist role, with more frequent on-call demands and significantly more time spent on the delivery of professional services and education and teaching but less time on medication supply than community pharmacists. Rural community pharmacists also reported 'more regular and closer relationships with customers, often being the first point of contact; better quality relationships with GPs; feeling more respected by their customers for the professional roles they performed; and were also less competitive regarding market share than their urban colleagues' (Smith et al., 2013).

SUPPORTING THE RURAL AND REMOTE WORKFORCE

Over the past two decades there have been numerous and significant initiatives to support the growth, education, scope of practice and different models of care of the rural and remote health workforce, which are reportedly having an impact (Sen Gupta et al., 2014). Several different models of service are also used in rural and remote Australia and these are slowly changing to ensure sustainability of services in the long run. Wakerman et al. (2008) have undertaken significant work in this area and have identified the essential elements for sustainable primary health care services for small rural and remote communities, which include: supportive policy, sustained funding, coordination of policy across national and state governments and community readiness for change.

Wakerman (2015) tells us that we have now moved beyond the deficit view of rural health. There is now a stronger recognition of our tough context that provides an 'incubator for developing and testing new models of care and expanded scope of practice' (Productivity Commission, 2005; Wakerman, 2015). While these are exciting times the recruitment, retention and distribution of the workforce remains a significant issue, so let us explore why they go, why they stay and why they leave.

Why do they go and why do they stay?

The World Health Organization tells us that approximately one-half of the global population live in rural areas, yet they are served by only 38 per cent of the nursing workforce and less than a quarter of the total medical workforce (Dolea, Braichet, & Shaw, 2009). Australia fits this trend with 31 per cent of the population living rurally, with 31 percent of nurses, 19 per cent of doctors and 23 per cent of allied health professionals serving these populations (Keane, Lincoln, & Smith, 2012).

While there are numerous reasons why health practitioners choose to work in rural and remote Australia, the most common reason given is their attraction to the 'rural lifestyle' (Keane et al., 2012; Smith et al., 2010; Smith et al., 2013; Strasser, 2002). Many get to enjoy their chosen lifestyle, love the challenging and different work that extends their scope of practice and develop close relationships with the community; and many choose to work there in the long term (Hays, Veitch, Cheers, & Crossland, 1997; Smith et al., 2013). However, this is not always the case with reports of a national doctor shortage, a global nurse shortage and a significant undersupply of health professionals in rural and remote Australia (Health Workforce Australia, 2012a, 2013). There has been much research into the area of recruitment and retention and much has been learnt with considerable models, approaches, incentives, scholarships and programs to address the issue (Australian Medical Workforce Advisory Committee, 2005; Battye & McTaggart, 2003; Department of Health and Ageing, 2008; Hays, 2012; Smith et al., 2013).

Who goes?

Rural background is the one most consistently reported factor associated with recruitment to rural practice, across all health professions including nurses, both in Australia and overseas (Allan, Crockett, Ball, Alston, & Whittenbury, 2007; Dalton, Routley, & Peek, 2008; Easterbrook, Godwin, & Wilson, 1999; Henry, Edwards, & Crotty, 2009; McAuliffe & Barnett, 2009; McDonald, Bibby, & Carroll, 2003; Somers, Strasser, & Jolly, 2007). Rural doctors (those born or raised in a rural area) are reportedly 2 to 2.5 times more likely to practise in a rural area than their non-rural counterparts (Laven & Wilkinson, 2003). In Victoria, about half of pharmacy students from a rural origin return to rural practice at some point after graduation and for varying lengths of time (Monash University, 2005). Medical students from the first seven graduating cohorts at James Cook University, where rural background is part of the selection process, are showing very positive results with 65 per cent of graduates undertaking a rural internship and future practice location (Sen Gupta et al., 2014). In contrast, graduates with a metropolitan background were found to be predominantly returning to metropolitan locations after postgraduate year seven (Sen Gupta et al., 2014).

Rural background is important because it provides health professionals with an understanding of rural values and familiarity with rural ways of life. Family and partner are cited by many health professionals as being one of the key factors in their overall career choice (Jutzi, Vigt, Drever, & Nisker, 2009), with having family or friends in rural areas or having a partner from a rural area being particularly important in the decision to take up rural practice (Devine, 2006; Lee & Mackenzie, 2003). Rural people fit easily back into rural life.

Recruitment and retention

However, when we talk about the '2 Rs' – recruitment and retention – people often see them as the same thing. Yet they are not. It is a little like putting rural and remote in the same category when we know they are significantly different from each other. Those factors that attract people to work rurally are different from those that impact on their decision to stay. This is partly because the decision to go – recruitment – is made outside a rural context, whereas the decision to leave or stay – retention – is made from within a rural context.

Research, both internationally and in Australia, has found two key factors that most strongly influence students to enter rural practice and to stay there (Dunbabin & Levitt, 2003; Strasser, Hays, Kamien, & Carson, 2000). The two key factors are: a rural background and a positive and meaningful rural placement during their undergraduate years, which was found to be one of the most important factors influencing career choices (Smith et al., 2013; Veitch, Underhill, & Hays, 2006).

Various other initiatives have been developed to encourage students to rural practice. These include rural scholarships for medical, nursing, pharmacy and allied health students, and the establishment of undergraduate multidisciplinary rural health clubs, university departments of rural health, rural clinical schools, rural workforce agencies and a rural incentive program for general practitioners. Many colleges and universities also include compulsory rural placements and Indigenous studies in an effort to prepare students for rural practice. As more students experience rural life, it seems that the rural health voice is being heard, the literature is being generated and the negative stigma of rural life is changing. These initiatives are proving to be slowly having an impact as more new graduates take up rural practice, and the long-term benefits are starting to trickle through into the next decade, as we wait for these students to complete and consolidate their learning.

Table 11.2 lists the 'pull and push' factors to rural and remote practice across the health disciplines, based on numerous reports over the past two decades. While there

TABLE 11.2 Recruitment and retention – the pull and push factors		
WHY THEY GO RURAL	WHY THEY STAY	WHY THEY LEAVE
Rural background	Rural background	Conflict with employer or
Rural spouse	Rural spouse	health department
Lifestyle	Lifestyle	On-call requirements
Positive rural placement	Good housing	Inadequate housing
Attractive location – coastal	Minimum of 3 health professionals	High workload; short-staffed;
	of the same discipline	solo practice
Financial incentives	Long-term employment contract	Short-term contract
	Private practice	Employed
	Financial incentives	No financial incentives
Employment package –	Good conditions – 6 weeks holiday,	Unable to take holidays and
relocation, extra holiday	2–4 weeks study leave,	study leave, poor access to
and study leave	remuneration, locum support	locums
Positive recruitment process	Supportive management, good	Inability to debrief
	relationships with the team	Poor management practices,
		conflict in a small team
		Safety issues
Sense of adventure	Joint academic appointment	Poor support systems
Good orientation	Good professional development	Poor access to professional
	opportunities	development
Friends or family there	Community engagement and	Culture shock – cross-cultural
	acceptance	issues
	Spouse employment	Spouse dissatisfaction
	Younger children – school	Children reach high school
	Resourcefulness	Dealing with bureaucracy
Buy a practice	Invested in infrastructure, e.g.	Sold their practice
Good housing	private practice, pharmacy	Poor maintenance of housing

are many similarities, there are also many differences between the disciplines. For example, rural community pharmacists often own the pharmacy as opposed to a government employed short-term doctor. Therefore, their decision to leave a community will involve different considerations.

Why they leave

One of the main factors that cause people to leave is conflict in the workplace, in small teams or with health departments, and poor management practices. A study undertaken in the Northern Territory reports issues to do with retention of remote area nurses may improve with better managerial practices (Weymouth et al., 2007).

They identified issues to do with effective communication and leadership, staffing replacement and leave, prompt attention to infrastructure issues and staff development with appraisal as the main 'pull factors'. They also found that it was important to ensure remote area nurses felt supported and valued and that, with systematic support, they may stay longer in remote practice. Many urban-based managers reportedly lack sufficient grassroots understanding of the rural and remote context. They have been found to have little understanding of what will work and what is needed in these work environments, where there is a strong community culture, and issues of access and support are paramount (Humphreys, Jones, Jones, & Mara, 2002). The stigma related to rural practice also serves as a barrier both to recruitment for all health professionals and to re-entry into metropolitan practice for those who may wish to update their skills after a long period of time.

The other reasons for leaving vary between the disciplines. In remote area nursing, where nurses are mostly female, work on call and live alone, safety and the risk of personal violence is also a trigger to leave (Lenthall, 2008). In predominantly Indigenous communities culture shock* is often the trigger that makes people leave, though many do not recognise what it is at the time.

Adequate relief and locum support is another key issue for all disciplines. Many informed administrators are now using successfully a hub-and-spokes model of service, whereby at least three practitioners of the same kind are based in regional centres and travel to those communities not large enough to justify resident services. They create regional, rather than specific, appointments and provide their own locum support within the team using a 'buddy' system with regional centres. It seems that, once the minimal group of three is achieved, long-term sustainability is more likely as the practitioners can relieve each other.

Are we in the right forest?

I do wonder whether we are looking at the issue of retention in remote Australia in the right way. When we measure retention it is based on 'length of stay' in a community. Yet many health professionals are employed on short-term contracts so when they leave it is recorded as resignation. To complicate the situation there is no consistent national approach to recording retention in most health professions except for doctors. What some studies have found is that those who leave rural and remote locations often move to another rural or remote location (Mitchell et al., 2015; Smith et al., 2013). Yet our data are not picking this up as retention. So why are we not looking at this as retention? If we looked at health workforce data from a national perspective instead of a local perspective it would give us a better picture of what movement is going on in the rural and remote landscape.

---

*Culture shock is that feeling of uneasiness, anxiety and stress that arises when suddenly all our familiar cues, languages, relationships and actions appear to be out of place, suspect or even inappropriate (Eckermann et al., 2012).

It seems time to do two things. The first is to get good workforce data on all health disciplines; currently the only decent data are on the general practice workforce, when the biggest profession is nursing where we cannot even establish what the turnover rate is within regions let alone statewide or nationally. The second is we need to make a paradigm shift in how we measure retention and the movement of the rural and remote health workforce.

National data-collecting systems

There is one further factor that deserves special mention and greatly impacts upon rural health services. The government allocates health resources for rural and remote health services according to a number of factors, which largely focus on the work of doctors. The Health Insurance Commission (HIC) collection of data is the largest and most complete source of information about what doctors do. However, it excludes those doctors who have different funding arrangements from the HIC's Medicare system. It also excludes other health professionals such as remote area nurses and nurse practitioners, and the substantial number of rural doctors who are salaried hospital employees, those who work for community controlled Aboriginal Medical Services. Both groups do not use the Medicare billing system, as the doctors are salaried employees who are paid from a government grant. As a result their consultations are not included in the HIC data. This could explain why the various reports state that the Indigenous patient encounter rate does not differ significantly between the rural and metropolitan sectors, when the incidence is reported elsewhere as being much higher than for metropolitan people. This information, therefore, presents a skewed view of rural and remote health work, yet resources are allocated on this basis.

CONCLUSION

Rural and remote practice can offer the best of worlds. But practitioners need to be well prepared for their role and have the required resourcefulness, clinical acumen, a sense of adventure and an open heart.

A workforce in balance is one that meets the population's needs – that is, enough health professionals, of the right kinds, in the right places. Yet this statement demonstrates the first of three striking features found on reviewing the health workforce literature. The first is the enormous amount of literature to be found relating to the medical workforce, which is enough to fill a semitrailer, compared to the minimal amount of literature to be found on all the other health disciplines combined, which is enough to fill a Holden Ute with room for the esky. This is in spite of the fact that nurses make up 50 per cent of all health professionals and, with Indigenous health practitioners in remote areas, they make up 95 per cent of the entire workforce in remote areas.

The second striking factor is the enormous recruitment and retention similarities between the disciplines. They all report shortages, difficulty in recruiting and lack of locum relief and professional development opportunities; many discuss trends like the ageing of their workforce, and how these staffing difficulties increase with geographical remoteness. There is little literature that looks at the workforce as a whole, and lip service is generally paid to multidisciplinary approaches. Is it time to ask why this is so?

The third striking factor is the huge diversity and enormous inequities in our systems. There is a widening gap between the haves and the have-nots. Minority groups such as allied health professionals are marginalised; the distribution of resources favours certain groups; and there is a total exclusion of some groups. With so many commonalities between the disciplines this situation begs the question: why are more multidisciplinary approaches not being used across the various disciplines in recruiting and educating the entire rural and remote workforce? Why aren't we looking at the workforce as a whole, rather than in bits?

It is fair to say that significant funds have been provided to rural and remote health over the past two decades and we are moving away from a deficit-focused approach through the use of innovation. While there has been some improvement in health status it is still well behind our urban cousins, especially for remote Indigenous people. Our focus and investment continue to be on the workforce, the general practice workforce in particular, due to their distribution issues. So are we in the right forest? Shouldn't we be focusing on those factors that affect health in the first place – poverty, level of education, housing, social support, early childhood development – the social determinants of health? And using interprofessional education to lead the way? The rural and remote workforce is a perfect position to do so. If we aspire to live in a perfect world, we need to look realistically at the problems. While this means adopting interprofessional approaches by the right kinds of health professionals in the right places, it also means getting real about focusing our work on those factors that affect health if we are to make any impact upon those we are there to serve.

Discussion Points

1   Use the internet to search the rural workforce agencies and government sources to identify three current initiatives to increase workforce supply in rural or remote Australia. Identify the disciplinary group, the type of initiative, how long it has existed and the impact it has had on increasing workforce numbers.

2   Were these initiatives for recruitment or retention of the workforce? Which different strategies need to be used for recruitment and which need to be used for retention? Discuss.

3   Discuss the skills and knowledge required to work in a remote or isolated practice.

References

Allan, J., Crockett, J., Ball, P., Alston, M., & Whittenbury, K. (2007). It's all part of the package' in rural allied health work: a pilot study of rewards and barriers in rural pharmacy and social work. *Internet Journal of Allied Health Sciences and Practice*, 5(3).

Australian Bureau of Statistics (ABS). (2013a). 3222.0 – *Population projections, Australia, 2012 (base) to 2101*. Canberra: ABS. <http://www.abs.gov.au/ausstats/abs@.nsf/Lookup /3222.0main+features52012%20%28base%29%20to%202101> Accessed 29.07.15.

Australian Bureau of Statistics. (2013b). *Australian social trends*, April 2013 (Vol. 41012.0). Canberra: ABS. <http://www.abs.gov.au/AUSSTATS/abs@.nsf/Lookup/4102.0Main +Features20April+2013> Accessed 29.07.15.

Australian Bureau of Statistics. (2014). 4727.0.55.001 – *Australian Aboriginal and Torres Strait Islander health survey: First results, Australia, 2012–13*. Canberra: ABS. <http:// www.abs.gov.au/ausstats/abs@.nsf/Lookup/39E15DC7E770A144CA257C2F00145A66 ?opendocument> Accessed 29.07.15.

Australian College of Rural and Remote Medicine (ACRRM). (2013). *Cairns consensus statement on rural generalist medicine*. Brisbane: ACRRM. <https://www.acrrm.org.au/ rural-generalist-medicine> Accessed 29.07.15.

Australian Government. (2015). *Review of Australian Government Workforce programs, 8.2 Allied Health*. Canberra: Department of Health, Australian Government. <http://www .health.gov.au/internet/publications/publishing.nsf/Content/work-review-australian -government-health-workforce-programs-toc~chapter-8-developing-dental-allied-health -workforce~chapter-8-allied-health-workforce> Accessed 20.06.15.

Australian Health Practitioner Regulation Agency (AHPRA). (2015). *AHPRA – Regulating Australia's health practitioners in partnership with the National Boards*. Canberra; AHPRA. <https://www.ahpra.gov.au/> Accessed 18.06.15.

Australian Institute of Health and Welfare (AIHW). (2001). *Nursing labour force 1999*, Cat. No. HWL 20. (National Labour Force Series No 20). Canberra: AIHW.

Australian Institute of Health and Welfare. (2003). *Pharmacy labour force to 2001: National health labour force series No. 25*. Canberra: AIHW. <http://www.aihw.gov.au/publication -detail/?id=6442467457> Accessed 29.07.15.

Australian Institute of Health and Welfare. (2012). *Nursing and midwifery workforce 2011*. Canberra: AIHW. <http://www.aihw.gov.au/WorkArea/DownloadAsset.aspx?id =10737422164> Accessed 29.07.15.

Australian Institute of Health and Welfare. (2013a). *Allied health workforce 2012, National health workforce series*. Canberra: AIHW. <http://www.aihw.gov.au/WorkArea/Download Asset.aspx?id=60129544590> Accessed 29.07.15.

Australian Institute of Health and Welfare. (2013b). *Employed nurses and midwives selected characteristics, remoteness area, 2009, 2013*. Canberra: AIHW. <http://www.aihw.gov.au/ workforce/nursing-and-midwifery/additional/> Accessed 29.07.15.

Australian Institute of Health and Welfare. (2013c). *Who are nurses and midwives?* Canberra: AIHW. <http://www.aihw.gov.au/workforce/nursing-and-midwifery/who-are-they/> Accessed 20.06.15.

Australian Institute of Health and Welfare. (2014a). *Australia's allied health workforce growing*. Canberra: AIHW. <http://www.aihw.gov.au/media-release-detail/?id=60129549972> Accessed 17.06.15.

Australian Institute of Health and Welfare. (2014b). *Medical workforce 2012*. Canberra: AIHW. <http://www.aihw.gov.au/WorkArea/DownloadAsset.aspx?id=60129546076> Accessed 29.07.15.

Australian Institute of Health and Welfare. (2015a). *Health workforce*. Canberra: AIHW. <http://www.aihw.gov.au/workforce/> Accessed 29.07.15.

Australian Institute of Health and Welfare. (2015b). *Medical practitioner workforce*. Canberra: AIHW. <http://www.aihw.gov.au/workforce/medical/> Accessed 29.07.15.

Australian Institute of Health and Welfare. (2015c). *Nursing and midwifery workforce*. Canberra: AIHW. <http://www.aihw.gov.au/workforce/nursing-and-midwifery/> Accessed 18.06.15.

Australian Institute of Health and Welfare. (2015d). *Pharmacy workforce*. Canberra: AIHW. <http://www.aihw.gov.au/workforce/pharmacy/> Accessed 17.06.15.

Australian Institute of Health and Welfare. (2015e). *Who are medical practitioners?* Canberra: AIHW. <http://www.aihw.gov.au/workforce/medical/who/> Accessed 18.06.15.

Australian Institute of Health and Welfare. (2015f). *Focus on midwives*. Canberra: AIHW. <http://www.aihw.gov.au/workforce/nursing-and-midwifery/midwives/> Accessed 19.06.15.

Australian Medical Workforce Advisory Committee (AMWAC). (2005). *The general practice workforce in Australia: Supply and requirements to 2013*; AMWAC Report 2005.6. Sydney: AMWAC.

Bachelor of Nursing Redevelopment Working Group (BNRWG). (2005). *Statement of intent for the redevelopment of the Bachelor of Nursing Program*. Adelaide: BNRWG, School of Nursing, University of South Australia, unpublished report.

Battye, K. M., & McTaggart, K. (2003). Development of a model for sustainable delivery of outreach allied health services to remote north-west Queensland, Australia. *Rural and Remote Health*, 3(online), 194. Available from: <http://rrh.deakin.edu.au>.

Blue, I. (2002). Characteristics for Australian rural health care professional practice. In I. Blue (Ed.), *The new rural health* (pp. 190–203). South Melbourne: Oxford University Press.

Bushy, A. (2002). International perspectives on rural nursing: Australia, Canada, USA. *The Australian Journal of Rural Health*, 10, 104–111. Available from: <www.rrh.org.au>.

CRANAplus. (2014). *Framework for remote and isolated professional practice*. Cairns: CRANAplus. <https://crana.org.au/advocacy/professional-issues/remote-practice/> Accessed 28.07.15.

CRANAplus. (2015). *Pathways to remote professional practice* (May 2015 ed.). Cairns: CRANAplus.

Curtin Indigenous Research Centre (CIRC). (2000). *Training re-visions. A national review of Aboriginal and Torres Strait Islander Health Worker training*. Canberra: CIRC, with Centre for Educational Research and Evaluation Consortium and Jojara and Associates, commissioned by the Office for Aboriginal and Torres Strait Islander Health.

Dalton, L., Routley, G., & Peek, K. (2008). Rural placements in Tasmania: do experiential placements and background influence undergraduate health science students' attitudes towards rural practice? *Rural and Remote Health*, 8, 962.

Dempsey, K. (1990). *Smalltown: A study of social inequality, cohesion and belonging*. Melbourne: Oxford University Press.

Department of Education, Science and Training (DEST). (2002). *National review of nursing education 2002: Our duty of care*. Canberra: DEST No 6880.

Department of Health and Ageing. (2008). *Report on the audit of health workforce in rural and regional Australia, April.* Canberra: Australian Government.

Devine, S. (2006). Perceptions of occupational therapists practising in rural Australia: a graduate perspective. *Occupational Therapy Journal*, 53, 205–210.

Dolea, C., Braichet, J.-M., & Shaw, D. M. (2009). Health workforce retention in remote and rural areas: call for papers. *Bulletin of the World Health Organization*, 87, 486.

Dunbabin, J., & Levitt, L. (2003). Rural origin and rural medical exposure: their impact on the rural and remote medical workforce in Australia. *Rural and Remote Health, 25 June 2003*, 1–17. Available from: <www.rrh.org.au>.

Easterbrook, M., Godwin, M., & Wilson, R. (1999). Rural background and clinical rural rotation during medical training: effect on practice location. *Canadian Medical Association Journal*, 160, 1159–1163.

Eckermann, A. K., Dowd, T., Chong, E., Nixon, L., Gray, R., & Johnson, S. (2012). *Binan Goonj: Bridging cultures in Aboriginal health*. Chatswood NSW: Elsevier International.

Fitzgerald, K., Hornsby, D., & Hudson, D. (2000). *A study of allied health professionals in rural and remote Australia*. Canberra: National Rural Helalth Alliance.

Garnett, S. T., Coe, K., Golebiowska, K., Walsh, H., Zander, K. K., Guthridge, S., et al. (2008). *Attracting and keeping nursing professionals in an environment of chronic labour shortage: A study of mobility among nurses and midwives in the Northern Territory of Australia*. Darwin: Charles Darwin University Press.

Hays, R., Veitch, P. C., Cheers, B., & Crossland, L. (1997). Why doctors leave rural practice. *The Australian Journal of Rural Health*, 5, 198–203.

Hays, R. B. (2012). Remote supervision of health professionals in areas of workforce need: time to extend the model? *Rural and Remote Health*, 12, 2322. Available from: <www .rrh.org.au>.

Health Workforce Australia (HWA). (2012a). *Health Workforce 2025: Doctors, nurses and midwives* (Vol. 1). Adelaide: HWA. <www.hwa.gov.au/sites/uploads/FinalReport_Volume1 _FINAL-20120424.pdf> Accessed 29.07.15.

Health Workforce Australia. (2012b). *Australia's health workforce series: Doctors in focus*. Adelaide: HWA. <https://www.hwa.gov.au/sites/uploads/australias_health_workforce_series _doctors_in_focus_20120322.pdf> Accessed 29.07.15.

Health Workforce Australia. (2013). *National rural and remote health workforce innovation and reform strategy*. Adelaide: HWA. <www.hwa.gov.au> Accessed 29.07.15.

Health Workforce Australia. (2014). *Australia's health workforce series: Aboriginal and Torres Strait Islander health workers/practitioners in focus*. Adelaide: HWA. <http://www.hwa.gov.au/ sites/default/files/HWA%20Aboriginal%20and%20Torres%20Strait%20Islander%20Health %20Workers%20in%20Focus_FINAL.pdf> Accessed 29.07.15.

Henry, J., Edwards, B., & Crotty, B. (2009). Why do medical graduates choose rural careers? *Rural and Remote Health*, 9, 1083. Available from: <www.rrh.org.au>.

Humphreys, J., Jones, M. P., Jones, J. A., & Mara, P. R. (2002). Workforce retention in rural and remote Australia: determining the factors that influence length of stay. *The Medical Journal of Australia*, 176, 472–476.

Humphreys, J., Wakerman, J., Kuipers, P., Wells, B., Russell, D., Siegloff, S., et al. (2009). *Improving workforce retention: Developing an integrated logic model to maximize sustainability of small rural and remote health care services*. Canberra: Australian Primary Health Care Research Institute, Australian National University; School of Rural Health, Monash University; Centre for Remote Health, Flinders University.

Humphris, D. (2005). *Integrating common learning in pre-registration health and social care professional programmes.* Southampton UK: University of Southampton. <http://www.common.learning.net/> Accessed 06.05.15.

International Council of Nurses (ICN). (2005). *ICN releases first series of issue papers on the global shortage of registered nurses.* Geneva: ICN.

Jones, J., Blue, I., Adams, M., & Walker-Jeffreys, M. (2003). *An evaluation of the Pathways to Professional Primary Health Care Practice for Remote Area Nurses program in the Central Australians network of the Northern Territory.* Whyalla: Spencer Gulf Rural Health School, University of South Australia.

Jutzi, L., Vigt, K., Drever, E., & Nisker, J. (2009). Recruiting medical students to rural practice: perspectives of medical students and rural recruiters. *Canadian Family Physician,* 55, 72–76.

Keane, S., Lincoln, M., & Smith, T. (2012). Retention of allied health professionals in rural New South Wales: a thematic analysis of focus group discussions. *BMC Health Service Research,* 12, 175.

Knight, S. (1997). Foreword. In L. Siegloff (Ed.), *Rural nursing in the Australian context* (pp. v–vi). Canberra: Royal College of Nursing Australia.

Koch, T. (2006). Dead baby born at roadside after hospital turns parents away. *The Australian.*

Laven, G., & Wilkinson, D. (2003). Rural doctors and rural background: how strong is the evidence? A systematic review. *The Australian Journal of Rural Health,* 11, 277–284.

Lee, S., & Mackenzie, L. (2003). Starting out in rural NSW: the experiences of new graduate occupational therapists. *The Australian Journal of Rural Health,* 11, 36–43.

Lenthall, S. (2008). *Back from the edge: reducing and preventing occupational stress in the remote area nursing workforce.* PhD dissertation. Alice Springs: Flinders University Centre for Remote Health.

Lenthall, S., Wakerman, J., Opie, T., Dollard, M., Dunn, S., Knight, S., et al. (2011). Nursing workforce in very remote Australia, characteristics and key issues. *The Australian Journal of Rural Health,* 19, 32–37.

Liaw, S.-T., & Kilpatrick, S. (Eds.), (2008). *A textbook of Australian rural health.* Canberra: Australian Rural Health Education Network.

McAuliffe, T., & Barnett, F. (2009). Factors influencing occupational therapy students' perceptions of rural and remote practice. *Rural and Remote Health,* 9, 1078. Available from: <www.rrh.org.au>.

McDonald, J., Bibby, L., & Carroll, S. (2003). *Recruiting and retaining rural general practitioners: A mismatch between research evidence and current initiatives?* Seventh National Rural Health Conference, March 1–4. Hobart: National Rural Health Alliance.

McEwan, K. (2001). *Discussion paper. Wanted: new rural workforce strategies for female doctors, findings from a survey of women in rural medicine.* Mascot NSW: NSW Rural Doctors Network.

Mitchell, C., Wellman, D., & Gullo, D. (2015). *Doctors in remote Queensland: they don't stay do they?* Paper presented at the 13th National Rural Health Conference People, places and possibilities, Darwin.

Monash University. (2005). *Graduate tracking project: Analysis of pharmacy workforce trends and the efficiency of rural student placements.* Final report: Pharmacy Guild of Australia Rural and Remote Pharmacy Workforce Development Program. Melbourne: Monash University.

National Aboriginal and Torres Strait Islander Health Worker Association (NATSIHWA). (2015). *What is a health worker/health practitioner?* Canberra: NATSIHWA. <http://www.natsihwa.org.au/what-health-worker> Accessed 20.06.15.

National Health Service (NHS). (2001). *Working together – Learning together: A framework for lifelong learning for the NHS.* London UK: Department of Health.

Productivity Commission. (2005). *Australia's health workforce, Position paper.* Canberra: Productivity Commission.

Remote Vocational Training Scheme (RVTS). (2015). *The Remote Vocational Training Scheme.* Albury: RVTS. <http://www.rvts.org.au/about/history> Accessed 17.05.15.

Royal Australian and New Zealand College of Radiologists (RANZCR). (2012). *Planning for the best: Tripartite national strategic plan for radiation oncology 2012–2022. Supporting regional and rural access to radiation oncology services.* Sydney: RANZCR.

Rural Doctors Association of Australia (RDAA). (2010). *The medical workforce shortage in rural and remote Australia: The facts.* Canberra: RDAA. <www.rdaa.com.au> Accessed 20.06.15.

Rural Health Workforce Australia (RHWA). (2015). *GP workforce trends, more than a numbers game.* Fact sheet April 2015. Melbourne: RHWA. <http://www.rhwa.org.au/site/index.cfm?display=32639> Accessed 29.07.15.

Sandhill, R. (2005). Dr Death in Bundaberg. *Quadrant*, December 2005. <http://www.rogersandall.com/doctor-death-in-bundaberg/. Accessed 14.07.15.

Sen Gupta, T., Woolley, T., Murray, R., Hays, R., & McCloskey, T. (2014). Positive impacts on rural and regional workforce from the first seven cohorts of James Cook University medical graduates. *Rural and Remote Health*, 14, 1. Available from: <www.rrh.org.au>.

Smith, J. D. (2006a). *Educating to improve population health outcomes in chronic disease* (2nd ed.). Darwin: Menzies School of Health Research.

Smith, J. D. (2006b). Start the revolution in thinking. *The Rural Nurse, Association for Australian Rural Nurses*, 14(1), 8–9.

Smith, J. D., & Hays, R. (2004). Is rural medicine a separate discipline? *The Australian Journal of Rural Health*, 12, 67–72.

Smith, J. D., Margolis, S. A., Ayton, J., Ross, V., Chalmers, E., Giddings, P., et al. (2008). Defining remote medical practice: a consensus viewpoint of medical practitioner working and teaching in remote practice. *The Medical Journal of Australia*, 188(3), 159–161.

Smith, J. D., White, C., Roufeil, L., Veitch, C., Pont, L., Patel, B., et al. (2013). A national study into the rural and remote pharmacist workforce. *Rural and Remote Health*, 13, 2214. Available from: <www.rrh.org.au>.

Smith, J. D., Wolfe, C., & Croker, F. (2010). *Northern Territory Review of Nursing and Midwifery Education and Training, confidential report.* Ocean Shores NSW: RhED Consulting Pty Ltd.

Somers, G., Strasser, R., & Jolly, B. (2007). What does it take? The influence of rural upbringing and sense of rural background on medical students' intention to work in a rural environment. *Rural and Remote Health*, 7, 706. Available from: <www.rrh.org.au>.

Strasser, R. (2002). Preparation for rural practice. In I. Blue (Ed.), *The new rural health* (pp. 204–220). South Melbourne: Oxford University Press.

Strasser, R., Hays, R., Kamien, M., & Carson, D. (2000). Is Australian rural practice changing? Findings from the national rural general practice study. *The Australian Journal of Rural Health*, 8, 222–226.

Teo, E., Lockardt, K., Pushparajah, J., Waynforth, D., & Smith, J. D. (2015). How do the specialty choices and rural intentions of medical students from Bond University (a full-fee paying, undergraduate-level medical program) compare with other (Commonwealth Supported Places – CSP) Australian medical students? *Australian Medical Student Journal*, 5(1), 47–52.

Van Der Weyden, M. B., & Chew, M. (2004). Arriving in Australia: overseas trained doctors. *The Medical Journal of Australia*, 181(11/12), 633–634.

Veitch, P., Underhill, A., & Hays, R. (2006). The career aspirations and career locations of James Cook University's first cohort of medical students: a longitudinal study at course entry and graduation. *Rural and Remote Health*, 6, 537. Available from: <www.rrh.org.au>.

Wainer, J. (2001). *Female rural doctors in Victoria: It's where I live*. Melbourne: Victorian Rural Workforce Agency.

Wainer, J., Bryant, L., Strasser, R., Carson, D., & Stringer, K. (1999). *A life not a wife*. Paper presented at the 5th National Rural Health Conference, Adelaide.

Wakerman, J. (2015). Editorial: Rural and remote health: a progress report. *The Medical Journal of Australia*, 202(9), 461–463.

Wakerman, J., Humphreys, J. S., Wells, R., Kuipers, P., Entwistle, P., & Jones, J. (2008). Primary health care delivery models in rural and remote Australia: a systematic review. *BMC Health Services Research*, 2, 276.

Wells, R. (2005). *The future health workforce: options we do and do not have*. Paper presented at the 8th National rural health conference, Central to Health: sustaining well-being in remote and rural Australia, Alice Springs.

Weymouth, S., Davey, C., Wright, J. I., Nieuwoudt, L. A., Barclay, L., Belton, S., et al. (2007). What are the effects of distance management on the retention of remote area nurses in Australia? *Rural and Remote Health*, 7, 652, (Online). Available from: <www.rrh.org.au>.

World Health Organization (WHO). (2002). *The world health report 2002: Reducing risks, promoting healthy life*. Geneva: WHO.

World Health Organization. (2005). *Preparing a health care workforce for the 21st century*. Geneva: WHO.

World Health Organization. (2015). *Health statistics and information systems*. Geneva: WHO. <http://www.who.int/healthinfo/global_burden_disease/estimates/en/index1.html> Accessed 11.06.15.

CHAPTER 12

REMOTE HEALTH PRACTICE

Sue Lenthall | Janie Dade Smith

Remote Australia makes up 78 per cent of the landmass of this great country. It is enormously diverse, from the huge central deserts, to the ski slopes in the south, the ochre-coloured mountains of the west, the crocodile-infested rivers of the north and Antarctica and the many surrounding islands. You know you are entering remote Australia when you drive from the cities, past small rural towns, along roads that become longer, straighter and dustier, and when you turn onto gravel or dirt and see cattle, sheep, emus and the odd camel wander across the road. In remote Australia the climate is one of extremes and the landscape is both intimidating and beautiful. As you travel for several hours to get from one town to the next, you get a sense that you have left 'rural' Australia and entered 'remote' Australia. Not only is the city far away, but everyone else is too. Only those who have never been to a remote area would be unable to differentiate between remote and rural areas as they are so very different from one another (Kelly & Smith 2007).

Remote areas are characterised by small and highly dispersed populations, higher proportions of Indigenous people and less access to all services. Remote communities

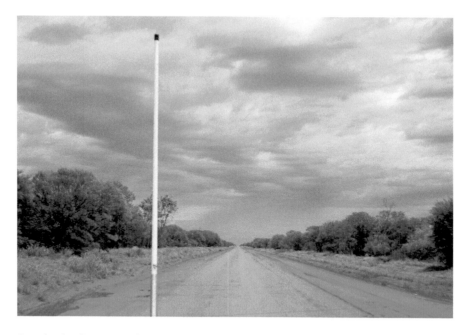

Reproduced with permission from: CRANAplus.

include: railway sidings, mining towns, cattle stations, pastoral leases, discrete Indigenous communities, outback towns, tourist resorts, detention centres, shipping and Australia's surrounding oceans, islands and Antarctica. All are remote, and all are different from one another and function in diverse ways.

While this speaks of the diversity found in remote Australia – geographically, climatically and culturally – it also speaks of the different models of health care and the different types of health professionals found in remote and very remote locations in Australia.

There is an old saying in remote areas that 'if you've seen one remote community, then you've seen one remote community'. This saying emphasises the uniqueness and differences found in each community. It also alerts remote health professionals to the issues they might need to consider when they move from one community to another, which could mean unlearning what they think they already know – especially if state boundaries are crossed. These issues may include learning: a different language, different cultural norms and practice; about differing health status and practical issues, such as dealing with water supply, travelling in certain weather conditions, knowing who to approach and other local oddities.

The previous chapter examined the roles, characteristics and workforce trends of the rural and remote health professionals in Australia. In this chapter we look at the differences and the commonalities between the disciplines in order to determine their scope of practice. We then apply this information to a case study on 'a day in the life of a remote area nurse' and present the different model of consultation they use in remote practice. This will assist the new remote health professional to understand the scope of practice, the cross-cultural context and the other personal and professional issues they will need to understand to work there. We then discuss the educational requirements to prepare for remote practice, which helps establish how we should go about educating and preparing the remote health workforce now and in the future.

PROFESSIONAL ROLES

Although there are many differences between what the various professions do, there are also many similarities when working in remote areas. In fact, remote health practitioners often have more in common with those they have morning tea with than they do with their colleagues of the same discipline in the city. All professions, whether physiotherapists, doctors or nurses or Aboriginal or Torres Strait Islander health practitioners, work in advanced and expanded levels of practice; and, the more remote the location, the more advanced the practice tends to be. Many practitioners also play multiple roles, which can often include those of administrator, educator, researcher and academic, veterinarian, social worker, ambulance driver and some may also provide outreach services and travel to numerous communities. This is particularly so for allied health professionals and doctors who mostly use fly-in fly-out and drive-in drive-out models of care, as well as care through tele-health.

Scope of practice

When we talk about remote practice we are talking about the practice of health professionals working in remote and very remote communities in Australia – as defined in Chapter 2. There are significant differences between remote and very remote

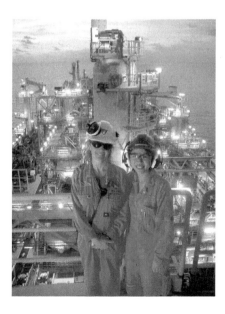

Reproduced with permission from: CRANAplus.

practice as a result of the geography, the types of health professionals available and the types of populations serviced (Smith et al., 2008). In very remote Australia the health practice is usually strongly cross-cultural and is undertaken by remote area nurses, Aboriginal and Torres Strait Islander health practitioners and via the phone to medical officers (Lenthall et al., 2011). This model of practice is significantly different from remote practice at a mine site, for example, where the population consists of mostly fit younger adults, where the health professional is usually a para-medic or occupational health and safety nurse, and it is based on an oil rig or a dusty mine site.

When we look at both situations we can see that the advanced practice and the multiple roles can mean that the remote practitioner requires a greater breadth and depth of knowledge and skills to work there than in the urban setting. This is called the practitioner's 'scope of practice'. For example, all doctors require a core set of knowledge and skills to be able to practise as a doctor. However, remote doctors need more advanced clinical skills, such as an ability to provide advice and guidance on renal dialysis, as well as knowledge of procedures and practices that in metropolitan practice would be the province of a specialist – a nephrologist managing complex medical conditions (Smith et al., 2008). They also need to be able to provide tele-phone advice without necessarily ever seeing the patient. A remote nurse would need to be able to suture, insert an intravenous infusion, provide health promotion advice and undertake the physical examination of a patient and consult with a doctor over the telephone regarding the management of the patient's conditions.

In this environment the remote doctor's or nurse's scope of practice requires a greater breadth and depth of clinical knowledge and skills that can be called upon when there is no access to a medical specialist or doctor. Therefore, all practitioners require a higher level of clinical acumen to diagnose and manage illness as there are often no pathology or radiology facilities and the usual clinical diagnostic support found in the tertiary setting is not available (Smith et al., 2008). Defining the doctor's or nurse's scope of practice helps to define the educational requirements to prepare them for these roles to practise as a remote area practitioner as we shall see.

KEY REMOTE HEALTH FACTORS

There are two key factors that differentiate educating a workforce for remote practice from educating a workforce for urban or city-based practice. They are:

1   the *context* in which the health professionals work
2   the additional and different educational *content* the health professional requires to work there.

The context

'Remote context' essentially means those things that vary due to the interrelated conditions in which they exist, such as the remote environment. For example, what is the difference between performing a Pap smear on a woman in an urban area and carrying out the same procedure on a woman in a remote area? The difference is the remote context – the remote practitioner may be performing the Pap smear on their next-door neighbour, their child's teacher or their friend. The practitioner may also be a doctor who has flown in to provide women's health services via the Royal Flying Doctor Service or may be a nurse who is specifically trained in women's health. Another context could be cross-cultural; for instance, the patient may not speak English, and may have brought her teenage daughter into the consultation to act as an interpreter. Therefore the interrelated conditions will be: 1) performing an intimate procedure and 2) using an interpreter who is 3) a family member, where 4) different cultural norms may exist. These four factors together put the procedure in a different context.

The context, therefore, changes everything about a normal situation. The remote context changes everything about the experience for both the practitioner and the patient.

Common context

Everything is amplified in the remote context: the temperature, the excitement of working in extreme situations, the higher levels of innovation required, the fascinating medicine and the rewards of working where few have dared to venture. It takes a special type of person to work remotely and it can be the 'best of worlds' for that reason. Health professionals will get to see some of the most beautiful and extraordinary landscapes and cultures; they will meet people they would have normally

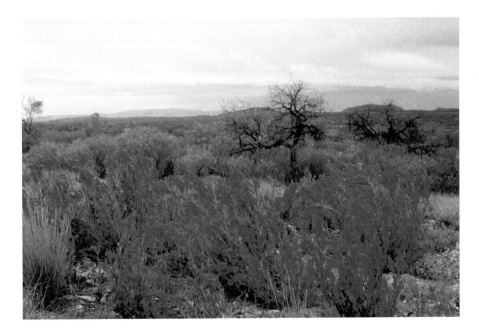

Reproduced with permission from: CRANAplus.

never come across and do some of the best fishing of all time. Those who get to work in remote Australia are in a very privileged position as they get to see a side of remote Australia that others only see on postcards, and they report high levels of job satisfaction (Lenthall, 2015). However, it can also be 'the worst of worlds' due to the climatic extremes, the health status of the populations served and the challenges and frustrations of clinical life.

There are some key contextual features that are common across the remote workforce, irrespective of the discipline, and they become increasingly significant with greater remoteness. These are important for all health professionals to understand as these are the things that change everything about what would ordinarily be a normal situation for most practitioners. They include the following:

- **Climatic extremes** – Most geographically remote communities experience climatic extremes with temperatures that can reach below zero and over 50 degrees, which can impact on both the practitioner and the population being served.

- **Relationship with the community** – The relationship between the community and the health professional tends to be closer and more personal in very small communities where everyone knows who you are even if you don't know them. This has been described as being like 'living in a fishbowl' (Austin, 2010). This means that the job does not finish at 5 p.m. and you will always be 'the nurse or the doctor' even if you are not on call, even if you are in the shop and even if you are out fishing.

- **Working in isolation** – Where practitioners work will define their degree of personal, professional and social isolation. Most very remote communities do not have the sporting facilities, restaurants, cafes or hairdressers found in most Australian towns and cities. Isolation aggravates access to locum relief, professional support and development, education for children and spouse employment. It also enhances the likelihood of burnout and reduces retention of the workforce (Opie et al., 2010; Lenthall et al., 2011).

- **Resourcefulness and infrastructure** – Whether it is fixing an ailing computer, undertaking maintenance on an X-ray machine or changing a tyre on a four-wheel drive, resourcefulness is a key attribute in remote areas where equipment is sometimes outdated (Australian Bureau of Statistics, 2013). Hence, all remote practitioners have to be flexible, self-reliant and resourceful.

- **Interprofessional teamwork** – A key feature of remote practice is the interprofessional nature of the work. The more remote the practice, the greater the need for interprofessional approaches, as a practitioner is more likely to be the only one of their discipline.

- **After-hours work** – Most clinical work, whether performed by a dentist, vet, doctor, nurse, radiographer, Indigenous health worker or psychologist, involves after-hours work in the remote context. After-hours work often also draws on the extended skills of other members of the multidisciplinary team, who are frequently called in to assist.

- **Workforce supply and organisation** – Remote health services often experience high turnover rates and there is a growing mix of short-term, casual and agency staff. This this turnover is referred to as the 'churn' factor, whereby workers churn though the cycle of staffing, which is challenging for employers and remote staff (Garnett et al., 2008; Cavanagh, 2014).
- **Survival skills** – As remote practitioners are members of the community in which they live, they need to know how to care for themselves as the work can be physically, emotionally and clinically challenging (Lenthall, 2015). This includes finding ways in which to live as members of the community and work as health professionals in an environment where everyone knows you. This raises issues of confidentiality, and the need to find ways to maintain a personal, professional and family life, and maintain that all-important sense of humour. Health professionals also need to know where to find support systems for themselves and to understand the different ways in which remote communities operate (see Chapters 1 and 2).

The common content

Irrespective of whether the professional is a physiotherapist, doctor or nurse, to work in a remote area they will need to have an understanding of the following common *content* areas:

- **Advanced clinical skills** – Every remote practitioner will require advanced and extended clinical skills in their discipline, plus those skills that would usually be referred to the next practitioner in the hierarchy. For example, a remote area nurse would need to be able to insert an intravenous infusion, manage chronic disease and perform routine preventive screening procedures that would normally be the responsibility of a doctor. Many find this aspect of their role challenging yet very rewarding.
- **Extended interprofessional skills** – It is often the combination of the team's advanced skills and their ability to practise those skills as part of a respectful and supportive team that can make the difference between life and death for a patient when an emergency occurs. For example, an Indigenous health professional who can recognise pre-eclampsia in a pregnant woman often makes the difference between whether the patient and her baby survive or not. It is important that all practitioners are adequately trained and updated in these skills (CRANAplus, 2015). Of greater importance is that practitioners know their own limitations, and when, how and to whom to refer (Smith et al., 2008).
- **Dealing with emergencies** – All remote practitioners will be exposed to emergency situations and will often need to deal with them without the required training, resources and support systems they might find in an urban setting. For example, a psychologist may have to deal with an acutely psychotic patient, or a doctor may have to deal with a multiple-vehicle road accident in the middle of the night. These unexpected situations happen more frequently in remote settings

and practitioners will need to draw on their own extended skills, plus those of the multidisciplinary team, to manage them. This is usually also the expectation of the community.

- **Tele-health** – Doctors in particular often work remotely from the patient and provide diagnostic and management advice over the telephone, radio or other electronic means (Smith et al., 2008). This requires an advanced level of skills for both the doctor and the referring remote health professional.

- **Indigenous issues** – All Australians have a responsibility to have some understanding of Indigenous history and culture and why things are the way they are, so as to be able to contribute to change. This is particularly true for remote health professionals because of their greater exposure to Indigenous peoples who make up 24 per cent of the population in remote Australia (Australian Institute of Health and Welfare, 2014). Health professionals also require knowledge of the Indigenous health issues related to their field, the social determinants of health and the state and local relevance, to be able to work in a culturally safe manner. For example, in remote and tropical areas it is essential to understand the importance of using contemporary approaches to ear health, and to know the causes, prevalence and prevention of diabetes and renal disease in the Indigenous community.

- **Cross-cultural communication skills** – Good communication skills are essential for all health professionals, especially in small communities, and particularly in Indigenous communities where English is often a second or third language and where different value and belief systems operate. This will also vary between disciplines. For example, an audiologist or psychologist may require a deeper level of understanding in this area than, say, an anaesthetist.

- **Public health work** – All remote practitioners need to understand the basic infrastructure in the community such as the water and sewerage supplies, garbage disposal processes, food storage systems and the disease prevention strategies and screening processes that are in place. This is particularly true for those living in tropical regions and remote areas.

- **Primary health care and health promotion** – The remote health workforce is largely educated in a biomedical model of health care. Yet to be effective in the remote setting they require practical information about how to apply the principles of primary health care to their daily practice (see Chapter 10). This includes an ability to negotiate culturally safe care and to educate, conduct programs and promote a healthy lifestyle within the whole community.

- **Associated legal and ethical issues related to their field** – When remote health practitioners extend their usual roles, as defined by metropolitan authorities, there may be occasions when the usual black-and-white legislative boundaries become blurred. For example, remote area nurses may supply and administer drugs. To do this, they need to understand the legislation and clinical practice guidelines under which they are employed and have successfully completed a pharmacotherapeutics course.

- **Professional development** – With limited access to resources and professional development opportunities, it is still vital for remote practitioners to be lifelong learners and find alternative ways to maintain and update their levels of knowledge, skills and competence. This includes knowing where and how to find information.
- **Research** – It is important that remote practitioners are able to undertake local research, critically analyse information and apply it to their local community's needs. It is also important to be participants in research to contribute to the evidence base.

Throughout this process we have discussed the numerous commonalities and the fewer differences between the remote health disciplines, and have argued that the degree of remoteness extends the breadth of skills required. To understand this more fully, let us take a look at remote practice in more detail.

REMOTE PRACTICE AS A SEPARATE DISCIPLINE

Wakerman (2004, p. 213) offers a working definition of remote health practice:

> Remote health is an emerging discipline with distinct sociological, historical and practice characteristics. Its practice in Australia is characterised by geographical, professional and, often, social isolation of practitioners; a strong interprofessional multidisciplinary approach; overlapping and changing roles of team members; a relatively high degree of GP substitution; and practitioners requiring public health, emergency and extended clinical skills. These skills and remote health systems need to be suited to working in a cross-cultural context; serving small, dispersed and often highly mobile populations; serving populations with relatively high health needs; a physical environment of climatic extremes and communications environments of rapid technological change.

For more than three decades health professionals in rural and remote Australia have argued that rural and remote practice is different and additional enough to justify its existence as a separate discipline (Smith & Hays, 2004; Smith et al., 2008). This has resulted in three key organisations being established and supported with government funding to educate, support and represent them. In particular, this includes: CRANAplus – established initially as a remote nursing organisation in 1981 and that now represents the whole remote health workforce; Services for Australian Rural and Remote Allied Health (SARRAH) – who represent rural and remote allied health professionals; and the Australian College of Rural and Remote Medicine (ACRRM) – who represent rural and remote doctors. ACRRM was accredited as a separate discipline for the first time in the world in 2008 with a curriculum and assessment program accredited by the Australian Medical Council to support it (Smith et al., 2007; Australian College of Rural and Remote Medicine, 2015).

The only nationally accredited remote vocational training program is the Remote Vocational Training Scheme, which provides training for medical practitioners in Aboriginal and Torres Strait Islander communities and in remote and isolated communities throughout Australia (Remote Vocational Training Scheme, 2015). Doctors who successfully complete this program gain Fellowship from the Royal Australian College of General Practitioners and ACRRM as well as vocational recognition with Medicare Australia. While the discipline with the highest number of practitioners in remote Australia is nursing, there is no similar scheme or vocational training requirements, though specific courses are recommended (CRANAplus, 2014b).

Remote practice is also seen by some as isolated practice, whereby it includes those who work in solo practice, such as nurses working in prisons and detention centres (CRANAplus, 2014a). It also includes those who are culturally isolated but who live on the urban fringes, such as doctors working in Western Sydney. Yet remote health is continually tagged onto rural health as an appendage and, like all minority groups, often loses its own voice and becomes the silent partner. When we examine the significantly different health status of remote populations, which are worse off by all health indicators, it becomes critical that we appreciate this difference so that we can treat these different groups differently within their own context.

THE REMOTE AREA NURSE

The remote area nurse (RAN) makes up the largest professional discipline working in remote Australia. Therefore, their role deserves special mention as it is significantly different from the role of a registered nurse in any other setting. In this section we will describe what a remote area nurse looks like, where they work, who they work for, what they do, how they do it and the challenges they face. We will then present a case study that describes a 'day the in the life of a RAN' and the consultation model they use in remote practice.

RANs – who are they?

The typical remote area nurse is female and around 44 years old or older. They are often people who have grown up kids and who have always wanted to work remotely and contribute to society with the skills they have. The typical RAN has a nursing degree, about a quarter have midwifery qualifications and a few have remote or rural qualifications. They have usually worked in a hospital or a community health setting for some years before deciding to go remote, and some worked remotely in their early years and always wanted to come back (Lenthall et al., 2011). In more recent times, especially since the Northern Territory Intervention in 2008, there have been increasing numbers of agency staff, short-term locums as well as what are called 'orbiting staff' who are often experienced remote practitioners who go in and out of communities on a needs basis (Wakerman, Curry, & McEldowney, 2012; Nursing and Allied Health Rural Locum Scheme, 2015).

Where are they?

Remote area nursing occurs in remote and very remote communities including: remote primary health care centres, mine sites, small towns, railway sidings, islands, detention centres, Antarctica, on snow slopes, on ships, on remote tourist resorts and in discrete remote Indigenous communities. In 2011 there were 1076 registered nurses working in 301 very remote health facilities, of whom about 43 per cent worked in remote Indigenous communities. Three-quarters of these nurses practised in very remote primary health care centres without in-patient facilities. The majority of these RANs were based in Western Australia, then Queensland and then the Northern Territory, which had the highest number of nurses working in Indigenous primary health care centres (Lenthall et al., 2011).

Who do they work for?

RANs are employed in a range of settings including, but not limited to:

- state and territory government health services
- community controlled health services
- Aboriginal Medical Services
- primary health care services/clinics
- multi-purpose centres
- private general practices
- mining and other industries
- mobile and fly-in fly-out and drive-in drive-out services
- private and non-governmental organisation (NGO) health providers (CRANA-plus, 2014b).

What do they do?

Unlike rural nurses RANs usually work in communities where there is no resident doctor and where they work as part of a multidisciplinary team. In 2001 most RANs were found to work in very remote areas in small teams of about six nurses, supplemented with Aboriginal and Torres Strait Islander health practitioners, though in some larger communities up to thirteen nursing positions have been recorded (Lenthall et al., 2011). So, what do they do?

Remote area nursing is based on the principles of primary health care, which is not so much about 'what' you do as about 'how' you do it. It involves diagnosing illness; prescribing and dispensing medications; undertaking community development, health promotion and public health activities; and managing chronic disease and treating emergencies through the use of clinical protocols. For those working in Indigenous health this can be for a population with the worst health status in the world on some indicators. For many RANs the work is challenging and interesting, and they value the high level of responsibility and flexibility they have (Australian Bureau of Statistics, 2013).

While it is advanced practice, RANs are not independent practitioners and do not have the autonomy or prescribing rights that doctors and nurse practitioners have. RANs practise using clinical protocols such as the Central Australian Rural Practitioners Association (CARPA) *Standard Treatment Manual* or the *Queensland Primary Care Manual*. This is an important point as it legally covers RANs for the extended role they perform (CRANAplus, 2015). CRANAplus also provides substantial training programs and a *Clinical Procedures Manual* to support RANs in their roles (CRANAplus, 2015).

To demonstrate what RANs do that is so different from urban practice, the following case study about a day in the life of a RAN has been developed.

CASE STUDY – A DAY IN THE LIFE OF A RAN

Mary is a 52-year-old registered nurse who comes from Newcastle; she has two grown up kids who still live there. She has had considerable experience in working in remote Indigenous communities as an orbiting health professional and has worked in about six different communities on and off over the past 15 years. For the past six months she's been working in Distmount in Central Australia, a community where she has worked previously. She knows many of the people and speaks some of the local Aboriginal language. Mary has a Masters degree in Remote Health Practice and a strong commitment to social justice and to improving Indigenous health.

Distmount is a remote Indigenous community with a population of about 500 people. The health care service is a remote primary health care service staffed by three registered nurses and three Aboriginal health practitioners, but only one of these positions is filled at the moment by Rosie, who is very experienced. The other two nurses are agency nurses on short-term contracts. A fly-in medical clinic is conducted every fortnight and medical support is provided via telephone consultations, as well as visiting specialist services.

Mary's working day starts at 8.30 a.m., with the opening of the clinic. She sees a variety of people including two mothers with sick kids; both have fevers with mild chest infections. She takes an opportunity to undertake growth assessments of the children and notes that one is due for an immunisation. She arranges for the mother to return with her little boy when he is feeling better. She also sees Emily who has diabetes and has come to get her medications refilled. Mary notes that Emily is overdue for her Adult Health Check* and she agrees to have the check now. Mary takes some blood and asks her how her kids are. She then talks to her about what she has been eating and how she is coping with her diet and exercise.

At 10.30, the visiting eye team arrives to conduct an eye clinic, but Mary didn't realise they were coming. She asks one of the agency nurses to work with them and they borrow the

*An Adult Health Check is an assessment process to identify the client's health status and their need for preventative health care and to provide opportunities for health education and health management and assists in the early detection of chronic conditions (Northern Territory Department of Health, 2015).

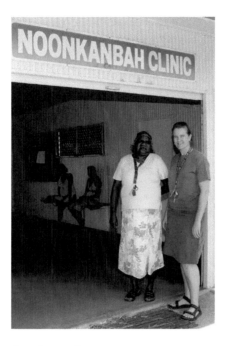

Reproduced with permission from: CRANAplus.

ambulance to go and pick up the clients. The rest of the morning Mary is busy seeing a variety of other people with a variety of illnesses and providing advice to the other nurses. In all of the consultations Mary follows the RAN Model of Client Consultation (see Table 12.1 later).

At 12.30 Mary goes home to have a sandwich for lunch. Ten minutes later she gets a call from the office in town to tell her that a new RAN, Kylie, is waiting at the airport. Apparently, Kylie has experience in accident and emergency and paediatrics, but has never worked in a remote Indigenous community before; she is very excited about going remote. Mary rolls her eyes, 'another newbie to orientate' she thinks. Mary drags out her orientation folder to find her paper on 'Don't move the furniture and other advice for new Remote Area Nurses (RANs)' (Lenthall, Gordon, Knight, Aitken, & Terrie, 2012)

After lunch, Mary and Rosie talk to the grade 3 and 4 students at the local school on the importance of cleaning their teeth. They found some useful teaching material from the internet. This is the part of the job that both Mary and Rosie love; they leave the school laughing and chatting.

On the way back to the clinic, they stop and get a cold drink at the local store and they run into Dawn who tells them that her dad Henry is crook again with his sugar. They stop and check in on Henry at his house. Henry is lying outside of the house on blankets beside the fire with the billy boiling, with two dogs beside him. Rosie calls across from the fence and waits to be invited into the yard. Henry's grandkids are playing in the yard and are covered

Continued

in red dust. Rosie talks to Henry in the local language and asks him about the football match last weekend and then she asks him how he is feeling, how his medications are going and where his dosette box is. She is relieved to find that it is on top of the cupboard so the kids can't get to it. Rosie takes Henry's blood sugar and blood pressure and talks to him about his tucker. Mary asks about the idea of him being seen by a renal physician in town, but Henry is reluctant to go. He knows that people who go into town often don't come home and he doesn't want to have to move there and go on one of those machines that his cousin, who now lives in Alice Springs, had to go on. Rosie updates Mary on the family situation. Henry has agreed to come to the clinic the next day for additional blood tests. Mary and Rosie drive around town and talk about the leaking toilet at Henry's house and agree to talk to the shire office to get it fixed. They give people a wave as they go. When they get back to the clinic there are lots of people waiting.

At 2.15 p.m. Emily Miller runs in with her 10-year-old son Tom in her arms. She tells Rosie and Mary that Tom fell over a 'wheelybin' about an hour ago, and is now complaining of pain to his back and tummy. Tom is pale, complaining of right-sided abdominal pain and crying, and Mary takes a history and a physical examination using the RAN Model of Client Consultation (see Table 12.2 later). Mary decides to ring the on-call doctor at Alice Springs Remote Health.

Audio of consultation. Audio access through Student Consult.

Telephone consultation – Mary and the Doctor

(Ivanhoe & Gordon, 2015)

RAN: *Hi Martine, it's Mary here at Distmount. I have a 10-year-old child here who has had a fall and I suspect he has an acute abdomen. He is in moderate to severe distress, curled up on the trolley, crying out that he has pain in his juni (meaning stomach). Can I discuss it with you?*

Dr: *Yes, go ahead.*

RAN: *It's Tom Miller, Emily's little boy – she is with him. His date of birth is 1st January 2003; his hospital registration number is 12456. Emily tells me that he had a fall – he was playing on the basketball court and he tried to hurdle a big rubbish bin that was lying on its side. He fell over the top of it on his right side. She tells me that it happened just after lunch at about 12:30 – it's now 14:30. She tells me he didn't seem badly hurt at the time and the other kids took him home. However, the pain increased and he became distressed so they called the clinic and asked for the Aboriginal Health Worker to pick him up.*

Dr: *Ok, so how is he now?*

RAN: *Rosie carried him in and he is lying on the trolley curled up on his side and in moderate to severe distress, crying, but lying still. I have examined him; he had no loss of consciousness at the time according to witnesses. He just seemed 'winded'. He is pale, no* *diaphoresis. Complaining of generalised right-sided abdominal pain, quiet when lying still but crying out with any movement; his pain seems to be coming in waves, sharp and strong. He has not vomited.*

- *Head – No injuries noted.*
- *Chest – No bruising, no pain on palpation, good air entry on both sides.*
- *Abdomen – Some bruising over his right side, tense but not rigid; bowel sounds are present; on palpation he has pain localised to his right side and right renal angle. He describes it as 'big pain'.*
- *Arms and legs – No injuries noted.*
- *Observations – Temperature is 36.5, pulse 120, blood pressure 114 over 75, respirations are 20 and his Sats (oxygen saturation) are 99 per cent.*
- *His urinalysis is brown red with macroscopic haematuria. He only passed a few drops.*
- *His haemoglobin is 127 g/L; and his weight is 35 kilograms.*

Dr: *I agree it sounds like an acute abdomen, a likely contused kidney. He will need evacuation today. Now, do you have a line in?*

RAN: *Yes, we have just got a 20G cannula in and we have him on 4 litres of oxygen. We also have 500 mL of normal saline ready. What would you like for pain?*

Dr: *I can't open my computer; can you tell me if he has any medical history or allergies?*

RAN: *Yes, he is normally a well 10-year-old child. Only history is CSOM (chronic suppurative otitis media) and presentations for skin infections. He has no allergies, he is on no medications and his immunisations are up to date.*

Dr: *OK, let's keep him on nil by mouth; give him 250 mL normal saline stat and 2 mg morphine intravenously stat. And I will ring the emergency department at Alice Springs Hospital and organise the evacuation. Is that OK?*

RAN: *Yes.*

Dr: *Once he has settled, can you re-examine him? Examine his chest and re-examine his right upper quadrant please. Keep him on half hourly observations, take a full blood count and put him on a fluid balance chart, and we may need an indwelling catheter depending on his progress. If you are happy with that I will ring you back in about 15 minutes.*

RAN: *Thanks Martine, can I repeat the morphine if needed?*

Dr: *Yes, titrate it to his blood pressure, you can give 2 mg every 10 minutes as needed.*

RAN: *OK, that's morphine 2 mg IV stat and repeat 10 minutely as long as systolic BP remains over 90?*

Dr: *Yes thanks, I will ring you back shortly.*

Continued

15 minutes later….

Dr: *Hi Mary, how is Tom?*

RAN: *He is much more settled now. Lying quietly, but easily roused. I have given 4 mg of IV morphine in total and 250 mL of normal saline is through.*

I have re-examined his chest – no pain on palpation, good air entry on both sides, no tracheal deviation, JVP (jugular venous pressure) is normal.

Abdomen – his pain seems to have settled in the right renal angle – he has developed bruising over the right side and the area is tense and slightly swollen, but not rigid, tender on light palpation, he has bowel sounds. There do not appear to be any other injuries. He has passed about 200 mL of rusty urine, macroscopic blood stained.

Dr: *OK, well it certainly sounds like a contused kidney at the very least. Can you tell me what his obs are now?*

RAN: *Yes, his pulse is 96, his BP 105 over 65, respirations are 20, haemoglobin is 115, Sats are 100 per cent on 4 litres of oxygen. His pain has settled and he is lying quietly but doesn't like being disturbed.*

Dr: *Good, you have done a good job. Let's get another IV line in and continue the fluids at maintenance dose. Ring me if you think he needs more pain relief or he may need a further bolus of fluids. I have called the Royal Flying Doctor Service (RFDS) and the emergency department (ED). They will call you shortly with an expected time of arrival. Is Emily going with him?*

RAN: *Yes, she is happy to go and family will look after the other children. She weighs 80 kilograms.*

Dr: *Good, the RFDS should not be too long, they have a plane ready to go.*

RAN: *Thanks Martine, just to summarise, I will continue normal saline at 125 mL per hour and ring you if there are any changes in his condition or if he requires further analgesia.*

Dr: *Yes, thanks Mary, I will fax the referral to ED – the computer is now up and running. Ring me if you are worried, OK?*

RAN: *Yes thanks – thanks for your help.*

Rosie and Mary talk to Emily about the problem and that Tom may have injured his kidney and needs to go into the hospital in town to see a specialist doctor. Emily is worried about who will look after the other kids as her sister Margaret has just had another baby and her mum is too sick to look after them all.

Rosie takes Emily back to her house to have a chat about who could look after her other kids and to pick up some clothes to go to hospital. Mary receives a call to hear that the plane will not be there at 5.30 p.m. as it is off doing a clinic in the other direction. She monitors Tom, taking his observations regularly and giving him some pain relief until the flight arrives. She has documented the situation in a referral letter to the hospital, and has notified the airstrip manager that an RFDS plane will be arriving. When Mary and Rosie hear the plane overhead they load up the ambulance with Tom, Emily and her other kids and an Aunty and they drive to the airstrip.

Mary hands over Tom to the RFDS nurse while Emily and Tom board the plane. Donald, Emily's youngest, cries as he will miss his mum. Rosie tells Mary that she'll check on how the kids are doing while Emily is away. About 6.30 p.m. both Rosie and Mary head home for their dinner. Mary listens to some music and rings her daughter in Newcastle for a chat. At 8.20 p.m. Mary is called out to Joanna Miles who is worried about her 3-year-old son Steven. Mary realises how tired she is and therefore she takes extra care in assessing Steven. Luckily, while he seems to have a cold, he is still eating, drinking and playing well. Mary and Joanna agree to give Steven some Panadol and see how he is in the morning. Finally Mary goes home. She's on call that night, but there are no further call outs. It's been a long and tiring day. Challenging, but also very satisfying.

This case study provides an overview of a day in the life of a RAN and draws out the breadth and depth of personal and professional skills required to work remotely. It also demonstrates the need for good orientation and preparation for the role. In the case study Mary used the RAN Model of Client Consultation. This model was developed by a group of highly experienced remote area nurses and academics in 2015 in order to support new and experienced remote area nurses to use a standard process of consultation (Lenthall et al., 2015).

How do they do it? – The RAN Model of Client Consultation

The RAN Model of Client Consultation is a client-centered, comprehensive, systematic approach to client assessment that manages the risk to the client, the nurse and the organisation. It has seven principles (see Table 12.1) and eight steps (see Table 12.2), and it offers one model that could be used by new and existing practitioners (Lenthall et al., 2015).

This consultation framework provides one process that RANs use to undertake a consultation in remote practice and offers novices and existing remote health practitioners a way forward. Other methods exist; one endorsed by CRANAplus is the SOODAF model:

Story or subjective assessment

Ongoing health problems or past history and management

Observation or objective assessment

Diagnosis or list of differentials

Actions or management plan

Follow-up (CRANAplus, 2014a).

Regardless of what you use, what is important is that you use an endorsed model, with endorsed processes and the standard treatment manuals for your state.

TABLE 12.1 The RAN Model of Client Consultation – Principles	
PRINCIPLE	CONSIDER
Culturally safe	• Who is the right person to undertake this consultation – gender and cultural issues?
	• How can I make the person feel comfortable?
	• Is there need for an interpreter?
	• Are appropriate family members present if necessary?
Holistic and comprehensive	• Consider the whole person – the context of their lives, their families and community
	• Ask the client about their experience of the illness, how it has impacted on them
	• Consider any chronic diseases or ongoing health problems
	• Remember, when someone presents, it may be for more than one reason and the first one is not necessarily the most important one
	• It is important to get a balance between thoroughness and focusing on the person's concerns
Systematic	• Obtain the history before taking the observations or performing the physical examination. The history will tell you what you need to examine
	• In examination, take a head-to-toe approach
Shares power with the client	• Negotiate with the client around history taking and the management plan
	• Encourage the client to share in the decision making so that they own their own health
	• Assist with building the client's self-reliance and health literacy
Provides coordination and continuity of care	• Use and update the client's records, both the progress notes AND clinical items (or the equivalent) – for the patient information system being used
	• Reflect on the consultation and collaborate/discuss with your colleagues – Aboriginal and Torres Strait Islander Health Practitioners, other Registered Nurses and Medical Officers
	• Contact other agencies as required
Encourages clinical reasoning	• Consider the age, place of the client and how this impacts on their risk of developing illnesses. Determine what is the most likely assessment; what can't you afford to miss?
	• Use a problem-solving approach that takes into account the clinician's knowledge, experience and attitudes in order to reach a hypothesis
Promotes clinical safety and quality	• Work within your individual scope of practice
	• Adhere to regionally developed and endorsed best practice treatment protocols for common presenting conditions
	• Adhere to quality policies and procedures within individual organisational structures

Adapted with permission from: Lenthall, S., Knight, S., Foxley, S., Gordon, V., Ivanhoe, T., & Aitken, R. (2015). Remote Area Nurse Model of Consultation. *International Journal of Advanced Nursing Studies, 4*(2), p. 149–152.

DESCRIPTION	STEP
	TABLE 12.2 The RAN Model of Client Consultation – Consultation steps
	1 Open the consultation Before seeing the client: • Review client records, note outstanding recalls or actions, ensure privacy When seeing the client: • Greet the client and establish rapport – the '4Fs' – family, football, fun and food (as in hunting) • Note general impressions • Check name, next of kin, chart number and date of birth are correct • Check if an interpreter or practitioner of other gender needed
S T O R Y	**2 Take a history** Reason for presentation: • Listen to the story; establish ideas, concerns, expectations Use the OLDCARTS method for each reason for presentation: **O**nset – when did it start? **L**ocation – where does it hurt, where is the problem? **D**uration – how long, have you had it before, what happened then? **C**haracteristics – description of the pain or the problem **A**ggravating factors – what makes it worse? **R**elieving factors – what makes it better? **T**reatments – what have they tried, what do they think it is, how it is impacting on them and others, anything else? **S**igns and symptoms (other) (CRANAplus, 2014a) • Ask questions relevant to the system involved, e.g. respiratory, cardiac Current health review: • Appetite, nausea, change in weight, sleep, energy/activity, bowels, 'waterworks', interest in life, periods, sexual health, emotional health – self harm; do you ever feel unsafe? • Drug and allergy history: current medications (prescribed, over the counter and traditional), allergies and immunisation status • Alcohol/other drugs/smoking Other history: • Past medical and surgical history: accidents, admissions to hospital, treatments at other clinics, accidents and injuries, chronic diseases, gynaecological and obstetric history including last Pap smear • Family medical history: general health • Personal and social history

Continued

DESCRIPTION	STEP
	TABLE 12.2 The RAN Model of Client Consultation – Consultation steps–cont'd

DESCRIPTION	STEP	
O B S E R V E	3	**Undertake a clinical examination** • Rapid physical (head-to-toe) assessment • General observations as indicated – may include body mass index (BMI), waist circumference • Temperature, pulse, respirations, blood pressure, urinalysis, oxygen saturation, blood glucose level, haemoglobin • Systematic assessment of relevant systems – LOOK …LISTEN …FEEL • Investigations: as indicated by the history, the client's age, where they live (place) and how their age and place increase their risk of developing illnesses or disease • Patient consent
A S S E S S	4	**Undertake assessment and discussion** • Make an assessment of 1) the reason for the presentation and 2) other health issues • Summarise findings from the history and clinical examination with the client and discuss the assessment with them • Explore the person's knowledge and clarify – including long- and short-term implications • Assess and use opportunities for brief interventions and health promotion as appropriate
P L A N	5	**Negotiate a management plan** • Follow best practice treatment manuals and protocols • Discuss goals and targets, and negotiate a management plan with the client and appropriate others as required • Refer as necessary for further investigation or management • Include when appropriate – long-term care, identified risk factors, public health screening and preventative health initiatives
	6	**Close the consultation** • Check the client's understanding and agreement with the management plan – 'what is your understanding of what you are going to do now?' and 'do you have any questions?'
	7	**Document the consultation** Update client's record using SOAP: **S**tory **O**bservations **A**ssessment **P**lan • Update progress notes and clinical items, recall system and, if appropriate, the personally controlled electronic health record

TABLE 12.2 The RAN Model of Client Consultation – Consultation steps–cont'd	
DESCRIPTION	STEP
	8 **Reflect on your own practice**
	• What went well?
	• What could be improved?
	• How are you?

Adapted with permission from: Lenthall, S., Knight, S., Foxley, S., Gordon, V., Ivanhoe, T. & Aitken, R. (2015). Remote Area Nurse Model of Consultation. Alice Springs: Centre for Remote Health, Flinders University.

OCCUPATIONAL STRESS

Working in remote practice can be stressful for all health professionals concerned as they are often working outside their usual scope of practice, where they need to be flexible, resourceful and innovative. Also Akers found that the role of remote health practitioners is often romanticised and that nurses, in particular, spend long hours on call, are often working alone, have poor orientation to the role, are responsible for a large number of patients and are more likely to experience traumatic events with little time to recover.

In 2009–10 a national analysis of occupational stress levels in the remote area nursing workforce was undertaken (Opie et al., 2010). The researchers found that nurses working in very remote Australia experience significantly higher levels of psychological distress and emotional exhaustion compared with other professional populations, including human service workers, police officers, psychiatric nurses and ward nurses (Opie et al., 2010). The four main stressors they identified were: 1) the remote context; 2) workload and scope of practice; 3) poor management; and 4) violence and safety concerns (Lenthall et al., 2011). They found:

1 **The remote context creates its owns stressors** – It can be emotionally exhausting, and the remote context contributes to other difficulties involving social issues, staffing, intercultural factors, isolation and difficulties with equipment and infrastructure (Opie et al., 2010).

2 **Workload and scope of practice** – The 'frontline' nature of remote area health work and the lack of medical and allied health presence dictate that nurses are subject to greater workloads, with high levels of responsibilities and expectations from the employer and the community. Many RANs reported a lack of preparation or orientation to their role. In a study of RAN occupational stress, 30 per cent of RANs reported not receiving any orientation to their current positions while, among those who did, less than half thought it was adequate (Lenthall,

2015). In particular, there was not sufficient cross-cultural education or training in advanced clinical skills, primary health care and public health.

3 **Poor management** – Poor management was identified by RANs as a problem (Lenthall et al., 2009; Wakerman & Davey, 2008). In remote Australia, there is a relatively small pool from which managers and leaders are drawn. Typically, clinicians are promoted to management positions without additional education or training and often it is because they are 'the last man standing'. Bullying by managers and by other remote staff has also been identified as a major problem (Akers, 2013). However, while there are stories about poor management, managers can be an 'easy target' when anything goes wrong and they rightly or wrongly are often blamed (Lenthall, 2015).

4 **Violence and safety concerns** – RANs were found to often be confronted by violence within the clinic or the community and, unfortunately, there has been an increase in reported violence in the workplace since 1995 (Fisher et al., 1995; Opie et al., 2011). However, this has been recognised and many employers and health services have introduced improved safety measures, such as the increased use of drivers during call outs at night and prevention (Australian Bureau of Statistics, 2013).

TIPS IN PREPARING FOR REMOTE HEALTH PRACTICE

In this chapter so far we have drawn out what happens in very remote Indigenous health practice and identified some of the challenges faced by remote health professionals. This section outlines some tips about preparing for remote practice in any setting, as it is vitally important that health professionals are well prepared for their remote roles, from which many make long careers. For those interested in 'going remote' there are several organisations that provide some very useful resources for students: CRANAplus, which provides a framework for, and pathways to, remote practice (CRANAplus, 2015); and the National Rural Health Students Network, which provides student placement information and resources (National Rural Health Students Network, 2015). The following tips have been adapted from Lenthall et al. (2012) and CRANAplus (2015). They provide some things to consider before and after you go remote; while they refer to the largest profession – remote nurses – the principles are the same for all disciplines.

- **Be prepared for advanced practice.** Learn about using a primary health care approach, know the social determinants of health, understand the health status of the population you will be serving and know how to practise in a culturally safe way. These concepts will enable you to achieve more than 'band-aid' care. Advanced clinical skills are also essential. We recommend prior experience in emergency, paediatrics, chronic disease management and midwifery or obstetrics. Many preparatory courses exist such as: the Remote Emergency Care or Remote Maternity Care short courses through CRANAplus; a variety of tertiary preparation courses such as the Flinders University Remote Health Practice program at

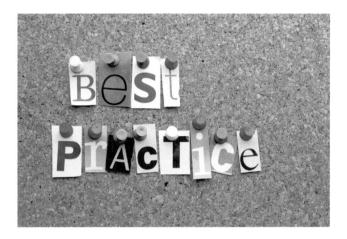

Reproduced with permission from: iStockphoto/Matt Jeacock.

the Centre for Remote Health in Alice Springs. The following tips do not replace the need for appropriate, formal preparation.

- **Before you go,** make sure you ask your potential employer at interview what orientation they have planned for you, how to update your skills, what support is available to do so and what the after-hours requirements are. Also ask about personal issues such as having pets, what to bring and what is in the community such as the store, a school, a police station; and what health services they offer (CRANAplus, 2015). Some communities provide basic health care services, and use hub and spokes models of care, whereas others have renal dialysis units and birthing facilities, so it is important prior to going to know what services are offered as you will need to appropriate skills.

- **When you get there,** introduce yourself to significant people in the community such as the elders, health council members, traditional healers, school teachers, store manager and appropriate others.

- **Find a mentor** or preferably two. Ask a health worker or community person to be a cultural and community mentor and ask another more experienced health professional from elsewhere to also be a mentor. CRANAplus offers a free national multidisciplinary mentoring program that you can access, so contact them and find out how to go about it (www.crana.org.au).

- **Expect culture shock.** If you are working in an Indigenous community it is normal to experience culture shock. This may include a variety of feelings in the first 12 months, which are normal. Firstly you may experience a period of excitement or fascination – the honeymoon phase; then a feeling of disenchantment – the 'what am I doing here?' phase. Gradually, you may begin to develop relationships with the community and start to feel you know what you are doing – the effective functioning phase, when you might experience what a privilege it is to be working within such a rich context. This is a normal process and it is important to identify and talk to your mentor about it.

- **Speak little and listen lots.** If you are working in an Indigenous community it is important to listen to Indigenous health professionals as they will often be your greatest support and teachers.
- **Engage in professional loitering.** Hang round the store and the large tree in front of the council offices and observe what goes on. Talk to the elders under the tree and get to know their families.
- **Learn about the local history**. It helps to understand the community and its people.
- If an **Indigenous language** is spoken, attempt to learn it. It's a great relationship builder.
- Recognise that **you are not the expert** and don't act as one. You are merely a tool being used by the community to achieve their goals – so listen, hear, respect, learn and contribute.
- **Develop relationships.** Relationships in remote Indigenous communities are vital and their importance cannot be overstated. It may be useful to use the four 'Fs' of family, food (hunting), football and fun to help establish and maintain relationships.
- Seek out and **use the best practice protocol manuals** always.
- **Give time to the team.** Consider strategies that improve team functioning such regular meetings and social events, and join in.
- **Be respectful.** Ask the Indigenous health professionals what the most respectful term is when addressing clients. Remember your manners when dealing with clients and staff. Be gracious to visitors and new staff, offer hospitality – a cup of tea, a meal and a friendly word.
- **Avoid burnout.** Keep a journal, ensure you have another interest or outlet and keep in touch with families and friends. Take a break before you REALLY need it. If you are feeling stressed, talk to someone or contact CRANAplus Bush Support Services, a free, confidential 24-hour support and debriefing service for health professionals and their families (1800 805 391).
- **Have an open heart.** You will make mistakes, both cultural and clinical, accept them, laugh at yourself with others and be open to change. If people can see that you are trying, and are being open to understanding, they will be open and accepting. This is how trust is established.
- **Don't move the clinic furniture** or rearrange the pharmacy when you first arrive. It is staking a claim to the clinic but is not welcome. An Aboriginal Health Professional once reported that each of the 18 new nurses in the past 12 months had moved the clinic furniture. Remember you are a guest.
- **Appreciate the experience**. RANs often live and work with people and in places that most Australians never get to experience. It's a privilege, enjoy it.

IMPLICATIONS FOR FUNDERS, MANAGERS AND EDUCATIONAL DESIGNERS

The above scenarios offer unique challenges for those who manage or develop programs for remote health professionals. While there have been significant positive changes in the general ways in which all health professionals have been educated over the past decade, the orientation and professional development programs for remote practitioners have not changed and are very discipline, state, regional and educator specific. Some useful initiatives have been the 'Pathways Program' in Central Australia that was found to improve retention (Jones, Blue, Adams, & Walker-Jeffreys, 2003; vanHaaren & Williams, 2000); the Transition to Remote Area Nursing program from the Centre for Remote Health; and the Pathways to Rural and Remote Orientation Training (PaRROT) program in north Queensland that is having some success (Queensland Health, 2015). However, lip service has generally been paid to the interdisciplinary approaches as each discipline is funded from its own siloed bucket.

Common learning – Interprofessional

We know that health professionals in remote practice have more in common with those they have morning tea with than those in their own professional disciplinary silos. If we look at what each professional learns, or needs to learn, we can see that this learning is 'common' in both content and context and that, if there are major differences, they largely fall into the category of depth and breadth of clinical content. We also know that the major 'stuff ups' we have in health are often directly related to poor communication between the disciplines. You know the old story – the specialist didn't tell the GP, who didn't tell the remote area nurse, who didn't tell the visiting physiotherapist, who didn't tell the patient, who didn't mention it to the specialist the last time they were flown out for their appointment! These communication issues are compounded by a lack of respected interprofessional processes for reporting disaffected or incompetent practitioners. The 'Dr Death' scenario in Bundaberg in 2005 provides a good example (Sandhill, 2005).

Common learning occurs in other countries such as Sweden, Canada and the United Kingdom and begins in the first undergraduate year. It is based on 'working together – learning together' through interdisciplinary education for all health professions over three undergraduate years (National Health Service, 2001). And it is very relevant for remote practice where all disciplines have to work together. This includes doctors, nurses, physiotherapists, pharmacists, social workers, dentists and the numerous other allied health and social care professionals, and it applies to the remote Australian context.

Interprofessional learning is proving to be very successful in improving communication between the health disciplines, who work better together, using patient-centred approaches that meet the population's needs (Humphris, 2005). Hence, it is very relevant to remote health professionals, who are in a prime position to take the lead. Research tells us that patient-centred care results in increased adherence to care plans, reduced morbidity and improved quality of life for patients, particularly in those low-resourced areas with reduced workforce – remote and rural areas (World Health Organization, 2005). This is an approach that will actually have an impact upon the health of the people, not just the workforce.

In Australia there are some moves towards a similar model, though these are like a gentle breeze rather than the cyclone of change that is required. Some Australian academics see this as all undergraduate students learning health content together, such as anatomy and physiology. This is *not* what this common learning process is about. It is about learning health and social care knowledge and skills, which are common across all disciplines, together – it is not about common subjects across the disciplines. These topics are often described in Australian education circles as domains of learning, such as communication skills, the health professional role, legal and ethical practice, interprofessional teamwork, social care roles, client-focused care and the education processes, including critical thinking, problem solving, clinical reasoning, educational theory, learning styles, mentoring and feedback.

The major barriers we have in Australia to introducing such a model of education relate to our historical culture of male medical hierarchies and power structures, which are supported by all levels of government, who organise and fund programs through disciplinary silos. For this necessary change to occur in Australia, it will require real leadership, policy change at the national level, significant curriculum revision, cultural change, innovative educational approaches and some significant thinking outside of the box regarding the scope of practice and new or enhanced roles, plus government investment in workforce innovation to make it happen. This is an ideal model for remote areas – let's seize the day!

Interdisciplinary approaches in remote Australia

There are some interesting interdisciplinary approaches being used in some Australian states. In Queensland the Mount Isa Centre for Rural and Remote Health conducts innovative interdisciplinary undergraduate student placements in rural, remote and Indigenous communities, which have been enormously successful (Mount Isa Centre for Rural and Remote Health, 2015). Many of these students commented that it was the first time they were treated as valued members of a health care team, and it was often that feeling of worth that made many of them go back for more (Mount Isa Centre for Rural and Remote Health, 2015). In the Northern Territory the Centre for Remote Health in Alice Springs conducts multidisciplinary graduate programs in remote health practice that have a strong Indigenous and remote flavour (Centre for Remote Health, 2015). Other universities run sessions through their Departments of Rural Health and Rural Clinical Schools.

The main strength of this approach is that it encourages and professionally supports the team; and it has the additional spinoff whereby the visiting health practitioner may be inspired by, and develop an understanding of, remote practice. This factor is important, as metropolitan practitioners are also being educated about the roles and resources of rural and remote practitioners, which becomes more important when referring a patient for tertiary care. When they do this their understanding of the advanced and highly skilled roles of remote practitioners will ensure that the stigma often associated with rural practice is eradicated, though this will not occur while most of the training continues in metropolitan hospitals.

Many educational programs that currently educate the future remote and rural health workforce, however, remain discipline-specific, and a great deal of the content is still historically grounded in defined medical and hospital-bound culture.

What is important is to find a balance that also addresses the serious levels of ill health experienced by rural and remote people and contributes towards improving them.

CONCLUSION

The remote landscape has changed over the past decade with droughts, floods and a speckling of fluorescent vests as miners dig out our future resources. The health care landscape in remote Indigenous Australia has also changed. It now consists of orbiting staff zapping from one place to another, short-term agency staff, small teams of organ-based health care providers in their white Toyotas looking at the eye, the ear and the kidney and fly-in fly-out health care providers. The number of nurses with midwifery qualifications has declined from 65 per cent in 1995 to 29 per cent in 2008 (Health Workforce Australia, 2012, cited in Lenthall, 2011). This leaves a dearth of experienced people to monitor and support our future – the mothers, babies and children. The resident staff are sometimes poorly orientated and educated for their roles and the concept of primary health care practice wafts in the breeze as acute care needs dominate (Lenthall, 2015). This places the person whose care is being acted upon in a vulnerable place… remaining on the lowest rung of the health care ladder.

The education of the future remote health workforce offers unique challenges, and the commonalities across the health professions scream for the use of more interprofessional educational approaches. Lip service is generally being paid to genuine interdisciplinary approaches; there is a widening gap between the haves and the have-nots; the minority groups are marginalised; and the distribution of resources favours the medical profession who, while having the greatest workforce distribution problems, make up the smallest remote workforce group (Smith et al., 2013). It seems time to re-examine the current ways in which we do what we do.

It is time that the various colleges and university programs look out from their disciplinary silos at the challenges the remote landscape offers. Remote areas provide rich learning environments where students have unparalleled access to clinical learning material and where practitioners are placed in privileged roles that hold considerable status within the community (Prideaux et al., 2001). The remote landscape is also a multidisciplinary one, where there are many solo practitioners all struggling to meet the health care needs of the local populations, plus their own disciplinary requirements that are largely based on metropolitan ways of thinking. This begs another question: if we are really trying to educate rural and remote practitioners, why is most of the education still occurring in metropolitan tertiary teaching hospitals?

It is time to set the benchmark for remote practice, whereby all remote practitioners have remote specific qualifications to work there. We do not expect non-midwives to deliver babies, so why is it that we expect remote health professionals, who work with some of the sickest people in our community, to do so without orientation and specific education? It is also time for our professions to take the lead and guide funders in how to do this better. To do this we need a change in our thinking, and this could start with a change in the language we use when talking about remote practice. When we describe remote practice in Australia we need to stop using negative terminology such as 'need', 'disadvantage', 'crisis', 'hardship' and 'incentives to go there'. We need to start using words that are inclusive and speak realistically about real remote practice. We could starting using words like 'fascinating medicine', 'culturally diverse', 'environmentally challenging', 'interprofessional', 'equitable' and 'government investment in unique bottom-up primary health care approaches that are community driven'. This is the responsibility of all remote practitioners, their managers, their educators, their colleges and universities.

To be able to implement these changes, we need to build an evidence base and find clear descriptions of remote practice that draw on the commonalities across the disciplines and award these practitioners with appropriate professional status for the extended roles they perform. Programs should be supported by nationally coordinated initiatives that exclude intermediaries, thus bypassing any conflict between state and federal funding, and build on the needs of the marginalised groups – Indigenous health practitioners. We also need to ensure that government investment is well spent, in the right places, to ensure that the entire remote workforce is in balance and meets the health care needs of the population. These actions will improve health outcomes for the people whose health is being acted upon and entice more health professionals to experience the exciting world of remote Australia that many only get to see on a postcard.

Discussion Points

1   This chapter has drawn out that there are many similarities across the disciplines. The question then is: why do we continue to divide the remote workforce into vertical disciplines, or educational silos, when each university or college struggles to offer core rural and Indigenous studies? And when generally the same problems are experienced by all professionals working in rural and remote communities? Discuss.

2   There are hundreds of reports on rural workforce issues, though there remain few on the health of rural and remote people. Why is this so? Is this because our governments see rural and remote health as *only* the provision of services? Discuss.

3   Does this mean that educational practices are influenced by workforce needs, rather than by the health care needs of rural and remote people? Discuss.

References

Akers, A. (2013). *Bullying in the bush: Perspectives on the remote area health workforce.* The No 2 Bullying Conference. Gold Coast, Qld.

Austin, J. (2010). *Remote ready: Preparing form work in remote locations of the Northern Territory.* Darwin: Department of Education, Employment and Workplace Relations, Australian Government.

Australian Bureau of Statistics (ABS). (2013). *Causes of death, Australia.* Canberra: ABS. <http://www.abs.gov.au/ausstats/abs@.nsf/mf/3303.0> Accessed 02.08.15.

Australian College of Rural and Remote Medicine (ACRRM). (2015). *About ACRRM.* Brisbane: ACRRM. <www.acrrm.org.au> Accessed 04.05.15.

Australian Institute of Health and Welfare (AIHW). (2014). *Remoteness and the health of Indigenous Australians.* Australia's health 2014 Australia's health series, no 14. Cat. no. AUS 178. Canberra: AIHW.

Cavanagh, G. (2014). *Inquest into the death of ...Daniels* [2014] NTMC 024. Darwin: Department of the Attorney General and Justice, Northern Territory Government.

Centre for Remote Health (CRH). (2015). *Postgraduate programs – remote health practice.* Alice Springs: CRH, Flinders University. <www.crh.org.au> Accessed 06.05.15.

CRANAplus. (2014a). *Clinical procedures manual for remote and rural practice.* Alice Springs: CRANAplus. <www.crana.org.au> Accessed 02.08.15.

CRANAplus. (2014b). *Framework for remote and isolated professional practice*. Cairns: CRANAplus. <www.crana.org.au> Accessed 02.08.15.

CRANAplus. (2015). *Pathways to remote professional practice*. Cairns: CRANAplus. <www.crana.org.au> Accessed 02.08.15.

Fisher, J., Bradshaw, J., Currie, B., Klotz, J., Robbins, P., Reid-Searle, K., et al. (1995). *The context of silence: Violence and the remote area nurse*. Occasional paper. Rockhampton: University of Central Queensland, Faculty Health Science.

Garnett, S. T., Coe, K., Golebiowska, K., Walsh, H., Zander, K. K., Guthridge, S., et al. (2008). *Attracting and keeping nursing professionals in an environment of chronic labour shortage: A study of mobility among nurses and midwives in the Northern Territory of Australia*. Darwin: Charles Darwin University Press.

Health Workforce Australia (HWA). (2012). *Health Workforce 2025: Doctors, nurses and midwives*. Adelaide: HWA.

Humphris, D. (2005). *Integrating common learning in pre-registration health and social care professional programmes*. Southampton: Innovations Workforce Unit, University of Southampton.

Ivanhoe, T., & Gordon, V. (2015). *Telephone consultation, Mary and the doctor*. Alice Springs: Centre for Remote Health, Flinders University.

Jones, J., Blue, I., Adams, M., & Walker-Jeffreys, M. (2003). *An evaluation of the Pathways to Professional Primary Health Care Practice for Remote Area Nurses program in the Central Australians Network of the Northern Territory*. Whyalla: Spencer Gulf Rural Health School, University of South Australia.

Kelly, K., & Smith, J. D. (2007). Chapter 5. What and where is rural and remote Australia? In J. D. Smith (Ed.), *Australia's rural and remote health: A social justice perspective*. Melbourne: Tertiary Press.

Lenthall, S. (2015). Back from the edge: Reducing stress among remote area nurses in the Northern Territory. PhD thesis. Adelaide: Flinders University.

Lenthall, S., Gordon, V., Knight, S., Aitken, R., & Terrie, I. (2012). Do not move the furniture and other advice for new remote area nurses (RANs). *Australian Journal of Rural Health*, 20, 44–45.

Lenthall, S., Knight, S., Foxley, S., Gordon, V., Ivanhoe, T., & Aitken, R. (2015). *Remote Area Nurse Model of Consultation*. Alice Springs: Centre for Remote Health, Flinders University.

Lenthall, S., Wakerman, J., Opie, T., Dollard, M., Dunn, S., Knight, S., et al. (2009). What stresses remote area nurses? Current knowledge and future action. *Australian Journal of Rural Health*, 17, 208–213.

Lenthall, S., Wakerman, J., Opie, T., Dollard, M., Dunn, S., Knight, S., et al. (2011). Nursing workforce in very remote Australia, characteristics and key issues. *Australian Journal of Rural Health*, 19, 32–37.

Mount Isa Centre for Rural and Remote Health (MICRRH). (2015). *Placements*. Mount Isa: MICRRH. <http://www.micrrh.jcu.edu.au/> Accessed 06.05.15.

Nursing and Allied Health Rural Locum Scheme (NAHRLS). (2015). *About NAHRLS*. Canberra: NAHRLS. <http://nahrls.com.au/about-us> Accessed 05.05.15.

National Health Service (NHS). (2001). *Working together – Learning together: A framework for lifelong learning for the NHS*. London UK: Department of Health.

National Rural Health Students Network (NRHSN). (2015). *National Rural Health Students Network*. Melbourne: NRHSN. <http://www.nrhsn.org.au/site/index.cfm> Accessed 17.06.15.

Northern Territory Department of Health (NTDH). (2015). *Remote health atlas: Adult health checks*. Darwin: NTDH. <www.health.nt.gov.au/Remote_Health_Atlas/index.aspx> Accessed 03.08.15.

Opie, T., Dollard, M., Lenthall, S., Wakerman, J., Dunn, S., Knight, S., et al. (2010). Levels of occupational stress in the remote area nursing workforce. *Australian Journal of Rural Health*, 18, 235–241.

Opie, T., Lenthall, S., Wakerman, J., Dollard, M., MacLeod, M., Knight, S., et al. (2011). Occupational stress in the Australian nursing workforce: a comparison between hospital -based nurses and nurses working in very remote communities. *Australian Journal of Advanced Nursing*, 23, 4.

Prideaux, D., Saunders, N., Schofield, K., Wing, L., Gordon, J., Hays, R., et al. (2001). Country report: Australia. *Medical Education*, 35, 495–504.

Queensland Health. (2015). *Pathways to rural and remote orientation training*. Cairns: Queensland Health Department. <https://www.health.qld.gov.au/parrot> Accessed 06.05.15.

Remote Vocational Training Scheme (RVTS). (2015). *The Remote Vocational Training Scheme*. Albury: RVTS. <http://www.rvts.org.au/about/history> Accessed 17.05.15.

Sandhill, R. (2005). Dr Death in Bundaberg. *Quadrant*. December 2005. <http://www .rogersandall.com/doctor-death-in-bundaberg/> Accessed 03.08.15.

Smith, J. D., & Hays, R. (2004). Is rural medicine a separate discipline? *Australian Journal of Rural Health*, 12, 67–72.

Smith, J. D., Margolis, S. A., Ayton, J., Ross, V., Chalmers, E., Giddings, P., et al. (2008). Defining remote medical practice: a consensus viewpoint of medical practitioner working and teaching in remote practice. *Medical Journal of Australia*, 188(3), 159–161.

Smith, J. D., Prideaux, D., Wolfe, C., Wilkinson, T. J., Gupta, T. S., DeWitt, D. E., et al. (2007). Developing the accredited postgraduate assessment program for Fellowship of the Australian College of Rural and Remote Medicine. *Rural and Remote Health*, 7, 805. <www.rrh.org.au>.

Smith, J. D., White, C., Roufeil, L., Veitch, C., Pont, L., Patel, B., et al. (2013). A national study into the rural and remote pharmacist workforce. *Rural and Remote Health*, 13(2), 2214.

vanHaaren, M., & Williams, G. (2000). Central Australian nurse management model (CAN Model): a strategic approach to the recruitment and retention of remote area nurses. *Australian Journal of Rural Health*, 8, 1–5.

Wakerman, J. (2004). Defining remote health. *Australian Journal of Rural Health*, 12(5), 215–219.

Wakerman, J., Curry, R., & McEldowney, R. (2012). Fly in/fly out health services: the panacea or the problem? *Rural and Remote Health*, 12, 2268.

Wakerman, J., & Davey, C. (2008). Rural and remote health management: the next generation is not going to put up with this. *Asia Pacific Journal of Health Management*, 3(2), 13–17.

World Health Organization (WHO). (2005). *Preventing chronic diseases: A vital investment*. Geneva: WHO. From: <http://www.who.int/chp/chronic_disease_report/full_report.pdf> Accessed 02.08.15.

CHAPTER 13

A RURAL FUTURE

Janie Dade Smith

The face of rural Australia has changed significantly for the past generation of rural Australians. Rural Australia no longer rides to prosperity on the sheep's back, and there is a continual trend for young rural people to move to the bright lights of the city to go to university or find work. While some rural communities are growing and thriving, many others feel under siege. They have declining populations, declining incomes, declining services, a declining quality of life and increasing suicide rates (Australian Institute of Health and Welfare, 2014a).

While some things have certainly improved since the last edition of this book the image of inequity and social disadvantage remains, in which rural and remote Australians have a poorer health status that is worsened by their geographical location and their culture. These factors are compounded by a lack of access to health care, limited transport availability and shortages of health facilities and professionals. Remote Australia presents a grimmer picture especially for its Indigenous inhabitants, compounded by continued poor data, bureaucratic blame-shifting and definitions of health that are not used by its residents. This raises several important questions.

In this chapter I explore a concept that may help rural communities find a road forward – social capital. I then explore the growth of the rural health movement in Australia and, from a social justice perspective, I examine the future priorities and

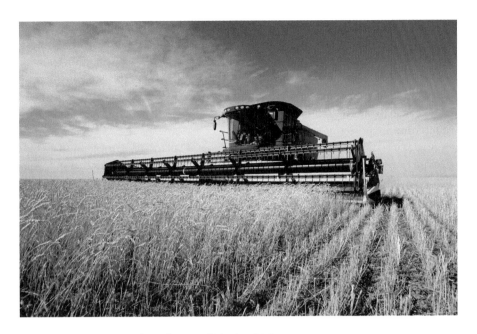

Reproduced with permission from: Shutterstock/Stephen McSweeny.

PAUSE AND THINK

Should rural people expect the same level of health as their metropolitan counterparts?

Should they expect to aspire equally to a retirement with good health, a long life and happiness in the town of their choice?

Should they expect to be treated as equal members of this great nation? If so, how can this be achieved?

---

barriers against the National Strategic Framework for Rural and Remote Health, which provides a national vision for health care for Australians living in rural, regional and remote Australia (Australian Health Ministers Advisory Council, 2012).

SOCIAL CAPITAL

Today there seems more to worry about than the 'man on the land', especially in an economic rationalist and political environment, where Australia's Governments are more concerned with international events, and where sport adds more to the GDP than wool or wheat (Government of South Australia, 2011). In response to the developments of the past two decades, a new ideology has emerged that may provide a glimmer of light on the rural horizon. This is the ideology of social capital.

'Social capital' is a term that has come into its own over the past two decades, in particular with business, economics, health, community, academic and political groups who argue about what it means and the ways in which to use the term. The Australian Bureau of Statistics defines social capital as being 'networks, together with shared norms, values and understanding which facilitate cooperation within or among groups' (Australian Bureau of Statistics, 2014b, p. 1). This is something we have always done in rural and remote Australia, probably without naming it, as we partake in activities in RSL halls and sporting clubs where mateship and small town country life are powerful cultural symbols.

To put it simply, social capital is 'the value' that we place upon 'the glue' that holds a community together in these settings. This is done through the work that individuals do together for the 'common good' of the people, their neighbourhood or the community. This notion of common good refers to those things that benefit the community and the person as part of that community (Cox & Caldwell, 2000). For example, during the bush fire season everyone, from the sandwich-maker to the firefighter, works together for the common good of the town. These activities build self-esteem, empathy, social support and trust, and give people a sense of purpose and pride in being part of their town – the place where they belong. The King Lake fire in Victoria in 2009 in which 120 people died and all the homes in the community were lost provides a good example of people continuing to work together to rebuild their community.

PAUSE AND THINK

Why is it when communities burn down that the people want to rebuild there?

What is it that holds them together?

What makes others help them in times of need?

The people involved in building the social capital in a community have a certain community connectedness, or glue, that binds them and their communities together. This may include the referee of the football club, the petition writer to the local council, the volunteer at the women's centre or the business person who provides training opportunities for long-term unemployed people. We all know of local organisations that have taken off due to the enthusiasm of a few parents, or after a new inspiring basketball coach arrives in town. It is the resulting social support, networking, communication, empathy, self-esteem and trust that build the social capital in that community.

Strong social capital in a community provides people with a sense of purpose and a sense of community, and it has been found to also make them healthier (Rocco & Suhrcke, 2012). Researchers have found that people who are isolated socially, culturally or geographically, and those without sufficient social networks, 'suffer two to four times the risk of mortality, independent of all other known risk factors' (Baum, Palmer, Modra, Murray, & Bush, 2000, p. 250). The evidence for this is building to the extent where the World Health Organization has named social support (one of the building blocks of social capital) as one of the social determinants of health (Wilkinson & Marmot, 2003). Let us examine in more detail some of the key factors that are necessary for good social capital to exist in a community.

Key factors for social capital

Social capital is a bottom-up phenomenon, which is essentially the 'space between people' and the 'glue that binds them together'. It is based on a number of key factors including:

- trust – having well established interpersonal relationships and social networks that include strangers
- level of education
- volunteering and working together for a common purpose
- social support and inclusion, decision-making processes, social unity, communication, relationship building and empathy
- mutual reciprocity and inclusiveness
- participation with others towards a common good (Australian Bureau of Statistics, 2014b; Cox & Caldwell, 2000).

Trust

The issue of trust is an important one in the Australian community, especially these days when the government focus is on international issues such as terrorism and 'stopping the boats' to win political points. In 2014, The Edelman Trust Barometer, which measures the nation's levels of trust in government, found that globally trust in government had fallen to an historic low of 44 per cent, whereas in Australia it had increased to 56 per cent (Pash, 2014). However, it also found that 60 per cent of Australians do not trust government leaders to tell the truth; and 40 per cent do not trust them to make ethical and moral decisions. Interestingly, it also found that the highest levels of trust were found in non-governmental organisations, who rated 70 per cent; and the lowest levels of trust were in the media, who rated 48 per cent (Pash, 2014).

So what is trust? 'Mutual trust is the glue that holds a good society together,' because it generates self-esteem and a sense of social belonging (Latham, 2000). It is this sense of belonging that many old-timers in rural Australia identify with when they say they would never think of leaving their town as 'it's where I belong' (Dempsey, 1990). Trust generally emerges through the familiarity that comes from face-to-face interactions, which occur more frequently in small communities where everyone knows your name (Latham, 2000). These communities also place greater value on the work that people do together for the common good, for example when the community is facing threats such as fires, floods and droughts, isolation and a lack of resources (Hughes, Bellamy, & Black, 2000). Trust also needs to be reciprocated as 'a family is unlikely to reach its full potential for nurturing its children and establishing systems of mutual support' without reciprocated trust (Hughes, Bellamy, & Black, 2000, p. 196).

In rural communities, researchers have found that there is a greater level of trust between members of the community, as well as higher levels of networks, civic participation and cohesion and better mental health (Ziersch, Baum, Darmawan, Kavanagh, & Bentley, 2009). However, previous studies have also found that rural people have a higher incidence of distrust of strangers and people of difference and a greater fear of the unknown and dislike of new ideas than their city counterparts; and that there is considerable racism (Baum cited in Winter, 2000). Simmons and Hsu-Hage (2002) argue that the high suicide rates in rural communities could be a result of negative social capital, which could be perceived as being due to lack of support, empathy, communication and trust. This form of negative social capital often occurs when town populations are highly stratified by gender, race, class and ethnic differences (Gray & Lawrence, 2001). This is often more apparent in a rural or remote community.

Business and civic-mindedness … 'bloody banks'

Thirty years ago in rural Australia the bank manager held an esteemed position in the community. 'He' was usually a member of the local Rotary Club; everyone knew him by name; parents introduced him to their sons and daughters when they applied for their first car loan; and he used a personal approach. People were loyal and trusting, and they usually stayed with the one bank for life.

Today banks are some of the most disliked institutions in our society. This could also be due to the fact that between 1993 and 2000, over 2000 banks were closed in Australia, followed in 2008 by the global financial crisis. Many of these bank closures were in rural areas, which greatly affected small business whereby residents travelled the extra distance to do their shopping and banking in larger regional towns. These bank closures could also be due to the banks' philosophy that 'the business of business is business' and that their whole focus and perceived level of responsibility is on increased shareholder value. While banks espouse the virtues of building social capital, in practice 'they have contributed to the erosion of social capital in many communities through closing down branches and sub-branches, and threatening community infrastructure, in their relentless pursuits of higher profits' (Murphy & Thomas, 2000, p. 145).

Ironically, the positive spin-off of this negative situation is that members of local communities have become very angry and have worked cooperatively to set up their own community banks. The Bendigo Community Bank is one such example of a national franchise driven by people in local communities, and it is currently experiencing enormous growth. This is a good example of social capital and financial capital at work: the community working cooperatively together for the common good of the people and their community. Since its inception in 1998 they have returned more than $51 million to support local initiatives and have completed over 1250 local community projects (Bendigo and Adelaide Bank, 2011).

Volunteering

Volunteering is another key factor in building social capital, as it makes an important contribution to national life. In 2010, 36.2 per cent of Australians volunteered; that is 6.1 million people (Volunteering Australia, 2015). Those who volunteered in the community had a higher rate of participation in sport, some 87 per cent compared with those who did not volunteer at some 67 per cent (Australian Bureau of Statistics, 2012). Most volunteers were over 35 years of age, with slightly more women than men, and were mostly partnered with children (Volunteering Australia, 2015). Volunteers mostly worked in sporting and recreation groups, community and welfare groups, education and training, youth development groups and religious groups (Australian Bureau of Statistics, 2012).

In small rural communities volunteering is often critical to their sustainability, where volunteers are often seen as 'the joiners'. In 2010, 41 per cent of volunteers lived outside cities (Volunteering Australia, 2015). Volunteers were also found to be more involved in a range of activities in addition to their volunteering, due to the social networks that this builds. Volunteering contributes to the stocks of social capital through the building of community life and the communities.

Rural community building

Driving through a small rural community you can often assess the level of social capital there by the general sense of the community, the school yard and the engagement of the people with one another. Therefore, as rural communities are smaller one would think that social capital would be stronger in rural communities because they are perceived as being close-knit, friendly, helpful and civic-minded places, where everyone knows who you are, even if you do not know them. However, while this does occur in some small towns, it is not always the case. All rural communities possess systems of social status that can be distinguished by wealth, longevity in the community and reputation for service (Stehlik, 2001). Rural people can marginalise 'newcomers' – those who may have a different political view, religion, class or cultural background, or who do not conform to community standards (Dempsey, 1990). Baum found that there were often very clear divisions between certain groups in small towns and that distrust of strangers and a fear of the unknown and of new ideas were common (cited in Winter, 2000).

If social capital is the value we place on the glue that holds our society together, then to keep it together communities need to make sure that they build upon what they have to make it strong and valuable and reduce those factors that may cause it to come apart, such as racism, distrust, exclusion and fear (Baum, 1999). This is especially so when different cultural groups of refugees are being settled in these communities, many of whom come with personal histories of trauma and torture. For healthy social capital to be built up in rural communities it is important that the negative aspects, which vary greatly between communities, can be brought into balance. This will help build upon the sense of community that comes from trust, cooperation, understanding, empathy, reciprocity, respect and being open to new

ideas and working with different cultural groups. These factors will then have a positive long-term effect on rural people's health.

To use an analogy, it is as if everyone were making a patchwork quilt together, in
which all the patches are woven to form the whole. The patches represent the diverse
social fabric of the community, the colours make up the local characters and the
design creates the roles they play, but it is the golden thread of mutual trust and
respect that holds it together.

GROWING HEALTH SERVICES

Now let us put rural communities together with health services in an effort to find a
future path. There are several important factors that affect the way in which health
services are provided and accessed in rural and remote areas in Australia. These relate
to the people, the policies, the data and the government processes. The rural health
movement in Australia is also relatively new, so many of the approaches used are in
their teenage years. While a few reports on rural health existed in the 1970s, it is only
since the early 1990s that there has been a significant national focus on, and government investment in, rural, remote and Indigenous health.

The rural health movement: two decades of action

While much of the groundwork was undertaken in the previous decade by passionate
rural health and Indigenous individuals and lobby groups, it was not until 1989 and
1994 that the first National Aboriginal Health Strategy (National Aboriginal Health
Strategy Working Party, 1989) and the first National Rural Health Strategy (Australian
Health Ministers Advisory Council, 1994), respectively, were developed.

The first National Rural Health Strategy grew as a result of the first National
Rural Health Conference held in Toowoomba, Queensland, in 1991. This conference
provided a forum for the first consensus agenda on rural health issues in Australia
(Nichols, Streeton, & Cowie, 2002). The Strategy espoused principles of equity and
access; a population focus based on needs and supported by evidence; workforce
issues; and a strategic focus with policies that were sensitive to social and cultural
differences, especially in the health of Indigenous Australians (Australian Health
Ministers Advisory Council, 1994). The hallmark characteristic of the Strategy was
the need for multidisciplinary approaches that focus on primary health care, health
promotion and illness prevention, and that are consistent with the national health
goals and targets (now known as the National Health Priorities) (Australian Institute of Health and Welfare, 2015). These were the heady days when terms like 'inter-
sectoral collaboration' were high on the agenda, and there was a sense of excitement
in the rural and remote health workforce because their voices were finally being
heard.

Since that time there has been enormous energy and activity – biennial rural
health conferences, national frameworks, rural policies, rural health research, rural
incentives, rural student scholarships, University Departments of Rural Health funded
from 1997, Rural Clinical Schools funded from 2001 and significant government

investment in the process. With it has developed a strong sense of camaraderie among the numerous personalities and disciplines, and new organisations have sprung up all around the nation and brought with them a new rural culture, industry, language and set of acronyms.

Planting the organisational seeds

The only remote health professional organisation to exist before this time was the Council of Remote Area Nurses of Australia Inc, established in 1982, followed in 1991 by the first rural health professional organisation, the Rural Doctors' Association of Australia. The following year saw the birth of the Association for Australian Rural Nurses (AARN), the establishment of the Commonwealth's Branch of Rural Health and the first Rural Health Support Education and Training (RHSET) to be offered by the Commonwealth government. Yet it was not until 1998 that the Commonwealth Government established its first Office of Rural Health.

Gradually over that decade a number of Rural Health Training Units were established and the first two Indigenous Health Worker Education Programs were accredited in the Northern Territory and Queensland. In 1993 the growing number of rural medicine, nursing, allied health and consumer groups combined under the umbrella of the National Rural Health Alliance, which now consists of 37 different national rural and remote organisations and supports the work of the *Australian Journal of Rural Health*. In 1996 the Service for Australian Rural and Remote Allied Health (SARRAH) was formed and in 1997 the Australian College of Rural and Remote Medicine (ACRRM, 2004) became the first rural and remote medical college in the world. In July 2006 the Council of Australian Governments (CoAG) announced that they would provide rural medicine with formal recognition under Medicare as a generalist discipline in April 2007, and the ACRRM curriculum and assessment process was accredited by the Australian Medical Council for the first time (Smith et al., 2007). Recognition of the profession has attracted more doctors to rural practice, which will ultimately improve safety by increasing the number of skilled practitioners and the overall quality of medical services provided to rural communities. That same year the Council of Remote Area Nurses broadened its focus to include all remote and isolated health professionals and, as a result, changed its name to CRANAplus (CRANAplus, 2014).

Growing the infrastructure

During the past two decades there has been a growing rural infrastructure. While it largely focuses strongly on the rural and remote medical workforce, general practitioners in particular, it has had some positive impact upon other disciplines. The Rural Divisions of General Practice were established in 1993. They were taken over by Medicare Locals in 2011; and in July 2015 they were taken over by 31 Primary Health Networks (PHNs). The aim of the PHNs is to increase the efficiency and effectiveness of medical services for patients at risk and to improve the coordination of care. A total of $842 million has been invested by the Australian Government over three years to do so (Australian Government, 2014c). One wonders if it is just a matter of moving the deck chairs around under another name.

The 2014 federal budget saw the axing of many of the national organisations that managed the intellectual capital and national infrastructure such as Health Workforce Australia, Australian General Practice and Training and the National Health Prevention Agency. A major cut was also made to rural and remote student scholarships from the total pool. All of the services provided by these organisations were returned to the Health Department along with their Indigenous health responsibilities; and many other organisations received reduced funding or were defunded.

Rural Workforce Agencies were established in 1997 funded by the Department of Health to implement medical workforce recruitment and retention programs in rural and remote Australia. They also have a national body, now known as the Rural Health Workforce Australia, which provides information and policy advice on rural health workforce issues through the provision of workforce data analysis, planning and research, and program development and evaluation (Rural Health Workforce Australia, 2015a). They manage the National Rural Health Students Network, which in 2015 had over 9000 student members from all health disciplines, who belong to 28 University Rural Health Clubs from all states and territories (National Rural Health Student Network, 2015).

A major part of the rural health infrastructure was the establishment of eleven University Departments of Rural Health (UDRH) in 2001, which are coordinated by their national body, the Australian Rural Health Education Network (ARHEN). The aim of the UDRHs is to provide leadership and strategic direction in rural health education and research and to improve rural experience for all students in the health professions, including medical, nursing and allied health undergraduate and post-graduate students (Australian Rural Health Education Network, 2015). Their presence also increases the intellectual capital in the region by providing training, jointly appointed clinical academics and support, and research and community capacity. These academics engender those rural-specific experiences, in particular public health, Indigenous health, mental health, simulation and student placement coordination (Australian Rural Health Education Network, 2015). They are often linked with Rural Clinical Schools, which were established around the same time to support medical students, and are coordinated by a national body – the Federation of Rural Australian Medical Educators (FRAME). In 2015 there were 17 Rural Clinical Schools across Australia managed by 16 universities, who all have multiple training locations and are funded by the Australian Government (Australian Government, 2014a). They provide significant medical training infrastructure such as educational facilities and student accommodation to enable medical students to undertake training in rural environments. Research tells us that students with a rural background and those who have had positive rural placements are more likely to return once graduated; therefore these placements are an initiative to increase the number of Australian medical students returning to rural and remote practice (Australian Government, 2014b). The results are promising with a reported increase in the number of general practitioners working rurally, increased numbers of women in rural practice and a decline in the mean length of stay, which is shorter for remote doctors (Rural Health Workforce Australia, 2015b).

ADVANCING RURAL AUSTRALIA'S HEALTH

Much has been achieved over the past two decades to bring rural and remote health workforce issues to the attention of government policymakers and other Australians. This includes two major reviews, the first being the Productivity Commission Review of the Health Workforce (2005). The second, undertaken by the Health and Hospitals Reform Commission, made over 100 recommendations on access and equity issues, how to redesign the health system and make a responsive health system for future generations (National Health and Hospitals Reform Commission, 2009). These reports and others informed the establishment of Health Workforce Australia, which was established by CoAG in 2008 with $1.6 billion over five years, and was one of the many agencies closed down as part of the 2014 federal budget. One of the many significant reports they produced was *Health Workforce 2025*, which estimated what was needed for a sustainable health workforce for this century. It is now time to ask the questions.

PAUSE AND THINK

What impact have all of these initiatives had?

Have they just put the right health professional in the right place at the right time in the area of workforce need?

Are they in line with the research reports about what is needed?

What impacts have these initiatives had on the health of rural and remote people?

Are we seeing improved health outcomes of rural and remote people?

Many of the activities listed above were based on the notion that increasing the workforce nationally, and particularly in rural and remote areas, and improving their educational preparation would also increase the health status of the people. However, the first national report that specifically examined the health of rural and remote people was only produced in 1998, and provided the first benchmark to build on (Strong, Trickett, Titulaer, & Bhatia, 1998). Since that time there have only been intermittent reports from the two core institutions, the Australian Bureau of Statistics and the Australian Institute of Health and Welfare, plus short annual rural health status chapters in *Australia's Health* reports, which still report a big divide between the health of metropolitan Australia and that of rural and especially remote Australians (Australian Institute of Health and Welfare, 2014a; Health Workforce Australia,

2013). All reports mention the health of the people worsening with geographical remoteness.

While all of these activities have taken place and infrastructure has blossomed, it now seems appropriate for this rural health culture to take time to reflect and refocus to ensure that the initiatives are actually contributing towards their intended aim – improving the health status of rural and remote people – and not just towards providing more workforce numbers, more incentives and more research papers. Rural populations are ageing, chronic disease in remote Indigenous populations is multiplying rapidly and remote Indigenous inhabitants still have unacceptable levels of disease and disadvantage. If we are to be prepared for the impact these changes will make, we need to take our eyes off ourselves as a workforce and focus on those factors that affect health. A new framework for rural health provides a way forward, though it strongly resembles the first rural health strategy and there is no direct mention of Indigenous Australians, which all of the previous strategies had as a number one initiative.

A FRAMEWORK FOR THE FUTURE

In 2012 the Australian Health Ministers Advisory Council replaced the Healthy Horizons Framework with a National Strategic Framework for Rural and Remote Health (Australian Health Ministers Advisory Council, 2012). Their vision was that rural and remote Australians would be as healthy as other Australians and they set out five goals; that rural and remote communities would have:

1   improved access to appropriate and comprehensive health care
2   effective, appropriate and sustainable health care service delivery
3   an appropriate, skilled and well supported health workforce
4   collaborative health service planning and policy development
5   strong leadership, governance, transparency and accountability (Australian Health Ministers Advisory Council, 2012, p. 25).

While each goal is important in its own right they are all interrelated, such as the use of e-health, which can be used for clinical purposes but can also be used for professional development, patient education and administration.

This framework prioritises a way forward for action, through the allocation of resources and guidance for communities and the organisations concerned to improve rural and remote people's health. There are, however, some barriers that need to be addressed as part of this process.

BARRIERS TO 'JUST' HEALTH SERVICES

Retarding rural health

We know that more doctors, nurses and hospitals do not make better health, while they are essential; they only provide health services and infrastructure. Good access to education, nutritious food, adequate income, control over one's life and factors that reduce disease, such as good sanitation, clean water, suitable housing and pest control, make better health – the social determinants of health (Wilkinson & Marmot, 2003). Yet rural health dollars continue to be spent on producing rural workforce reports, providing medical workforce incentives and running innovative programs for health professionals. This is because those key factors that make for better health – housing, education and employment – are funded from other government departments outside the health department. As has already been seen, despite numerous initiatives to stop the 'blame game', there is a lack of coordination between the Commonwealth, state and regional health departments, which all focus around triennial election cycles, so when we try to make an impact upon these other departments, the problem compounds (National Health and Hospitals Reform Commission, 2009). Additionally, if Indigenous health is involved, the tiers of bureaucracy still seem to multiply despite targets in the Closing the Gap initiative to reduce them (Australian Government, 2015a). This often leaves a situation where those most in need miss out – both those who provide the services and those who receive them. It then becomes easy to see that the health of rural, remote and Indigenous Australians will not be equal to those in metropolitan areas while the responsibility for funding rests on a bureaucracy that is bogged in poorly coordinated multiple tiers of decision making. As Australians we have a responsibility to question this system.

Accessible definitions and data

Another significant barrier is the way in which we define 'rural' and 'remote' in Australia. These have recently been reviewed but mainly to focus on the allocation of incentives for doctors to work there (Australian Government, 2015b). This leaves the current quantifiable narrow classification systems to define rural and remote with gaps, inconsistencies and estimations that imprecisely define and understate the extent of the most disadvantaged communities and their health and socioeconomic status. These can distort the data that are provided and upon which governments allocate resources. New systems should also include at least the health and cultural status of that particular population, their morbidity and mortality data, their access to healthy food and good education, their levels of employment and the availability of real opportunities for change. This will enable a more accurate allocation of scarce resources and focus on those whose health is being acted upon.

Health policy in Australia is largely developed from international definitions of health. While this is most certainly credible for the Australian population at large, these definitions do not reflect those used by the rural, remote and particularly Indigenous peoples. For health programs to be effective and accessible, it is essential that their foundations be built upon the values and belief systems of the people they target. Hence definitions of health should be those that are used by the people and for the people.

The current system of collecting Health Insurance Commission data as the major source of health information relates directly to the work of doctors, and provides a distorted view of the health of rural, remote and Indigenous people. The systems that collect Indigenous health data remain substantively incomplete in providing a true national picture of the health of the sickest people in this country. Most reports state that there are variations, probable underestimations and difficulty in pointing to trends with confidence, and they only include four or five states, hence they are incomplete (Australian Bureau of Statistics, 2014a; Australian Institute of Health and Welfare, 2014b). This inequitable situation is an issue of natural justice, since health information is vital to informing our society and workforce about health priorities and about how resources are distributed. This lack of data increases the risk that attention and resources will be directed at the problems measured, instead of at those communities that constitute the greatest burden of disease (Couzos & Murray, 2003).

Appropriate education

For change to occur, the way in which we educate the future rural health workforce also requires further re-examination. Rural and remote areas offer rich learning environments in which students have unparalleled access to clinical learning material and numerous opportunities for innovations exist (Smith et al., 2007; Smith et al., 2008). The establishment of the Rural Clinical Schools and the University Departments of Rural Health is having some impact but the majority of health professional training still occurs in disciplinary silos in major tertiary teaching hospitals, which maintain hierarchies and metropolitan hospital-based ways of thinking. Excellent examples are also found in other countries such as the United Kingdom and Canada, which are also experiencing similar issues of ageing populations, chronic disease and a need for radical workforce change. For rural and remote Australia we need to look at each profession and determine if they can expand their scope of practice to take on certain skills of other professions, as well as checking to see if there are any gaps. Many are already practising in this way, especially in remote areas where advanced and extended skills are required. If there are gaps we need to examine the best ways of filling them, perhaps with new roles, generic roles or expanded roles. We need to develop national policy to bring about reform and health system change. This might include such things as foundational programs for generic health workers, expanding nurse practitioner roles in rural and remote practice, developing educational benchmarks for the rural and remote workforce and developing interdisciplinary education programs (Smith, 2006). Several recent reports provide some great ideas about how this could take place (Health Workforce Australia, 2013; Productivity Commission, 2005).

Conquering the stigma

Another major impediment is the mindsets and attitudes of those who make decisions about rural health policy, education and resource allocation. Many metropolitan-based governments, universities, training and professional organisations remain generally ignorant about rural and remote issues and have a perception that working in rural and remote areas is somehow second rate. However, the opposite is often true as rural and remote health practitioners need an advanced and extended scope of practice. To overcome this stigma rural health work needs to be promoted as a distinctive, legitimate, credible and an important endeavour, one that fully acknowledges the importance and value of the contribution rural communities make to the national economy and to the development of rural communities (Humphreys, 1999).

CONCLUSION – ADVANCE RURAL AUSTRALIA

History has shown that the most effective initiatives are those that are community-led (Jensen, 1997). Therefore, developing 'policies for change' with strong rural leadership, which strengthen social capital networks, and with real government commitment and investment, provides a way forward. This involves working collaboratively together with all players and making a conscious effort to walk away from the old and to develop the new rural cultures of the future (Jensen, 1997).

Leadership is changing in rural areas. Rural women's groups are developing rapidly and have government support. Positive change requires activities that are strategic, communicative and participatory. Perhaps it is time for rural leadership to come from those 'whose hands have rocked the cradle'* for this real change to occur.

Critical to success is a celebration of the diversity of this great nation. We need to accept that there are different viewpoints, cultures and lifestyles, and we can use this diversity to enrich rural policy for the future generations of Australians. Practical approaches could include using words that describe rural and remote health work in the real rural Australia: words like 'technologically rich', 'policy poor', 'exciting', 'culturally diverse', 'multicultural', 'innovative', 'fascinating medicine', 'environmentally challenging', 'equitable' and 'unique'.

The challenge is to find ways of preserving those aspects of rural culture that will sustain it, and initiatives that have strong rural leadership, grassroots approaches and participation by all parties, especially by those whose health is being acted upon.

For health providers a national approach that looks at health from a primary health care perspective, the tenets of which lie in social and economic justice based on the social determinants of health and the national health priorities, represents a way forward. These are the very principles espoused in the first National Rural Health Strategy in 1994.

To do this we need to be courageous enough to question in whose hands health lies; to be humble enough to work with others in a multidisciplinary way to achieve change; and to be sensitive enough to celebrate diversity and be open to the world, yet think for ourselves. This is what will make our society richer in spirit, more diverse in nature and more just in the long run. We may then find rural, remote and Indigenous Australians standing strongly together on their level field saying: 'We get a fair go, mate.'

---

*'The hand that rocks the cradle rules the world' is a saying about women.

Discussion Points

1 Having read this book and this chapter, list three key points that you think need to change that would improve the health of rural and remote Australians.

2 Discuss these points with other members of your group.

3 Establish how you as a health professional could put positive action into place to bring about change.

4 What factors would need to be in place for this to occur?

References

Australian Bureau of Statistics (ABS). (2012). *Sport and social capital, Australia 2010.* Canberra: ABS. <http://www.abs.gov.au/ausstats/abs@.nsf/Products/2E7D482DF1BA1D4FCA2579CD000CF784?opendocument> Accessed 30.07.15.

Australian Bureau of Statistics. (2014a). 4727.0.55.001 – *Australian Aboriginal and Torres Strait Islander Health Survey: First results, Australia, 2012–13.* Canberra: ABS. <http://www.abs.gov.au/ausstats/abs@.nsf/Lookup/39E15DC7E770A144CA257C2F00145A66?opendocument> Accessed 30.07.15.

Australian Bureau of Statistics. (2014b). *Topics at a glance: Social capital.* Canberra: ABS. <http://www.abs.gov.au/websitedbs/c311215.nsf/web/social+capital+-+overview> Accessed 30.07.15.

Australian College of Rural and Remote Medicine (ACRRM). (2004). *AMC Submission.* Brisbane: ACRRM.

Australian Government. (2014a). *Rural clinical training and support.* Canberra: Department of Health. <http://www.health.gov.au/clinicalschools> Accessed 30.07.15.

Australian Government. (2014b). *Rural clinical training and support (RCTS) 2011–2014: Operational framework.* Canberra: Department of Health and Ageing. <http://www.health.gov.au/internet/main/publishing.nsf/Content/596169EBA9E6B92DCA257BF0001BDA31/$File/RCTS%20Operational%20Framework%202011-2014.pdf> Accessed 30.07.15.

Australian Government. (2014c). *Primary Health Networks, grant program guidelines.* Canberra: Department of Health and Ageing. <http://www.health.gov.au/internet/main/publishing.nsf/Content/phn-guidelines> Accessed 30.07.15.

Australian Government. (2015a). *Closing the Gap: Prime Minister's Report 2015.* Canberra: Department of the Prime Minister and Cabinet. <http://www.dpmc.gov.au/pmc-indigenous-affairs/publication/closing-gap-prime-ministers-report-2015> Accessed 30.07.15.

Australian Government. (2015b). *Rural classification reform: Frequently asked questions.* Canberra: Department of Health. <http://www.doctorconnect.gov.au/internet/otd/publishing.nsf/Content/Classification-changes> Accessed 30.07.15.

Australian Health Ministers Advisory Council (AHMAC). (1994). *National rural health strategy.* AHMAC, Commonwealth of Australia, Canberra: Australian Government Publishing Service.

Australian Health Ministers Advisory Council. (2012). *National strategic framework for rural and remote health*. AHMAC, Commonwealth of Australia, Canberra: Australian Government Publishing Service. Retreived 4.8.15 from: <http://www.ruralhealthaustralia.gov.au/internet/rha/publishing.nsf/Content/NSFRRH-homepage> Accessed 04.08.15.

Australian Institute of Health and Welfare (AIHW). (2014a). *Australia's health 2014*. Canberra: AIHW. <http://www.aihw.gov.au/workarea/downloadasset.aspx?id=60129548150> Accessed 30.07.15.

Australian Institute of Health and Welfare. (2014b). *Remoteness and the health of Indigenous Australians: Australia's health 2014*. Canberra: AIHW. <http://www.aihw.gov.au/workarea/downloadasset.aspx?id=60129548150> Accessed 30.07.15.

Australian Institute of Health and Welfare. (2015). *National health priority areas*. Canberra: AIHW. <http://www.aihw.gov.au/national-health-priority-areas/> Accessed 30.07.15.

Australian Rural Health Education Network (ARHEN). (2015). *What is ARHEN?* Deakin ACT: AHREN. <http://www.arhen.org.au/about-us/what-is-arhen.html> Accessed 30.07.15.

Baum, F. (1999). *Social capital and health: Implications for health in rural Australia*. Paper presented at the 5th National Rural Health Conference, Adelaide.

Baum, F., Palmer, C., Modra, C., Murray, C., & Bush, R. (2000). Families, social capital and health. In I. Winter (Ed.), *Social capital and public policy in Australia* (pp. 250–273). Melbourne: Australian Institute of Family Studies.

Bendigo and Adelaide Bank. (2011). *In the community: A report into the community activities of Bendigo and Adelaide Bank*. Bendigo Vic: Bendigo and Adelaide Bank. <http://www.bendigoadelaide.com.au/public/in_the_community/pdf/In-the-Community-Report_20110322.pdf> Accessed 30.07.15.

Couzos, S., & Murray, R. (2003). *Aboriginal primary health care: An evidence based approach* (2nd ed.). Melbourne: Oxford University Press.

Cox, E., & Caldwell, P. (2000). Making public policy. In I. Winter (Ed.), *Social capital and public policy in Australia* (pp. 43–73). Melbourne: Australian Institute of Family Studies.

CRANAplus. (2014). *Framework for remote and isolated professional practice*. Cairns: CRANAplus. <https://crana.org.au/files/pdfs/Revised_Framework_Remote_Practice_Aug2014.pdf> Accessed 30.07.15.

Dempsey, K. (1990). *Smalltown – A study of social inequality, cohesion and belonging*. Melbourne: Oxford University Press.

Government of South Australia. (2011). *Trends in recreation and sport*. Adelaide: Office for Recreation and Sport, Government of South Australia. <https://www.recsport.sa.gov.au/sport-active-recreation/documents/Trends%20in%20Recreation%20and%20Sport%20Participation%20Final.pdf> Accessed 30.07.15.

Gray, I., & Lawrence, G. (2001). *A future for regional Australia*. Cambridge UK: Cambridge University Press.

Health Workforce Australia (HWA). (2013). *National Rural and Remote Health Workforce Innovation and Reform Strategy*. Adelaide: HWA. <http://www.hwa.gov.au/sites/uploads/HWA13WIR013_Rural-and-Remote-Workforce-Innovation-and-Reform-Strategy_v4-1.pdf> Accessed 30.07.15.

Hughes, P., Bellamy, B., & Black, A. (2000). Building social trust through education. In I. Winter (Ed.), *Social capital and public policy in Australia* (pp. 225–249). Melbourne: Australian Institute of Family Studies.

Humphreys, J. (1999, March 14–17). *Keynote address. Past conference, future strategies*. Paper presented at the 5th National Rural Health Conference, Leaping the boundary fence – using evidence and collaboration to build healthier communities, Adelaide.

Jensen, R. (1997, July 1997). *Rural Australia: past, present and future*. Paper presented at the Rural Australia: Towards 2000 conference, July, NSW.

Latham, M. (2000). If only men were angels: social capital and the third way. In I. Winter (Ed.), *Social capital and public policy in Australia* (pp. 192–223). Melbourne: Australian Institute of Family Studies.

Murphy, J., & Thomas, B. (2000). Developing social capital: a new role for business. In I. Winter (Ed.), *Social capital and public policy in Australia* (pp. 136–163). Melbourne: Australian Institute of Family Studies.

National Aboriginal Health Strategy Working Party. (1989). *National Aboriginal Health Strategy*. Commonwealth of Australia, Canberra: Aust Government Printing Service.

National Health and Hospitals Reform Commission (NHHRC). (2009). *A healthier future for all Australians: Final report June 2009*. Canberra: NHHRC. <http://www.health.gov.au/internet/nhhrc/publishing.nsf/content/1AFDEAF1FB76A1D8CA257600000B5BE2/$File/Final_Report_of_the%20nhhrc_June_2009.pdf> Accessed 30.07.15.

Nichols, A., Streeton, M. J., & Cowie, M. (2002). Australian College of Rural and Remote Medicine: identity, consensus and recognition: a decade of growth in rural medicine. *Australian Journal of Rural Health*, 10(5), 263–264.

National Rural Health Student Network (NRHSN). (2015). *About the NRHSN*. Melbourne: NRHSN. <http://www.nrhsn.org.au/about-us/about-the-nrhsn/> Accessed 30.07.15.

Pash, C. (2014). Australian trust in government is suddenly rising faster than anywhere in the world. *Business Insider Australia*. <http://www.businessinsider.com.au/suddenly-australian-trust-in-government-is-rising-faster-than-anywhere-in-the-world-2014-1> Accessed 30.07.15.

Productivity Commission. (2005). *Australia's health workforce: Position paper*. Canberra: Productivity Commission.

Rural Health Workforce Australia (RHWA). (2015a). *About us*. Melbourne: RHWA. <http://www.rhwa.org.au/site/index.cfm> Accessed 30.07.15.

Rural Health Workforce Australia. (2015b). *GP workforce trends, more than a numbers game*, Fact sheet April 2015. Melbourne: RHWA. <http://www.rhwa.org.au/site/index.cfm?display=32639> Accessed 30.07.15.

Rocco, L., & Suhrcke, M. (2012). *Is social capital good for health? A European perspective*. Copenhagen: WHO Regional Office for Europe. <http://www.euro.who.int/__data/assets/pdf_file/0005/170078/Is-Social-Capital-good-for-your-health.pdf> Accessed 30.07.15.

Simmons, D., & Hsu-Hage, B. (2002). Determinants of health, disease and disability: differences between country and city. In I. Blue (Ed.), *The new rural health* (pp. 79–90). South Melbourne: Oxford University Press.

Smith, J. D. (2006). *Educating to improve population health outcomes in chronic disease* (2nd ed.). Darwin: Menzies School of Health Research.

Smith, J. D., Margolis, S. A., Ayton, J., Ross, V., Chalmers, E., Giddings, P., et al. (2008). Defining remote medical practice: a consensus viewpoint of medical practitioner working and teaching in remote practice. *Medical Journal of Australia*, 188(3), 159–161. <http://www.ncbi.nlm.nih.gov/pubmed/18241174> Accessed 30.07.15.

Smith, J. D., Prideaux, D., Wolfe, C., Wilkinson, T. J., Gupta, T. S., DeWitt, D. E., et al. (2007). Developing the accredited postgraduate assessment program for Fellowship of the

Australian College of Rural and Remote Medicine. *Rural and Remote Health*, 7(4), 805. <http://www.ncbi.nlm.nih.gov/pubmed/17953499> Accessed 30.07.15.

Stehlik, D. (2001). Out there: spaces, places and border crossings. In L. Bourke (Ed.), *Rurality bites* (pp. 30–42). Altona Vic: Pluto Press Australia Pty Ltd.

Strong, K., Trickett, P., Titulaer, I., & Bhatia, K. (1998). *Health in rural and remote Australia: The first report of the Australian Institute of Health and Welfare on rural health*, Cat No PHE 6 (pp. 1–131). Canberra: AIHW. <http://www.aihw.gov.au/WorkArea/DownloadAsset.aspx ?id=6442459022> Accessed 30.07.15.

Volunteering Australia. (2015). *Key facts and statistics about volunteering in Australia.* Canberra: Volunteering Australia. <http://www.volunteeringaustralia.org/wp-content/ uploads/VA-Key-statistics-about-Australian-volunteering-16-April-20151.pdf> Accessed 30.07.15.

Wilkinson, R., & Marmot, M. (Eds.), (2003). *Social determinants of health: The solid facts* (2nd ed.). Geneva: World Health Organization. <http://www.euro.who.int/document/ e81384.pdf> Accessed 30.07.15.

Winter, I. (2000). Major themes and debates in the social capital literature: the Australian connection. In I. Winter (Ed.), *Social capital and public policy in Australia* (pp. 17–39). Melbourne: Australian Institute of Family Studies.

Ziersch, A., Baum, F., Darmawan, I., Kavanagh, A., & Bentley, R. (2009). Social capital and health in urban and rural communities in South Australia. *Australian and New Zealand Journal of Public Health*, 33(1), 7–16. <http://www.ncbi.nlm.nih.gov/pubmed/19236353> Accessed 30.07.15.

INDEX

Page numbers followed by "*f*" indicate figures, "*b*" indicate boxes, and "*t*" indicate tables.